MW01406511

# *Botulinum Neurotoxin Injection Manual*

# *Botulinum Neurotoxin Injection Manual*


**Editors**

**Katharine E. Alter, MD**
Medical Director
Rehabilitation Programs
Mount Washington Pediatric Hospital
Baltimore, Maryland

Senior Clinician
National Institutes of Health
Bethesda, Maryland

**Nicole A. Wilson, PhD, MD**
Principal
Roth Affinity LLC
St. Louis, Missouri

Special Volunteer
Rehabilitation Medicine Department
National Institutes of Health
Bethesda, Maryland



demosMEDICAL
New York

**Visit our website at www.demosmedical.com**

*ISBN:* 9781620700426
*e-book ISBN:* 9781617052095

*Acquisitions Editor:* Beth Barry
*Compositor:* diacriTech





**Library of Congress Cataloging-in-Publication Data**

Botulinum neurotoxin injection manual / editors, Katharine E. Alter, Nicole A. Wilson.
p. ; cm.
Includes bibliographical references and index.
ISBN 978-1-62070-042-6 — ISBN 978-1-61705-209-5 (e-book)
I. Alter, Katharine E., editor. II. Wilson, Nicole A., editor.
[DNLM: 1. Botulinum Toxins. 2. Injections. 3. Nervous System Diseases—drug therapy. 4. Neuromuscular Agents—therapeutic use. QW 630.5.B2]
RL120.B66
615.7'78—dc23

2014033134



14 15 16 17 / 5 4 3 2 1

*Dedicated to our patients, from whom we receive daily inspiration. To Terry for his encouragement and heroic efforts in making this text as close to perfect as we could hope and to Foster for his unending patience and the reminder that "all work and no play make Katharine and Nicole dull girls."*

# *Contents*

**Anatomic Illustrations**

# *Contributors*

**Katharine E. Alter, MD** Medical Director, Rehabilitation Programs, Mount Washington Pediatric Hospital, Baltimore, Maryland; Senior Clinician, National Institutes of Health, Bethesda, Maryland

**Zachary Bohart, MD, MS** Associate Director, Spasticity Program; Director, Neurorehabilitation Clinic, Braintree Rehabilitation Hospital, Braintree, Massachusetts; Clinical Instructor, Physical Medicine and Rehabilitation, Tufts University School of Medicine, Boston, Massachusetts

**Sherry A. Downie, PhD** Professor, Departments of Anatomy and Structural Biology and Physical Medicine and Rehabilitation, Albert Einstein College of Medicine, Yeshiva University, Bronx, New York

**Elie Elovic, MD** Director of Physical Medicine and Rehabilitation, HealthSouth Rehabilitation of Utah, Sandy, Utah

**Pritha Ghosh, MD** Assistant Clinical Professor, Co-Director, Movement Disorders Program, Department of Neurology, George Washington University/Medical Faculty Associates, Washington, DC

**Barbara I. Karp, MD** National Institute of Neurological Disorders and Stroke, Bethesda, Maryland

**Stephen Koelbel, MD** Director, Spasticity Program, Braintree Rehabilitation Hospital, Braintree, Massachusetts

**Dallas A. Lea II, MD** Principal Partner, Lea Medical Partners LLC; Medical Director, Lea Medical Therapies, Silver Spring, Maryland

**Codrin Lungu, MD** Clinical Fellow, Human Motor Control Section, Division of Intramural Research, National Institute of Neurological Disorders and Stroke, Bethesda, Maryland

**John McGuire, MD** Associate Professor, Froedtert Hospital, Medical College of Wisconsin, Milwaukee, Wisconsin

**Michael C. Munin, MD, FAAPMR** Professor, Department of Physical Medicine and Rehabilitation, University of Pittsburgh School of Medicine, Pittsburgh, Pennsylvania

**Fatta B. Nahab, MD** Departments of Neurology and Neuroscience, University of Miami Miller School of Medicine, Miami, Florida

**Stephen Nichols, MD** Attending Staff Physician, Mt. Washington Pediatric Hospital, Baltimore, Maryland

**David Simpson, MD, FAAN** Professor of Neurology, Director, Clinical Neurophysiology Laboratories; Director, Neuromuscular Division; Director, NeuroAIDS Program, Department of Neurology, Mount Sinai Medical Center, New York, New York

**Nicole A. Wilson, PhD, MD** Principal, Roth Affinity LLC, St. Louis, Missouri; Special Volunteer, Rehabilitation Medicine Department, National Institutes of Health, Bethesda, Maryland

# *Preface*

The past two decades have seen an almost exponential increase in the number of approved, accepted, and investigational uses of botulinum neurotoxins (BoNTs) in clinical practice. At the same time, the number of FDA-approved BoNTs has expanded from a single serotype A toxin to three serotype A toxins and one serotype B toxin. Clinicians who prescribe and inject BoNTs must be familiar with an ever-expanding list of clinical applications and with the unique properties of each of the available BoNT products, including a thorough understanding of the approved and unapproved indications and differences in the preparation/dosing for each of the commercially available BoNT products. Clinicians must also be aware of the potential risks and benefits of BoNT therapy, be skilled in various guidance techniques (e.g., imaging, electromyography), and be aware of strategies that are used when performing BoNT therapy. The purpose of this handbook is to provide a concise overview of the currently approved BoNTs and their use for specific clinical conditions, including the approved and published dosage ranges for the BoNT products (where available). Anatomic illustrations are provided to enhance localization of muscles and other target structures. We hope this information will be useful for clinicians and will ultimately enhance patient care.

*Katharine E. Alter, MD*
*Nicole A. Wilson, PhD, MD*

# Section One

## Botulinum Neurotoxin: Basic Science and Reconstitution

# 1

# *Pharmacology of Botulinum Neurotoxins*

*Katharine E. Alter, MD*
*Fatta B. Nahab, MD*
*Barbara I. Karp, MD*

Botulinum neurotoxins (BoNTs) are biological products produced by various strains of *Clostridium botulinum*, which are gram-positive, obligate anaerobic bacteria. BoNTs are widely recognized as the most potent toxin known to man. It is somewhat surprising that BoNTs are also used in clinical practice for an ever-expanding list of approved and off-label indications. Despite their deadly nature, BoNTs have an excellent safety profile when used in minute quantities by experienced clinicians. This chapter provides a review of the pharmacology of BoNTs, an understanding of which is essential for clinicians who use these agents to treat patients (1, 2).

## Normal Neurotransmitter Release

At presynaptic nerve terminals (NTs), neurotransmitters (NrTrs) (e.g., acetylcholine) are stored in synaptic vesicles (SVs). The arrival of an action potential at NTs leads to the mobilization of SVs through exocytosis, resulting in the release of a quanta of NrTrs contained within the SV (3). The release of NrTrs through exocytosis is a multistep process that includes binding and fusion of the SV with the neuronal membrane, followed by the release of NrTrs into the synaptic cleft (Figure 1.1). This process of binding and exocytosis requires the interaction of a suite of intracellular polypeptides, the soluble *N*-ethylmaleimide-sensitive receptor (SNARE) proteins. Different SNARE proteins are located in the cytosol, on the SV, and on the presynaptic membrane of NTs. Membrane-associated SNARE proteins include SNAP25 and syntaxin. Vesicle-associated SNARE proteins include synaptobrevin (also known as vesicle-associated membrane protein [VAMP]) and synaptotagmin. Following exocytosis, the NrTrs diffuse across the synaptic cleft and bind to the specific postsynaptic receptors. Postsynaptic activation of target structures results in the activation of target structures,

*FIGURE 1.1 Botulinum toxin pathway. Reprinted with permission from BioCarta.*

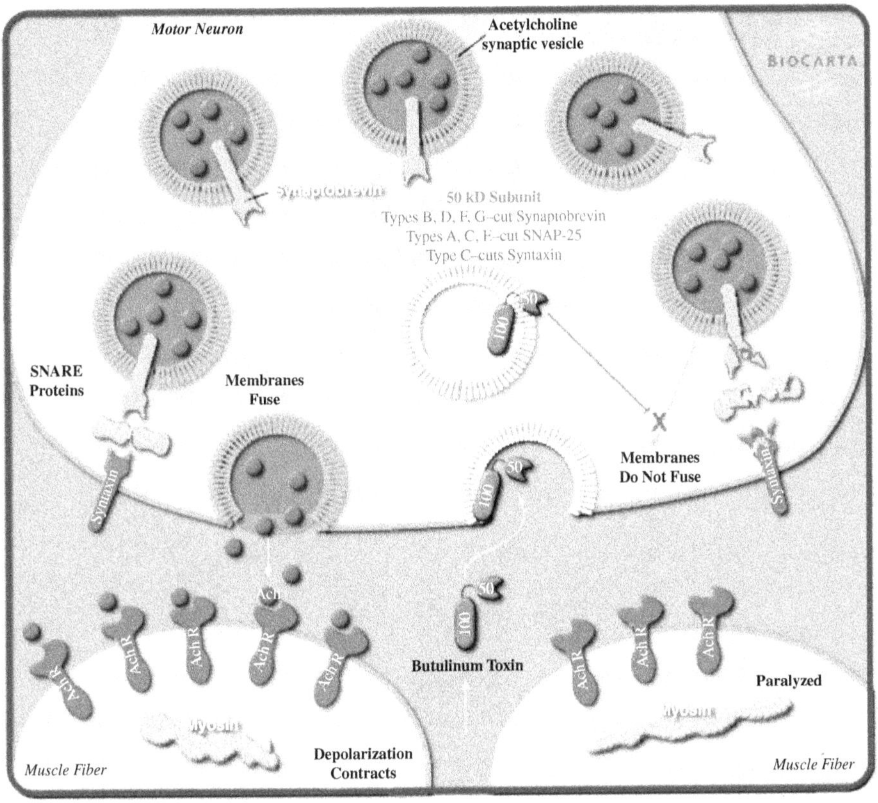


including muscle contraction at neuromuscular junctions (NMJs), glandular secretion (e.g., eccrine and salivary), and other sites (4).

## BoNTs Synthesis and Structure

BoNTs are synthesized as inactive, single 150-kDa polypeptide chains that are released, along with nontoxic proteins, from the cytosol from *Clostridium* bacterium following bacterial autolysis (1). Different strains of *Clostridium* produce different BoNT serotypes A to G, which vary in amino acid sequence. There are also amino acid variations within serotypes, creating subtypes within a given serotype (e.g., serotypes A1 and A2) (5).

The active BoNT molecule is composed of a 50-kDa light chain (LC) and a 100-kDa heavy chain (HC) linked by a disulfide bond. BoNTs are activated, or "nicked," by proteolytic cleavage to create the active disulfide chain molecule. The HC is responsible for receptor-mediated binding and membrane translocation. The LC, the catalytic domain, is responsible for blocking the action of BoNT at the synapse (6). BoNTs have a complex three-dimensional (3D) conformation that is required for site-specific binding and other actions of BoNTs (Figures 1.2A and B).

***FIGURE 1.2*** *(A) Botulinum neurotoxin molecule. Reproduced with permission from Annual Review of Biochemistry, Volume 79, 2010. (B) Botulinum neurotoxin molecule functional domains. Reprinted with permission from Raj Kumar and Bal Ram Singh, Botulinum Research Center, Institute of Advanced Sciences.*

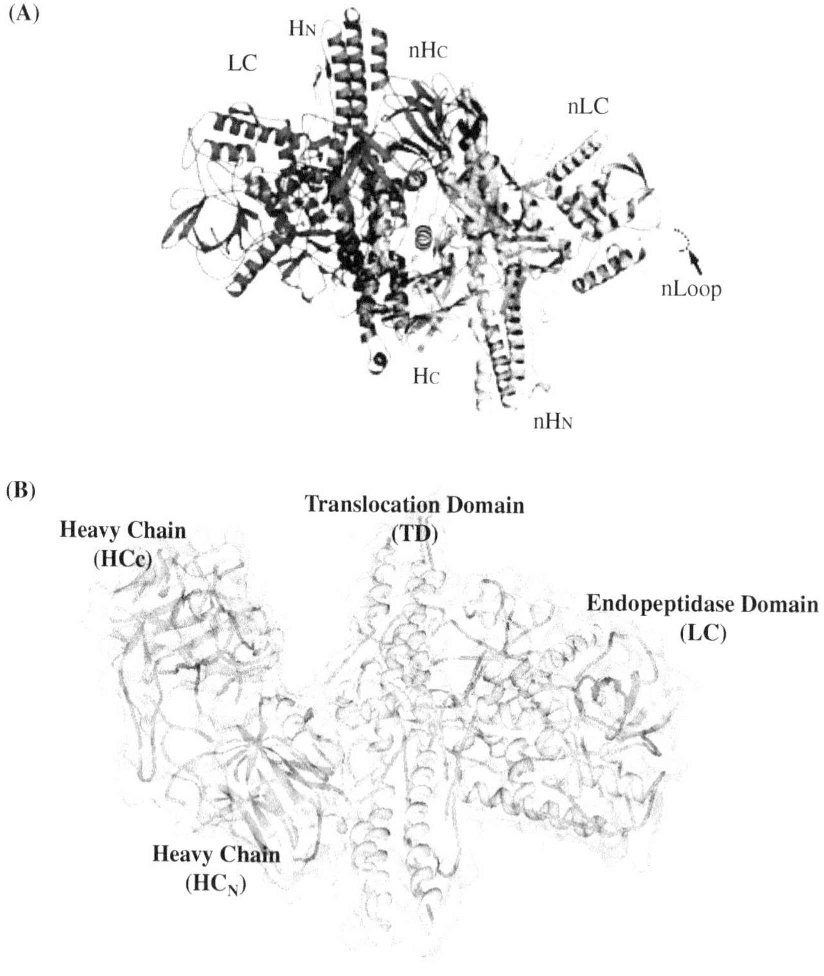


BoNTs, in their natural state, are associated with various nonhemagglutinating and hemagglutinating proteins, called complexing proteins (CPs). CPs increase the overall size of the neurotoxin complex to 300 to 900 kDa. Although little is known about the biological function of CPs, they are believed to protect or stabilize BoNT following ingestion and to prevent degradation following exposure to gastric proteases in the mammalian stomach (5, 7).

## BoNT Binding/Blocking

At cholinergic NTs, SNARE proteins are the intracellular targets of BoNTs. These intracellular nanomachines are involved in the intracellular transport and release of acetylcholine and other NrTrs (2, 7–11). The action of BoNT at presynaptic cholinergic NTs has been studied extensively and is understood in some detail. BoNTs, like other bacterial exotoxins, block their intracellular targets in a complex, multistep process. Step one of this process is uptake of the toxin into the presynaptic NT via site-specific binding of the HC-binding domain to a receptor on the presynaptic membrane. Following binding, the toxin is internalized by the process of receptor-mediated endocytosis. The LC is then cleaved from the HC by a process that has yet to be identified. To reach the SNARE targets in the cytosol of the neuron, the LC must then exit the endosome.

There are at least two proposed mechanisms for how the LC exits or translocates the endosome and both implicate the HC in this process. The translocation domain of the HC may act as a chaperone for the LC, facilitating its movement through the lipid bilayer. The other prevailing theory is that the HC creates a membrane pore through which the LC exits the endosome (12, 13). In this pore theory, conformational changes in the shape of the globular BoNT LC are required to allow it to exit the endosome. Under the influence of the acidic pH of the endosome, the LC unfolds and exits the endosome though the pore. Once in the cytosol, the LC must again refold into its original 3D conformation to allow it to bind to its SNARE target (13). This process of unfolding and refolding is influenced by a pH differential between the endosome (acidic) and the cytosol (neutral). Some researchers debate whether these conformational changes are required (12). Recent studies have revealed additional details about the HC and LC structure, including specialized regions of the HC. These specialized regions include a binding domain, translocation domain, and a belt region. The belt region surrounds the catalytic domain of the LC, which is buried deep in a cleft within the BoNT molecule. The belt region may serve to protect the LC catalytic moiety, although its exact function has yet to be elucidated (1).

After entering the cytosol of presynaptic neurons, the LCs of the various BoNT serotypes exert their action by blocking their respective SNARE proteins (Table 1.1). Once the LC binds to its SNARE protein target, the SNARE protein can no longer

**TABLE 1.1 BoNT Serotypes and SNARE Protein Targets**

| Serotype | SNARE Protein Target |
|---|---|
| A | SNAP25 |
| B | Synaptobrevin |
| C1 | Syntaxin |
| D | Synaptobrevin |
| E | SNAP25 |
| F | Synaptobrevin |
| G | Synaptobrevin |

function to release vesicular NrTrs. The action of that SNARE protein is permanently blocked. Although this blocking process is permanent and the poisoned nerve terminus degenerates, the toxin does not kill the neuron (1). The chemodenervation effects of BoNT are temporary because, eventually, the internalized BoNT is metabolized and the SNARE proteins and effected NTs regenerate. Once this process is complete, the function at the NT is restored, neural transmission resumes, and the function of the end organ is restored. This process of NT regeneration typically takes several months (2, 5).

## BoNT Potency and Dosing

BoNTs, being biological agents and not drugs, are measured in units of bioactivity, not by weight, mass, or volume. BoNT is measured and dosed in mouse units (MU or U), where 1 MU or U equals the median lethal dose (LD 50) for an intraperitoneal injection in a particular size, sex, and breed of mouse. For example, the MU of onabotulinumtoxinA is based on lethality in a 30-g female Swiss Webster mouse, following intraperitoneal injection of the neurotoxin. The potency, and therefore the recommended dose in units, for each serotype and each commercially available BoNT product is unique. Further differences among the products accrue from variances in the strain of *Clostridium* used to manufacture the toxin, as well as proprietary manufacturing practices. Therefore, these products are not interchangeable. This topic will be covered in detail in Chapter 2.

## Clinical Implications of BoNT Pharmacology

As noted earlier, BoNTs inhibit the release of NrTrs by blocking the action of one or more SNARE proteins required for NrTr vesicle exocytosis. Although the action of BoNTs at cholinergic NMJs was identified decades ago, their action is not limited to the NMJ. BoNTs also affect neuroglandular junctions, pain signaling, and other sites (2). BoNTs produce a sustained blockade of NrTr release, which at cholinergic NTs leads to chemodenervation. In clinical use, physicians exploit the effects of the chemodenervation produced by BoNTs through injection into specific muscles, glands, or other sites to selectively decrease the output of overactive neurons. The resultant decrease in neuronal activity thereby reduces overactivity in the target end-organ, such as muscle contraction, gland secretion, pain signaling, or others. By careful manipulation of the injected dose of BoNT, physicians can effectively titrate the extent of BoNT blockade on a specific target.

The uptake of BoNT is reportedly higher at active NTs. Hence, NTs that are pathologically overactive (i.e., those most active in the condition being treated) may have the highest uptake of BoNT and thereby be preferentially affected by the toxin. This bias toward a BoNT effect in overactive structures is potentially beneficial for patients and useful for clinicians in maximizing efficacy and minimizing side effects (14).

Following injection of BoNT for hypersecretion, pain, or muscle overcontraction, the clinical effects are typically first apparent within a few days and peak between 4 and 6 weeks after injection. The duration of effect may be influenced by the dose, target end-organ, severity of the condition being treated, and individual patient factors, but generally lasts 10 to 12 weeks. Although the duration of effect in aesthetic uses is generally 10 to 12 weeks, the response of overactive bladder to BoNT may last as long as 5 to 6 months (15, 16). Currently, most expert clinicians recommend re-injection when the patient's symptoms return, but no more frequently than every 12 weeks (15, 17). The limitation on the frequency of injections arises from concerns about the potential for antigenicity and antibody formation.

## Antigenicity, Antibody Formation, and Nonresponsiveness to BoNT

Some individuals or conditions do not respond well to BoNT (i.e., they have limited benefit or effect following BoNT injection). If there is no response to the first injection of BoNT, the patient is deemed a primary nonresponder. Primary nonresponse may be due to a variety of factors, either alone or in combination, including failure to properly target or inject the intended muscle/structure, selecting the wrong target or muscles, insufficient dosing, or injection of limbs with fixed contracture or other deformities that are not amenable to treatment with BoNT (17, 18).

Following injection, BoNTs, being foreign proteins, may induce neutralizing antibody formation rendering the toxin ineffective, which is called secondary nonresponse. Secondary nonresponse occurs rarely with current BoNT formulations. The presence of antibodies to BoNT can reduce or eliminate responsivity to BoNT injection. Although antibodies may form against either the toxin polypeptide itself or the accompanying CPs, it is likely that only some of these antibodies are neutralizing antibodies that contribute to reduced efficacy. Nonneutralizing antibodies may be present, but probably do not reduce the activity or clinical efficacy of BoNT (19).

Although BoNTs can induce an antibody response, they are only weakly antigenic in comparison to other biological toxins. When BoNT was first developed for clinical use, it was common for patients to receive an initial injection followed by "booster injections" every 2 to 4 weeks until response was achieved. Such booster injections, however, may foster the development of antibodies. To minimize the likelihood of antibody production and subsequent loss of clinical response, the practice of "booster injections" is now generally not advised. This recommendation is strengthened by early analyses showing that antibody formation was more likely in patients receiving high doses of BoNT or in those receiving injections more frequently than every 12 weeks (20). The initial reports on antigenicity were based on observations with an early preparation of onaboulinumtoxinA (1979 Botox®) that reported an antibody rate of 4% to 10% in patients being treated for cervical dystonia. The higher protein load of that preparation, compared to that of the currently available toxin (1997 Botox®), may have made it more antigenic. The current incidence of neutralizing antibodies is lower (2). A meta-analysis in 2000 revealed an overall antibody incidence of 0.49% in 2,240 patients with mixed diagnoses and indications for injection. Only 3 of 11 patients with antibodies were clinically unresponsive (21).

To reduce the risk of immunoresistance, the current expert consensus opinion is to use the smallest effective dose of BoNT, wait as long as possible between injection cycles, and avoid booster dosing (11).

## Safety

BoNTs have been used in clinical practice since the 1970s with an excellent safety profile when administered by physicians familiar with the risks and benefits of BoNTs (2, 11, 15, 17). When injected therapeutically in humans, the lethal dose of the various BoNT preparations is not known, and the doses required to cause systemic side effects are difficult to predict. Rare serious generalized adverse events, particularly neuromuscular weakness with respiratory compromise, have been reported following BoNT injections, most commonly with high doses and in compromised pediatric patients. However, similar life-threatening reactions can potentially occur in noncompromised patients at therapeutic doses. The serious nature of the potential risk prompted the Food and Drug Administration to add boxed warnings to all BoNT products in 2009 (Figure 1.3).

***FIGURE 1.3*** *Food and Drug Administration–approved boxed warning for BoNT products (Botox® example).*

WARNING: DISTANT SPREAD OF TOXIN EFFECT

Postmarketing reports indicate that the effects of BOTOX® and all botulinum toxin products may spread from the area of injection to produce symptoms consistent with botulinum toxin effects. These may include asthenia, generalized muscle weakness, diplopia, ptosis, dysphagia, dysphonia, dysarthria, urinary incontinence, and breathing difficulties. These symptoms have been reported hours to weeks after injection. Swallowing and breathing difficulties can be life threatening, and there have been reports of death. The risk of symptoms is probably greatest in children treated for spasticity, but symptoms can also occur in adults treated for spasticity and other conditions, particularly in those patients who have an underlying condition that would predispose them to these symptoms. In unapproved uses, including spasticity in children, and in approved indications, cases of spread of effect have been reported at doses comparable to those used to treat cervical dystonia and at lower doses.

*Source:* From Ref. (34). Botox PI [package insert/prescribing information]. Irvine, CA: Allergan. Available at http://www.allergan.com/assets/pdf/botox_cosmetic_pi.pdf

Fortunately, serious reactions to therapeutic BoNT injections are rare. The most common adverse events following BoNT injection are local and attributable to an "excessive effect" of the toxin or to pain and bruising from the injection itself. The "excessive effects" include problematic weakness in the target muscle, unintended weakness in adjacent muscles, and other toxin effects in nearby or distant toxin-sensitive glands or muscles. For example, in the treatment of cervical dystonia, the most commonly reported adverse events are dysphagia and dry mouth (15). The risk of these side effects in patients with cervical dystonia may be minimized by meticulous attention to injection targeting as far as possible from the oropharynx and avoiding excessive doses of BoNT (22).

## Central Effects of BoNTs

In addition to local effects in target or distant peripheral structures, there is mounting evidence that BoNTs are transported from peripheral sites into the central nervous system, including spinal motor neurons and the brain. Most of the data on retrograde transport and central effects arise from animal studies on pain reduction (5). Central or retrograde transport of BoNT to pain centers in the brainstem, particularly the trigeminal system, may be partly responsible for the antinociceptive effects of BoNT observed in animal studies and clinical practice.

## Summary

The use of BoNTs in clinical practice requires that physicians understand BoNTs mechanism of action to realize the potential benefits and to minimize the risks of these potent biological agents.

BoNTs are complex biologic molecules, and although much is now known about their structure and function, future research is likely to reveal additional information relevant to their clinical use. The versatility of BoNTs is likely to lead to the expansion of their use for as yet unidentified clinical problems and indications.

# 2

# *Comparison of Botulinum Neurotoxin Products*

*Katharine E. Alter, MD*
*Fatta B. Nahab, MD*

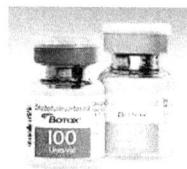

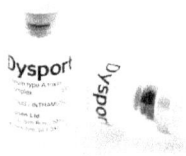

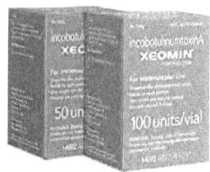

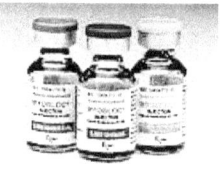


There are currently four botulinum neurotoxin (BoNT) products approved by the Food and Drug Administration (FDA) for clinical use in the United States: three serotype A BoNT products and one serotype B BoNT product. Worldwide, other BoNT products are also approved for clinical use (23–27). Each product has unique characteristics and carries specific labeling, approvals, and dosage recommendations (6, 28, 29). To reduce the risk of dosing errors, a unique generic name has been assigned to each commercially available BoNT product approved for clinical use (Table 2.1). These unique generic names also emphasize that BoNT products are not interchangeable. The four BoNT products currently approved for use in the United States are onabotulinumtoxinA (OBTA; Botox®), abobotulinumtoxinA (ABTA; Dysport®), incobotulinumtoxinA (IBTA; Xeomin®), and rimabotulinumtoxinB (RBTB; Myobloc®).

**TABLE 2.1A Commercial Botulinum Neurotoxin (BoNT) Products Available in the United States**

| Serotype | Generic Name | Brand Name | Manufacturer | First U.S. Approval | Indications (United States) | Indications (Outside the United States) | Composition |
|---|---|---|---|---|---|---|---|
| A | OnabotulinumtoxinA | Botox | Allergan | 1989 | 1,2,3,4,5,6,7,8,9 | 2,3,4,5,6,8,9,10,12 | Dimerized with two 300-kDa accessory proteins |
| A | AbobotulinumtoxinA | Dysport | Ipsen | 2009 | 3,4 | 2,3,5,8,9,10,11 | Dimerized with two 300-kDa accessory proteins |
| A | IncobotulinumtoxinA | Xeomin | Merz | 2011 | 2,3,4,9 | 2,3,8,9 | Serotype A BoNT only, without complexing proteins |
| B | RimabotulinumtoxinB | Myobloc (in the United States) Neurobloc (Outside the United States) | US WorldMed Eisai Limited | 2000 | 3 | 3 | Dimerized with two 150-kDa accessory proteins |

Note: Clinical indications for serotype A BoNT and serotype B BoNT products:

1. strabismus, 2. blepharospasm, 3. cervical dystonia, 4. moderately severe glabellar lines, 5. hyperhidrosis, 6. chronic migraine, 7. overactive bladder, 8. upper limb spasticity, 9. blepharospasm in patients previously treated with onabotulinumtoxinA (OBTA; Botox®), 10. hemifacial spasm, 11. calf muscles/equinus in patients with cerebral palsy ≥2 years of age, 12. pediatric lower limb spasticity, gastrocnemius.

**TABLE 2.1B Characteristics of Commercial Botulinum Neurotoxin (BoNT) Products**

| Product | Complex Size | Protein Load (ng BoNT/unit) | Vial Size (units) |
|---|---|---|---|
| OnabotulinumtoxinA (Botox) | 900 kDa | 2.4–~5 ng/100 units | 100<br>200 |
| AbobotulinumtoxinA (Dysport) | 300 kDa L complex<br>600 kDa M complex | 3.24–4.35 ng/500 units | 300<br>500 |
| IncobotulinumtoxinA (Xeomin) | 150 kDa | 0.6–0.73 ng/100 units | 50<br>100 |
| RimabotulinumtoxinB (Myobloc) | 700 kDa | 25 ng/2,500 units | 2,500<br>5,000<br>10,000 |

*Sources:* Refs. 50, 174.

**TABLE 2.2 Properties of Botulinum Neurotoxin (BoNT) Products Available in the United States (from Manufacturer's Package Insert/Prescribing Information)**

| BoNT Products | Product Details |
|---|---|
| AbobotulinumtoxinA | **Product:** Purified by series precipitation, dialysis, and chromatography steps. Neurotoxin-complex contains BoNT-A, hemagglutinin proteins, nontoxic, nonhemagglutinin proteins. Complex size 300–900 kDa. Protein load 4.54 ng<br>**Supplied:** ABTA (Dysport) is supplied in single-use, sterile 3-mL glass vials. Vial sizes: 300 units and 500 units containing lyophilized ABTA, 125 mcg human albumin, 2.5 mg lactose<br>**Reconstitution:** Sterile, preservative-free 0.9% NaCl.<br>**Storage/handling:** Store unopened vials at (2°C–8°C or 36°F–46°F). Protect from light. Administer within 4 hr of reconstitution; store reconstituted toxin in the refrigerator for up to 4 hr. Do not refreeze after reconstitution<br>**U.S. FDA-approved indications:** Cervical dystonia, glabellar lines<br>**Indications outside the United States:** Hemifacial spasm, upper limb spasticity (adults), dynamic equinus/calf muscles in ambulatory patients with cerebral palsy ≥2 y of age |
| IncobotulinumtoxinA | **Product:** Vials contain only IBTA (Xeomin), which has been separated from accessory proteins, yielding a pure form of lyophilized BoNT-A in a sterile, white to off-white powder. Complex size 150 kDa, protein load 0.6 ng<br>**Supplied:** 50-U or 100-U vials containing 1 mg human albumin and 4.7 mg sucrose<br>**Reconstitution:** Preservative-free, sterile 0.9% saline for injection<br>**Storage/handling:** Store unopened vials at room temperature 20°C–25°C (68°F–77°F), in a refrigerator at 2°C–8°C (36°F–46°F), or freeze at -20°C–10°C (-4°F–14°F) for up to 36 months. Administer reconstituted toxin within 24 hr |

*(continued)*

**TABLE 2.2 Properties of Botulinum Neurotoxin (BoNT) Products Available in the United States (from Manufacturer's Package Insert/Prescribing Information) (*continued*)**

| BoNT Products | Product Details |
|---|---|
| IncobotulinumtoxinA | **U.S. FDA-approved indications:** Cervical dystonia, blepharospasm in patients previously treated with OBTA/Botox, glabellar lines<br>**Indications outside the United States:** Poststroke upper limb spasticity (adults) |
| OnabotulinumtoxinA | **Product:** OBTA (Botox) is a sterile lyophilized BoNT-A, purified by acid precipitation. Crystalline complex containing toxin and other proteins (human albumin). Complex size 900 kDa. Protein load 5 ng<br>**Supplied:** Single-use glass vials, 100- or 200-unit vials Contents: 100-unit vial: 100 U OBTA neurotoxin complex, 0.5 mg human albumin, 0.9 mg NaCl, vacuum-dried powder without preservative; 200-unit vial: 200 U OBTA neurotoxin complex, 1 mg human albumin, 1.8 mg NaCl, vacuum-dried powder without preservative<br>**Reconstitution:** Sterile, preservative-free 0.9% NaCl for injection<br>**Storage/handing:** Unopened vials: refrigerate at (2°C–8°C), 100-U vials up to 36 months, 200-U vials up to 24 months. Once reconstituted, administer within 24 hr. Store reconstituted Botox in a refrigerator for up to 24 hr<br>**U.S. FDA-approved indications:** Blepharospasm, strabismus, cervical dystonia, primary axillary hyperhidrosis, chronic migraine, upper limb spasticity (adults), overactive bladder, detrusor overactivity, glabellar lines, lateral canthal lines<br>**Indications outside the United States:** Pediatric spasticity (gastrocnemius), focal poststroke spasticity (adults) |
| RimabotulinumtoxinB | **Product:** RBTB (Myobloc) is a sterile liquid formulation of a purified neurotoxin produced by fermentation of the bacterium *Clostridium botulinum* type B (Bean strain) and exists in noncovalent association with hemagglutinin and nonhemagglutinin proteins as a neurotoxin complex. The neurotoxin complex is recovered from the fermentation process and purified through a series of precipitation and chromatography steps. Myobloc is provided as a clear and colorless to light-yellow sterile injectable solution pH 5.6<br>**Supplied:** In single-use 3.5-mL glass vials. 5,000 U BoNT-B per 1 mL with 0.05% human serum albumin, 0.01 M sodium succinate, 0.1 M NaCl. Available as 2,500-U (0.5 mL), 5,000-U (1 mL), and 10,000-U (2 mL) vials.<br>**Storage/handling:** Refrigerate at 2°C–8°C (36–46°F). Do not freeze or shake. May be diluted with normal saline. Once opened, the product must be used within 4 hr as the formulation does not contain a preservative<br>**U.S. FDA-approved indications:** Cervical dystonia<br>**Indications outside the United States:** Cervical dystonia |

*Sources:* Refs. 34, 36, 38, 44.

## BoNT Approvals

The following is a brief review of the individual neurotoxins and their current U.S. indications. Information regarding non-U.S. indications is also provided in Table 2.1. Readers should be aware that although approvals/indications listed in this text are up to date as of the time of publication, approvals for additional BoNT products and indications for currently approved BoNT products are anticipated. Prior to prescribing/administering any BoNT product, clinicians must be familiar with the approved indications, pharmacology, handling, and dosing for that product (28, 30, 31).

### *OnabotulinumtoxinA (Botox)*

OBTA was the first BoNT product licensed worldwide and carries the longest list of approvals in the United States and abroad (32). The OBTA-toxin complex is a crystalline complex containing neurotoxin, human albumin, and NaCl as a vacuum-dried powder without preservative. The complex size is 900 kDa (active BoNT-A molecule size: 150 kDa) (34). The BoNT protein load is approximately 5 ng per 100 units. It should be noted that the current formulation of OBTA (designated BCB 2024) has a lower total protein load than the earlier formulation that was discontinued in 1997 (batch 79-11), with a subsequently reduced incidence of neutralizing antibody formation (21, 33). OBTA is approved in the United States for treatment of strabismus, blepharospasm, cervical dystonia, glabellar lines, lateral canthal lines, hyperhidrosis, migraine, overactive bladder, and upper limb spasticity in adults. In the United Kingdom, OBTA is also approved for hemifacial spasm, additional upper limb muscles in adults with spasticity, and the gastrocnemius muscle in children with cerebral palsy (34, 35).

### *AbobotulinumtoxinA (Dysport)*

AbobotulinumtoxinA was first approved in 1991 in the United Kingdom. It is currently approved in 75 countries, including the United States (where it has been approved since 2009), Ireland, the United Kingdom, and New Zealand. AbobotulinumtoxinA is a serotype A BoNT. The molecular mass of the neurotoxin complex is 300 to 900 kDa. The complex includes accessory proteins, human albumin, and the 150-kDa active BoNT-A neurotoxin. ABTA is distributed in 300- and 500-unit vials. In the United States, ABTA is currently approved for adult patients (≥18 years of age) for the treatment of cervical dystonia and moderately severe glabellar lines. In other countries (e.g., the United Kingdom), ABTA is also approved for blepharospasm/hemifacial spasm, upper limb spasticity in adults (clenched fist/wrist flexion), and equinus foot deformity in children with cerebral palsy (≥2 years of age) (36, 37).

### *IncobotulinumtoxinA (Xeomin)*

IBTA was introduced in 2005 and approved in the United States in 2012. IBTA is currently approved in 20 countries, including the United States, Canada, the United Kingdom, Austria, Denmark, Finland, France, Germany, Italy, Luxembourg, Norway, Poland, Portugal, Spain, Sweden, Argentina, and Mexico. It is derived from a wild-type strain of *Clostridium botulinum* neurotoxin serotype A (ATC 3502). During the manufacturing process, complexing proteins (CPs) associated with the BoNT are removed, leaving only the 150-kDa BoNT that is free of CP. The removal of these CPs may lead to a decreased antigenicity of the toxin complex and reduced antibody formation. IBTA is a lyophilized powder and is available in 50- and 100-unit vials. IBTA is approved in the United States for blepharospasm in patients previously treated with OBTA, cervical dystonia, and glabellar lines (31, 38–41). Worldwide, IBTA is approved for a variety of other conditions, including upper limb spasticity (in adults) in Europe, Canada, Mexico, and Argentina (40). Xeomin is the only BoNT that is stable for 3 years at room temperature (42).

### *RimabotulinumtoxinB (Myobloc/Neurobloc)*

Each vial of rimabotulinumtoxinB (RBTB; Myobloc in the United States, Neurobloc outside of the United States) contains BoNT-B complexed in noncovalent association with hemagglutinin and nonhemagglutinin accessory proteins. The complex size is 700 kDa and the active neurotoxin is 150 kDa. The protein load is 25 ng. The preparation comes as a prediluted, clear, colorless to light-yellow sterile injectable solution, with a pH of 5.5. RBTB is available in 2,500-, 5,000-, and 10,000-unit vials and was first approved in the United States in 2000 for the treatment of cervical dystonia. It is also approved in other countries for the treatment of cervical dystonia (43–45).

## BoNT Products: Antigenicity, Dilution, and Diffusion

### *Antigenicity*

BoNT products are foreign proteins and are therefore immunogenic and may trigger the production of neutralizing antibodies (NA) that can block the action of the neurotoxin, as well as non-NA directed at nontoxic proteins within the BoNT complex (46). NA to BoNT lead to antibody-induced treatment failure. There is a low overall risk of NA-induced treatment failure in patients receiving BoNT injections ranging from 1.28% in patients with cervical dystonia to 0.32% in patients with poststroke spasticity to 0% in patients treated for overactive bladder (21). Factors that may contribute to NA production include the protein load/dose, number of injection sites, and treatment interval (25). The risk of NA-associated treatment failure is relatively low with all of the currently approved BoNT products. The risk of NA production can be minimized further by reducing the BoNT dose to the minimum required for treatment effect, increasing the treatment interval, perhaps by avoiding booster dosing, and by meticulous handling of BoNT products to avoid inactivating the toxin. BoNT products can be inactivated during manufacturing, storage, reconstitution, and handling. Inactivated toxin will produce no clinical effect, but it remains antigenic and will contribute to antibody formation. Theoretically, the lower the protein load of the toxin, the less antigenic it may be (25). Patient-related factors may also influence antibody production, including the patient's ability to mount an immune response. Many clinicians empirically recommend avoiding immunizations within 2 weeks of BoNT injections to avoid stimulating the patient's immune system (18). This practice has not been studied nor has it proven to reduce the risk of NA treatment failure.

### *Dilution and Diffusion*

There remains a paucity of information on the effects of dilution on diffusion, clinical efficacy, and adverse events following BoNT injections. The general consensus is that more dilute solutions diffuse further (47). A variety of factors may influence the diffusion characteristics of BoNT following injection, including dose, concentration, muscle characteristics (mass), the number of neuromuscular junctions, and individual patient characteristics. Some studies indicate that the dose at the site of injection is the most important factor (48). Additional research is needed to determine the optimal dilution for each clinical indication and BoNT product.

## BoNT Products: Potency and Dose

The potency of all BoNT products is measured in mouse units (MU), where 1 MU or U equals the median lethal dose (LD 50) for an intraperitoneal injection in a particular size, sex, and breed of mouse. Because BoNT products are biological agents, not drugs, the potency and dosing of each BoNT product are unique. The observed differences in potency, both within and between BoNT serotypes, may be due to many factors including different strains of *Clostridium botulinum* used to produce BoNT products and proprietary manufacturing differences (29, 30).

When calculating the dose of BoNT, clinicians must remain acutely aware of product-specific dose recommendations. The manufacturers of each BoNT product explicitly state that these products cannot be interchanged and that the units used to calculate a dose for a given patient are unique for each BoNT product. In the prescribing literature, clinicians are advised that when switching a patient to a new brand (even if the patient is not naïve to BoNT and has a previously stable dose regimen on another product), they should initiate the treatment at the lowest recommended dose for a given product (34, 36, 38, 44).

## Converting Units/Dose Among BoNT Products

Despite the aforementioned recommendations, there is considerable interest in and have been numerous articles related to dose equivalency and/or dose conversion ratios among the various BoNT products (30).

### *Evidence Questioning the Practice of BoNT Dose Conversion Ratios*

In the past 15 years, a number of articles have detailed the dose or dose range, in units, for OBTA and ABTA for various clinical indications. From these published dose ranges, an apparent dose ratio of 2 to 4 units of ABTA for each 1 unit of OBTA has been observed. However, a number of authors have continued to question the practice of dose ratios, concluding that the available toxins are not bioequivalent (49–54). Many researchers question the use of these dose ratios as they were not obtained from controlled trials with head-to-head product comparisons (55). Many experienced clinicians and researchers report inherent differences within BoNT products that limit the usefulness of bioequivalent doses and that dose ratios are not reliable. These experts recommend dose calculation(s) based on the individual product (49, 51, 52, 54).

Of note, the majority of the studies mentioned derived a dose ratio based on clinical measures (i.e., clinical effects and/or adverse events) after the use of various BoNT products at specific conversion ratios. Clinical measures are less sensitive to change than objective measures, such as neurophysiologic or electromyographic measures. Ideally, future studies evaluating dose conversion should include objective measures (30, 56).

When considering dose ratios, one possibility is that conversion ratios should be condition- and/or population-specific (57, 58). For example, a different dose conversion ratio should be used for cervical dystonia than for glabellar lines and for adults versus children. Another possibility when considering a conversion ratio is that there is less room for error in certain conditions. For example, treatment of focal hand dystonia or injections for esthetic purposes has less room for error compared with treatment for muscle hypertonia from an upper motor neuron syndrome.

### *Evidence Supporting the Practice of BoNT Dose Conversion Ratios*

Despite recommendations from manufacturers and questions by researchers, clinicians frequently ask whether the use of dose conversion ratios is safe, and if so, how best to convert among the various serotype A neurotoxins or between serotype A and serotype B products. There are a number of articles dating from the late 1990s on this topic, and the majority describe ratios converting other BoNT products to OBTA (53, 55, 57–71). The following sections summarize the current evidence.

### *Dose Conversion Ratios for Converting ABTA to OBTA*

A number of recent open label, crossover, and double-blind studies describe a conversion ratio ranging from 1 to 6 units of ABTA for each 1 unit of OBTA. The majority of these articles report conversion ratios of 2 to 3 units of ABTA for each 1 unit of OBTA (53, 55, 57, 58, 60, 61, 62, 65, 67, 69, 71).

### *Dose Conversion Ratios for Converting IBTA to OBTA*

When comparing IBTA to OBTA, the published ranges of dose ratios were 1 to 1.7 units IBTA for each 1 unit of OBTA. In the majority of studies, a 1:1 dose ratio was used when converting or comparing the dose of these two products (59, 63–65, 68).

### *Dose Conversion Ratios for Converting RBTB to Serotype A BoNT Products*

Several published studies have compared the serotype B BoNT to various serotype A BoNT products. Schlereth et al. reported that serotype A BoNT products (ABTA and OBTA) were 20 to 50 times more potent than the serotype B BoNT (70). A 2011 study compared RBTB to ABTA when treating adult patients with sialorrhea and reported a dose ratio of 10 units of RBTB for every 1 unit of ABTA (2,500 units of RBTB vs.

250 units of ABTA) (66). Although expert clinicians report using a conversion ratio of 20 to 30 units of RBTB for every 1 unit of OBTA, the evidence to support this practice is limited.

## Summary

The published data on dose conversion remain limited and should be interpreted with caution. Additional controlled trials with head-to-head comparisons of individual preparations should be conducted to determine whether conversion ratios may be safely used in clinical practice and if so, to establish the optimal dose conversion ratio. When these studies are performed, the dose conversion information should be published and reported in the full prescribing information/BoNT product literature. At the time of publication, regulatory agencies and the manufacturers of BoNT products continue to discourage the use of conversion ratios. When treating a neurotoxin-naïve patient or when switching from one BoNT product to another, clinicians are advised to follow the manufacturer's recommendations on initial dose for the specific condition. Given the limited evidence on this topic and the recommendations from both manufacturers and regulatory agencies, clinicians who use conversion ratios should do so with caution.

# 3

# *Neurotoxin Storage, Reconstitution, Handling, and Dilution*

*Katharine E. Alter, MD*
*Codrin Lungu, MD*

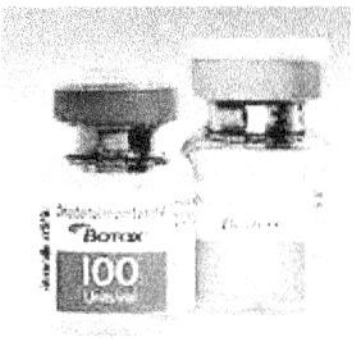

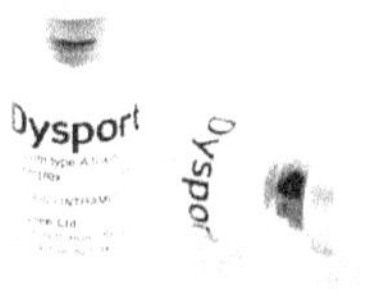

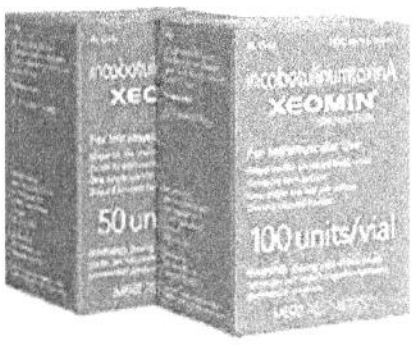

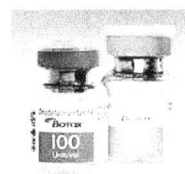

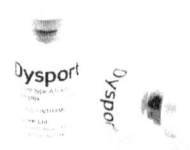

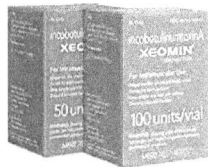

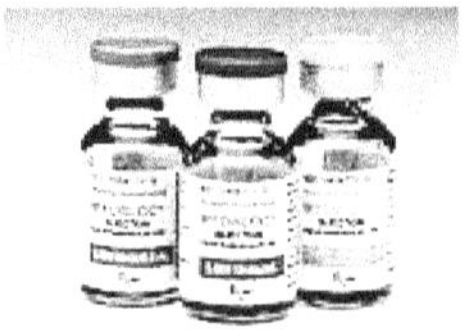

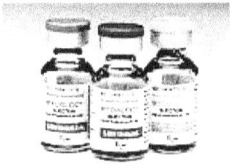

As noted in previous chapters, the four Food and Drug Administration (FDA)–approved botulinum neurotoxin (BoNT) formulations are not identical, nor are they interchangeable. The manufacturers of each BoNT product have published specific instructions for reconstitution/preparation of the product prior to administration and storage after reconstitution.

## Serotype B BoNT

RimabotulinumtoxinB (RBTB, Myobloc®), the only available serotype B BoNT, is also the only product available in the United States that is supplied as a ready-to-use solution. Therefore, RBTB does not require reconstitution but can be further diluted, as desired, with normal saline (NS, 0.9%) (44).

## Serotype A BoNTs

The three available serotype A BoNTs, onabotulinumtoxinA (OBTA, Botox®), abobotulinumtoxinA (ABTA, Dysport®), and incobotulinumtoxinA (IBTA, Xeomin®), require reconstitution prior to administration (34, 36, 38). The manufacturers of each of the serotype A BoNTs recommend preservative-free normal saline (PFNS) for injection (0.9% NS or PFNS) as the diluent. This recommendation is based on theoretical concerns that BoNTs are fragile and could possibly be denatured by preservatives in NS diluents.

Published studies have evaluated the effects of reconstitution using other diluents (NS plus benzol alcohol, NS plus hyaluronidase, sterile water, 1% and 2% lidocaine, bupivacaine, and 1% albumin) on the activity of the BoNTs and have found that the toxin remains active with diluents other than PFNS (47). However, none of these diluents has been rigorously studied, nor are they recommended by manufacturers of any of the available BoNT products. Clinicians should be aware of a single published report of a patient death due to anaphylaxis when 1% lidocaine was used as the diluent, although it is unclear whether the anaphylactic reaction was due to the lidocaine, the BoNT, or the combination of both (72). The authors' recommendation is that clinicians follow manufacturer's guidelines for reconstitution of BoNTs with PFNS until such time as other diluents are approved by the given manufacturer.

For all BoNT procedures with products requiring reconstitution, the medication should be prepared *immediately before* administration, but only after the patient has been examined, has been counseled, and has provided informed consent. Patients should not be treated with BoNT if they are ill, febrile, or if there is active infection at the site of injection. Therefore, examination of the patient is mandatory before reconstitution to avoid costly wastage.

There is little information published on dilution of BoNTs, nor is there a consensus on the optimal dilution for the individual BoNT products. Therefore, the topic of dilution requires additional study (73). Diffusion appears to be affected by dilution and dose, but not by molecular weight, complex size, or the presence of complexing proteins. There are also differences among BoNT products and, in particular, RBTB may have a greater diffusion than OBTA (74). It is likely that the optimal dilution of BoNT is dependent on the condition being treated, the size of the target, and the desired spread of the toxin. A higher dilution theoretically leads to greater diffusion or spread. In a study of OBTA for the treatment of blepharospasm, a higher dilution was equally effective, but led to more pain and larger local reactions (75). Kim et al. evaluated the effect of dilution on outcomes following treatment of spasticity with higher volumes resulting in marginally better treatment outcomes (76). Other studies revealed no difference in clinical outcome with varying dilution when treating children or adults with spasticity (77, 78). When treating small muscles with IBTA, dilution did not appear to influence efficacy (79).

## OnabotulinumtoxinA (Botox®) Reconstitution and Handling

OBTA is provided in single-use, sterile vials containing either 100 or 200 units of vacuum-dried powder. Reconstitute only with sterile PFNS immediately prior to injection. Once reconstituted, the product should be used within 24 hours.

Reconstituted product should be kept in the refrigerator at 2°C to 8°C. To reconstitute OBTA, the desired quantity of PFNS diluent is drawn into the appropriate-size syringe using a sterile large-gauge needle and the needle is then inserted into the vial (Tables 3.1A and B). Each vial of OBTA should have a partial vacuum. The negative pressure of this vacuum should pull the PFNS into the vial. If the vacuum is absent, the vial should be discarded and returned to the manufacturer (34). The contents of the vial should then be mixed with the NS diluent by gently rotating the vial. Do not shake or agitate the vials. (This may denature or deactivate the BoNT product.) Clinicians are advised to avoid turning the vial upside-down as the diluted product will stick to the stopper making it difficult to recover the entire contents of the vial (34, 80).

The volume of diluent added to the vial is determined by the condition being treated (Tables 3.1A and B). A dilution of 100 units with 1.0-mL PFNS (concentration 10 units/0.1 mL) is a typical dilution when treating patients with cervical dystonia. A dilution of 100 units in 1.0 to 2.0 mL (5 or 10 units/0.1 mL) is common when treating patients with spasticity, where higher volumes and larger muscles are targeted. In conditions where a small number of units and precise dosing are required (e.g., strabismus or blepharospasm), a higher volume of diluent is used, typically 100-units BoNT diluted with either 2.0- or 4.0-mL PFNS (concentration 5 units/0.1 mL or 2.5 units/0.1 mL). For urologic conditions, even larger dilutions are recommended (see Chapter 16). This allows precise dosing with a relatively small number of units.

As noted earlier, a partial vacuum will draw the PFNS into the vial. If the volume of diluent added to the vial is not sufficient to equalize the negative pressure vacuum, the air–fluid interface in the vial will create bubbles that will make it difficult to draw the toxin up into a syringe. To eliminate the bubbles, this partial vacuum must be equalized. To equalize the remaining vacuum, while leaving the needle in the vial, detach the syringe from the needle. The remaining vacuum/negative pressure will be equalized as air is drawn into the vial and the bubbles will dissipate. The syringe is then reconnected to the needle and the desired dose of diluted BoNT may be drawn up into the syringe. Any air bubble in the syringe barrel should be expelled and the syringe is attached to an appropriately sized sterile needle for injection. Patency of the needle should be confirmed by depressing the syringe plunger.

The manufacturer recommends that the toxin be administered within 24 hours of reconstitution, during which time it should be stored at 2°C to 8°C. It is worth noting that in practice, OBTA efficacy is preserved longer than these conservative guidelines suggest (81), and studies have demonstrated efficacy for cosmetic applications after storage for up to 2 weeks (82).

The choice of dilution depends on the therapeutic target. If a large dose is injected (e.g., for cervical dystonia or spasticity), the usual approach is to use 1 mL of PFNS/100 units of neurotoxin, resulting in a concentration of 10 units/0.1 mL. When better control over small doses is required (e.g., facial muscle injections), dilutions of 2-mL PFNS/100-units BoNT or 4-mL PFNS/100-units BoNT can be used, resulting in concentrations of 5 and 2.5 units/0.1 mL, respectively.

**TABLE 3.1A OnabotulinumtoxinA/Botox Manufacturer Reconstitution Instructions**

| PFNS (mL) | 100-Unit Vial: Dose per 0.1 mL (Units) | 200-Unit Vial: Dose per 0.1 mL (Units) |
|---|---|---|
| 1 | 10 | 20 |
| 2 | 5 | 10 |
| 4 | 2.5 | 5 |
| 6 | 1.66 | 3.33 |
| 8 | 1.25 | 2.5 |
| 10 | 1 | 2 |

Note: The dilutions and dose calculations shown in the table are for an injection volume of 0.1 mL. An increase or decrease in the Botox dose is also possible by administering a smaller or larger injection volume. For example, when 100 units is diluted in 1 mL, 0.05 mL = 5 units or 0.15 mL = 15 units.

When treating adult patients with Botox for one or more indications, the manufacturer's maximum cumulative dose should not generally exceed 360 units in a 3-month interval.

*Abbreviation:* PFNS, preservative-free normal saline (0.9%) for injection.

*Source:* Ref. 34. Botox PI [package insert/prescribing information]. Irvine, CA: Allergan. Available at http://www.allergan.com/assets/pdf/botox_cosmetic_pi.pdf

**TABLE 3.1B Manufacturer-Recommended Dilutions for Specific Indications for OnabotulinumtoxinA (Botox)**

| | |
|---|---|
| Axillary hyperhidrosis | The recommended dilution is 100 units in 4-mL PFNS.<br>Recommended dose is 50 units/axilla. |
| Detrusor overactivity | Total recommended dose is 200 units.<br>One 200-unit vial or two 100-unit vials are diluted with 6-mL PFNS. Additional dilution is then required as follows:<br>**For 200-unit vials**: Draw 2 mL of diluted OBTA into three 10-mL syringes. Draw an additional 8-mL PFNS into each syringe. The resulting dilution is 67 units/10 mL or 6.7 units/1 mL.<br>**For two 100-unit vials**: Draw 4 mL from each vial into a 10-mL syringe. Draw up the remaining 2 mL from each vial into a third 10-mL syringe. Then draw 6-mL PFNS into each of the three 10-mL syringes. This results in a concentration of 67 units/10 mL or 6.7 units/1 mL. |
| Overactive bladder | Recommended dilution: 100 units in 10-mL PFNS<br>Total dose: 100 units |
| Cervical dystonia | Recommended dilution:<br>100-unit vial with either 1-or 2-mL PFNS<br>200-unit vial with either 2- or 4-mL PFNS<br>Mean dosage: 236 units/treatment session (75th percentile: 198–300 units) |
| Chronic migraine | Recommended dilution: 100 units in 2-mL PFNS or 200 units in 4-mL PFNS for a concentration of 5 units/0.1 mL<br>Recommended dosage: 155 units/treatment session |

(*continued*)

**TABLE 3.1B Manufacturer-Recommended Dilutions for Specific Indications for OnabotulinumtoxinA (Botox) (*continued*)**

| | |
|---|---|
| Ophthalmologic indications | Blepharospasm and strabismus: Depending on desired dose, recommended dilution is either 100 units in 8-mL PFNS or 100 units in 4-mL PFNS. |
| Spasticity, upper limb (adults) | Recommended dilution: 100 units with 2-mL PFNS or 200 units with 4-mL PFNS.<br>Maximum recommended dosage: 360 units/treatment session |

*Abbreviations:* OBTA, onabotulinumtoxinA; PFNS, preservative-free normal saline (0.9%).

*Source:* Ref. 34. Botox PI [package insert/prescribing information]. Irvine, CA: Allergan. Available at http://www.allergan.com/assets/pdf/botox_cosmetic_pi.pdf

## AbobotulinumtoxinA (Dysport®) Reconstitution and Handling

ABTA is available in the United States in 300- and 500-unit vials, containing lyophilized powder for reconstitution (36). Each vacuum-dried vial is reconstituted with sterile PFNS (see Table 3.2). Using a sterile, large-bore needle, the PFNS diluent is drawn into an appropriately sized syringe and the needle is inserted into the vial. A partial vacuum should draw the diluent into the vials. Any vial that does not have a negative pressure vacuum should be discarded and returned to the manufacturer. Mix the PFNS diluent and the dried powder by gently rotating the vial. Do not shake, agitate, or turn the vial upside down, as cautioned earlier.

ABTA should be used within 4 hours of reconstitution. The toxin should be stored at 2°C to 8°C, away from direct light during this 4-hour period. A consensus panel in 2010 suggested that the preparation remains active/potent for up to 3 weeks (83). Until there are more data to support the practice of deviating from the manufacturer's guidelines, it is recommended that clinicians adhere to the 4-hour window-of-use following reconstitution of ABTA. In addition, there is a theoretical risk of infection given that ABTA is reconstituted in PFNS.

Manufacturer guidelines on reconstitution are provided in Table 3.2. The volume of diluent is determined by the clinical indication/target structures. Higher dilutions not only allow more precise dose calculations but also may lead to greater diffusion or spread of the toxin (73, 84). When treating glabellar lines, a 300-unit vial is typically diluted with 2.5-mL PFNS, resulting in a concentration of ABTA of 60 units/0.5 mL or 10 units/0.08 mL—this dilution allows precise administration of the small dose of ABTA required to treat these muscles. When treating larger muscles in patients with cervical dystonia, a 300-unit vial is reconstituted with 0.6-mL PFNS or a 500-unit vial is diluted with 1.5-mL PFNS, resulting in a concentration of 50 units/0.1 mL.

Higher dilutions may be considered for large muscles, and a common approach in clinical practice is to reconstitute a 500-unit vial with 2.5 mL of PFNS (85). When used for off-label indications, such as spasticity, higher volume dilutions are reported to be more effective and/or to have a greater area of spread (86). High-volume dilution of ABTA, as with other preparations, appears to lead to greater spread, but this also increases the potential risk of spread both locally (to adjacent nontargeted structures) and to distant sites (73, 86).

**TABLE 3.2 AbobotulinumtoxinA (Dysport) Manufacturer Reconstitution Instructions**

| Volume PFNS (mL) | 300-Unit Vial | | 500-Unit Vial | |
|---|---|---|---|---|
| 0.6 | 250 units/ 1 mL[1] | 25 units/ 0.1 mL[1] | N/A | N/A |
| 1.0 | 300 units/ 1 mL | 30 units/ 0.1 mL | 500 units/ 1 mL[1] | 50 units/ 0.1 mL[1] |
| 1.5 | 200 units/ 1 mL[2] | 10 units/ 0.05 mL[2] | | |
| 2.5 | 120 units/ 1 mL[2] | 10 units/ 0.08 mL[2] | 200 units/ 1 mL[3]* | 20 units/ 0.1 mL[3]* |

Manufacturer's recommended dilutions for: [1]cervical dystonia, [2]glabellar lines, and [3]spasticity.

*Treatment of spasticity with abobotulinumtoxinA is off-label. Manufacturer's recommended dilution for cervical dystonia: 300 units diluted in 0.6 mL or 500 units in 1-mL PFNS.

Manufacturer's recommended dilution for glabellar lines: 300 units in 3.5-mL PFNS.

*Abbreviation:* PFNS, preservative-free normal saline (0.9%).

*Source:* Ref. 36. Dysport PI [package insert/prescribing information]. Basking Ridge, NJ: Ipsen Biopharmaceuticals, Inc. Available at http://pi.medicis.us/printer_friendly/dysport.pdf

## IncobotulinumtoxinA (Xeomin®) Reconstitution and Handling

IBTA is supplied as a lyophilized powder in 50- and 100-unit vials (38). The manufacturer recommends reconstitution with sterile PFNS for injection. Using a sterile large-bore needle and the appropriately sized syringe, the PFNS diluent is drawn up and the needle inserted into the vial. The manufacturer recommends cleaning the exposed portion of the vial's rubber stopper with alcohol (70%) prior to needle insertion. The partial vacuum in the vial should pull the diluent into the vial. If the diluent is not drawn into the vial by the negative pressure vacuum, the vial should be discarded and returned to the manufacturer. The diluent and dried powder should then be mixed by gently rotating the vial. Avoid shaking, agitating, or turning the vial upside down. Unreconstituted vials of IBTA can be stored at room temperature. Once reconstituted, IBTA should be stored at 2°C to 8°C and used within 24 hours of reconstitution (38).

The volume of dilution is determined by the clinical indication for treatment and the size of the target muscle/structures. The manufacturer recommendations for dilution are presented in Table 3.3. At least for the treatment of glabellar lines, there are no specific data to suggest that higher volume/lower concentration of IBTA affects treatment outcome/efficacy (79).

**TABLE 3.3 IncobotulinumtoxinA (Xeomin) Manufacturer Reconstitution Instructions**

| Volume PFNS (mL) | 50-Unit Vial: Resulting Dose/0.1 mL (Units) | 100-Unit Vial: Resulting Dose/0.1 mL (Units) |
|---|---|---|
| 0.25 | 20 | — |
| 0.5 | 10 | 20 |
| 1.0 | 5 | 10 |
| 1.25 | 4 | 8 |
| 2.0 | 2.5 | 5 |
| 2.5 | 2 | 4 |
| 4.0 | 1.25 | 2.5 |
| 5.0 | 1 | 2 |
| 8.0 | — | 1.25 |

Reconstituted incobotulinumtoxinA solution should be administered within 24 hours after dilution. During this period, reconstituted IBTA should be stored in a refrigerator at 2°C to 8°C (36°F–46°F). Reconstituted IBTA is intended for intramuscular injection only. After reconstitution, IBTA should be used for only one injection session and for only one patient.

*Abbreviation:* PFNS, preservative-free normal saline (0.9%).

*Source:* Ref. 38. Xeomin PI [package insert/prescribing information]. Greensboro, NC: Merz Pharmaceuticals. Available at http://www.xeomin.com/files/Xeomin_PI.pdf

## RimabotulinumtoxinB (Myobloc® in the United States, NeuroBloc® Outside the United States) Reconstitution and Handling

As noted earlier, RBTB is provided in a ready-to-use solution (44) (Table 3.4). Each single-use vial contains RBTB in a concentration of 5,000 units/1 mL with 0.05% human serum albumin, 0.01 M sodium succinate, and 0.1 M sodium chloride. RBTB is available in vials of 2,500 units (0.5 mL), 5,000 units (1 mL), and 10,000 units (2 mL). RBTB should be stored at 2°C to 8°C, protected from light. Although the product is ready to use without further reconstitution, it can be further diluted with PFNS. This author's practice is provided in Table 3.5. If diluted, RBTB should be used within 4 hours of dilution. Because RBTB is sold in solution, the concentration cannot be increased beyond 5,000 units/1 mL (87, 88).

Complaints of a burning sensation or pain are common following injection of RBTB. On injection, RBTB is reported to cause more pain than serotype A BoNTs. The pH of RBTB is approximately 5.6 and this acidic pH is likely responsible for the reports of pain on injection (89).

## Injection Supplies

As with all patient contacts and invasive procedures, physicians should wash/clean their hands before and after patient contact or a procedure. The skin over the injection site should be inspected and cleansed with ethyl alcohol or other skin cleanser, per

TABLE 3.4 RimabotulinumtoxinB (Myobloc/NeuroBloc)*

| RimabotulinumtoxinB | 2,500-Unit Vial: Dose (Units) per 0.1 mL | 5,000-Unit Vial: Dose (Units) per 0.1 mL | 10,000-Unit Vial: Dose (Units) per 0.1 mL |
|---|---|---|---|
| Undiluted | 500 | 500 | 500 |

*RimabotulinumtoxinB (Myobloc) is supplied as a sterile solution of 5,000 units/1 mL. RimabotulinumtoxinB does not require reconstitution or dilution. If dilution is desired, the product can be diluted with 0.9% normal saline for injection (see Table 3.6).

*Source:* Ref. 44. Myobloc [package insert/prescribing information]. Louisville, KY: Solstice Neurosciences (US WorldMeds). Available at http://www.myobloc.com/hp_about/PI_5-19-10.pdf

the protocol of the physician and/or institution. If required by the institution, a "time out" should be performed prior to the procedure—this is good practice even if not formally required. This ensures the correct patient, product, dose, location, and position of the patient. Particular attention should be paid to these factors when repositioning a patient from prone to supine or vice versa as left–right confusion for a target can occur.

If desired, the dose for each target/structure can be drawn into separate syringes. Having a separate syringe for each muscle or target can speed the procedure at the bedside, as the clinician is not required to look at the markings on the syringe during BoNT administration. This is particularly helpful for pediatric or less cooperative patients. The recommended dose of each product is covered in subsequent chapters of this text covering specific indications. When initiating treatment, the lowest recommended dose should be used (34, 80).

## Needle Selection

The choice of needle size is dependent on the structures being targeted. For facial muscles, most clinicians use 30-gauge, 0.5-inch needles (80). For the off-label treatment of sialorrhea, a 30-gauge, 0.5- or 1-inch needle is typically used (18). When injecting muscles such as in the arm, forearm, superficial thigh, or calf, needles with lengths of 1 to 1.5 inches are often sufficient. When treating muscles of the hip girdle or when treating obese patients where the muscles may be quite deep, a needle length of 2.5 to 5 inches may be required (17, 18, 90). Insulated needles for injection (for electromyography [EMG] or electrical stimulation [e-stim]) are available in 20 to 70 mm, and spinal needles are available in 25-gauge at lengths of 2.5 to 5 inches. Generally speaking, most clinicians (and patients) agree that smaller needles confer less pain with injection. Therefore, using the thinnest needle possible that is of adequate length should be considered, with a preferred size of 25 to 30 gauge (18, 80). Monopolar EMG–injection electrode needles are available in sizes 24 to 30 gauge. When using ultrasound guidance for BoNT injections, standard hypodermic needles can be used. These needles are often thinner, penetrate the skin more easily, and, therefore, cause less pain than the insulated needles that are required when using EMG or e-stim to guide injections (18). When performing urologic procedures or off-label gastrointestinal procedures, additional equipment is also required.

**TABLE 3.5 RimabotulinumtoxinB (Myobloc/NeuroBloc) Dilution Instructions Using Preservative-Free 0.9% Normal Saline for Injection**

| RimabotulinumtoxinB vial | Dilution: 0.5-mL PFNS | | Dilution: 1-mL PFNS | | Dilution: 1.5-mL PFNS | | Dilution: 2-mL PFNS | | Dilution: 4-mL PFNS* | |
|---|---|---|---|---|---|---|---|---|---|---|
| Resulting concentration per 1 or 0.1 mL | Units per 1.0 mL | Units per 0.1 mL | Units per 1.0 mL | Units per 0.1 mL | Units per 1.0 mL | Units per 0.1 mL | Units per 1.0 mL | Units per 0.1 mL | Units per 1.0 mL | Units per 0.1 mL |
| 2,500-unit vial containing 0.5 mL | 2,500 | 250 | 1,667 | 167 | 1,250 | 125 | N/A | N/A | N/A | N/A |
| 5,000-unit vial containing 1.0 mL | N/A | N/A | 2,500 | 250 | 2,000 | 200 | 1,667 | 167 | N/A | N/A |
| 10,000-unit vial containing 2.0 mL | N/A | N/A | N/A | N/A | N/A | N/A | 2,500 | 250 | 1,667 | 167 |

Note: RimabotulinumtoxinB does not require reconstitution or dilution. If dilution is desired, the product can be diluted with 0.9% NS for injection as follows:

*Because RBTB is provided in 3.5-mL vials, reconstitution of a 10,000-unit vial of RBTB (2 mL) with 4-mL PFNS requires reconstitution in a 10-mL syringe. If this dilution is desired, draw 2-mL RBTB into a 10-mL syringe, then draw 4-mL PFNS, and finally draw 1- to 2-mL air into the syringe. Recap needle and invert syringe several times to mix RBTB and PFNS. With the syringe held vertically with the needle in the up position, depress plunger of syringe to remove air from the syringe.

*Abbreviations:* NS, normal saline; PFNS, preservative-free normal saline; RBTB, rimabotulinumtoxinB.

*Source:* Ref. 44. Myobloc [package insert/prescribing information]. Louisville, KY: Solstice Neurosciences (US WorldMeds). Available at http://www.myobloc.com/hp_about/PI_5-19-10.pdf

**Properties of Botulinum Neurotoxin Products Available in the United States (from Manufacturer's Package Insert/Prescribing Information)**

| BoNT Product | Product Details |
|---|---|
| **OnabotulinumtoxinA** | **Supplied:** Single-use, 100- or 200-unit vials. Contents (100-unit vial): 100 units onabotulinumtoxinA neurotoxin complex, 0.5 mg human albumin, 0.9 mg NaCl, vacuum-dried powder without preservative. Contents (200-unit vial): 200-units onabotulinumtoxinA neurotoxin complex, 1 mg human albumin, 1.8 mg NaCl, vacuum-dried powder without preservative.<br>**Reconstitution:** Sterile, preservative-free normal saline (PFNS) (0.9%) for injection.<br>**Storage/handing:** Unopened vials: Refrigerate at 2°C–8°C. 100-unit vials up to 36 months and 200-unit vials up to 24 months. Once reconstituted, administer within 24 hours. Store reconstituted OBTA in a refrigerator for up to 24 hours. |
| **AbobotulinumtoxinA** | **Supplied:** Single-use, sterile 3-mL glass vials. Vial sizes: 300 or 500 units contain lyophilized abobotulinumtoxinA, 125 mcg human albumin, 2.5 mg lactose.<br>**Reconstitution:** Sterile, preservative-free normal saline (PFNS, 0.9%) for injection.<br>**Storage/Handling:** Store unopened vials at (2°C–8°C or 36°F–46°F). Protect from light. Administer within 4 hours of reconstitution. Store reconstituted toxin in the refrigerator for up to 4 hours. Do not refreeze after reconstitution. |
| **IncobotulinumtoxinA** | **Supplied:** Single-use, 50- or 100-unit vials containing lyophilized BoNT as a sterile white to off-white powder, 1 mg human albumin, 4.7 mg sucrose.<br>**Reconstitution:** PFNS for Injection.<br>**Storage/handling:** Store unopened vials at room temperature (20°C–25°C, 68°F–77°F) or refrigerate at 2°C–8°C (36°F–46°F) or freeze at (20°C to 10°C ((4°F to 14°F) for up to 36 months. Administer reconstituted toxin within 24 hours. |
| **RimabotulinumtoxinB** | **Supplied:** Single-use, 3.5-mL glass, single-use vials. Clear, colorless to light yellow, sterile injectable preservative-free solution. 5,000-units BoNT/1 mL with 0.05% human serum albumin, 0.01 M sodium succinate, 0.1 M NaCl. Approximate pH: 5.6<br>**Available in:** 2,500 units (0.5 mL), 5,000 units (1 mL), and 10,000 units (2 mL)<br>**Storage/handling:** Refrigerate at 2°C–8°C (36°F–46°F). Do not freeze or shake. May be diluted with normal saline. Once opened, use within 4 hours. |

*Abbreviation:* BoNT, botulinum neurotoxin.

*Sources:* Refs. 34, 36, 38, 44.

4

# Guidance Techniques for Botulinum Neurotoxin Injections

*Katharine E. Alter, MD*
*Michael C. Munin, MD, FAAPMR*

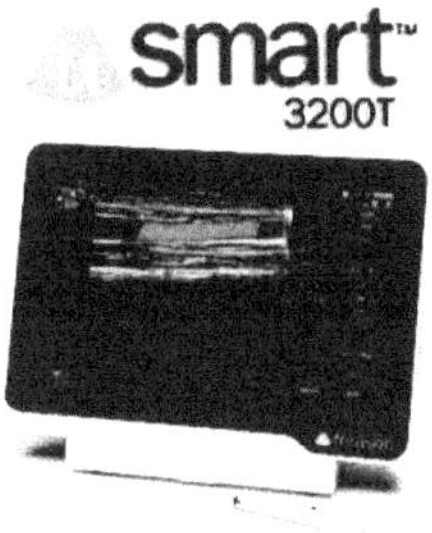


When performing botulinum neurotoxin (BoNT) injections, physicians may choose from an array of techniques to localize target structures. These techniques include anatomic reference guides (which rely on surface anatomy and palpation), electromyography (EMG), electrical stimulation (e-stim), high-frequency B-mode ultrasound (US), fluoroscopy, computed tomography (CT) guidance, and combinations of these (17, 91–93). Each technique has advantages and disadvantages. The following is a brief review of the commonly used guidance techniques.

## Anatomic Reference Guides, Surface Anatomy, and Palpation Guidance

Regardless of whether supplemental techniques for procedural guidance are used, every physician uses his or her knowledge of surface anatomy and palpation when performing BoNT injections. Many, if not most, physicians who perform BoNT injections also perform needle EMG and are therefore familiar with a number of anatomic reference guides on this topic (77, 94, 95). Such texts provide guidance on muscle localization based on palpation and surface landmarks. They were not intended to be guides for BoNT injections, but rather as reference guides for clinicians performing needle EMG. However, there are at least 2 anatomic reference guides that were explicitly written to provide guidance to physicians performing BoNT injections (96, 97).

Although some clinicians rely solely on anatomic reference guides, surface anatomy, and/or palpation (ARG/SA/P) to guide BoNT injections, due to the limitations of each technique when used alone, many clinicians also use supplementary targeting technique(s). For example, the accuracy of ARG/SA/P is limited by a number of patient factors and may also be limited by physician-related factors (Tables 4.1 and 4.2). All these factors may compromise the accuracy of targeting with palpation/landmarks. In addition, there is increasing evidence that calls into question the accuracy of ARG/SA/P when performing BoNT injections. A 2011 cadaver study compared the accuracy of wire placement in 14 lower limb muscles using anatomical guidance techniques versus US-guided wire placement (verified by CT) (98). The overall accuracy was 39% for blind needle placement and 96% for placement with US guidance. There was no difference in accuracy between the experienced clinician and a resident with 6 months of EMG training. Clinical studies in lower limb muscles have also reported limited accuracy of ARG/SA/P in targeting the medial and lateral gastrocnemius muscles, and in upper limb studies, there were substantial differences between reference guides in muscle fascicle location (99–101). Many studies show greater accuracy and efficacy of BoNT injections when using supplemental techniques, compared to use of ARG/SA/P alone (100–105).

**TABLE 4.1 Physician Factors that May Limit the Utility of Conventional Guidance Techniques (Anatomic, EMG, e-stim) for BoNT Injections**

| Limitations | Advantages |
|---|---|
| Limited training in gross anatomy, surface anatomy, palpation techniques | All physicians receive some training in anatomy |
| Limited grasp of 3D cross-sectional anatomy | Requires no equipment other than anatomical reference guides and the physicians skills in palpation |
| Limited knowledge of biomechanics and kinesiology | Some muscles may be easily localized and palpated |
| It may be difficult or impossible to palpate deep muscles | Injections can be performed with standard hypodermic needles<br>• Less pain than EMG electrode needles<br>• Less expensive than EMG electrode needles |
| It may be difficult to palpate/isolate muscles in regions with complex overlapping anatomy (forearm, neck, calf) | |

*(continued)*

**TABLE 4.1 Physician Factors that May Limit the Utility of Conventional Guidance Techniques (Anatomic, EMG, e-stim) for BoNT Injections (*continued*)**

| Limitations | Advantages |
|---|---|
| Difficulty palpating/isolating muscles in obese patients or in patients with muscle atrophy (disuse or postinjection) | |
| Contractures, deformity, and or pain may limit the use of PROM or AROM to isolate muscles | |
| Co-contraction in multiple muscles may confound localization when using palpation to localize muscles | |
| Not useful for localizing motor points/ motor endplates | |
| Contractures/tone may limit positioning the patient as described in anatomic reference guides; this may limit the use of these reference manuals to guide BoNT injections | |

*Abbreviations:* AROM, active range of motion; BoNT, botulinum neurotoxin; EMG, electromyography; e-stim, electrical stimulation; PROM, passive range of motion.

**TABLE 4.2 Patient Factors that May Limit the Utility of Conventional Guidance Techniques (Anatomic, EMG, e-stim) for BoNT Injections**

| |
|---|
| Anatomic variations or rearrangements |
| Involuntary movements |
| Contractures |
| Deformity |
| Muscle atrophy |
| Obesity |
| Impaired selective motor control |
| Cooperation |
| Pain |

*Abbreviations:* BoNT, botulinum neurotoxin; EMG, electromyography; e-stim, electrical stimulation.

## EMG Guidance

EMG is only useful when performing BoNT injections where muscles are the primary injection target(s). Equipment options for EMG-guided BoNT procedures include small portable audio amplifiers and/or audio–visual units. Alternately, physicians may use the needle EMG programs available on an EMG machine used for electrodiagnostic procedures. EMG-guided injections require single-use, sterile, insulated injecting needle electrodes. These injecting needle electrodes are available from several manufacturers in an assortment of sizes and lengths. The depth of the target muscle(s) determines the choice of needle.

When using EMG guidance for BoNT procedures, the procedure starts with inspection and the use of ARG/SA/P. The physician then inserts the injecting electrode through the skin, advancing the needle to the target while listening for audible EMG activity. If the patient has voluntary motor control, then the physician should instruct the patient to either relax or contract the target muscle to help with localization. If the patient has paresis or plegia in the injected limb, the examiner should passively move the joint associated with muscle attachment to identify insertional activity generated during passive movement. When the recording needle electrode is advanced into the target muscle, the tone associated with EMG activity will change from a low-pitch or "dull" tone to a high-pitch tone, characterized as "crisp." This indicates that the needle is near a depolarizing muscle fiber or motor unit that is firing. If the EMG tone remains dull as the patient contracts the target muscle, the needle position should be adjusted or repositioned to achieve a crisp tone. Due to impaired reciprocal inhibition, muscles with spasticity may contract even when positioned in an antagonist direction. For example, in spastic hemiplegia from stroke, firing of motor units within the biceps muscle can be seen at rest when the elbow is placed in full extension. In many conditions requiring BoNT injections, involuntary muscle activity can either assist or hinder muscle localization. Although patients with cervical dystonia (CD) may demonstrate increased motor-unit firing in a muscle due to overactivity (i.e., dystonia), increased activity may also be due to compensatory activity in muscles (i.e., co-contraction) in an attempt to resist dystonic muscle contraction. Careful inspection of abnormal postures is required to determine which muscle is the primary problem. In patients with impaired motor control from upper motor neuron syndrome, since all muscles in the vicinity can generate motor-unit potentials, co-contraction and synergy patterns often limit the usefulness of EMG when attempting to isolate a specific muscle (92).

EMG has many advantages in that it provides auditory feedback as to the level of activity or overactivity in a muscle. The limitations of EMG guidance for BoNT procedures are listed in Tables 4.1 and 4.3. One of the most important limitations

**TABLE 4.3 Limitations and Benefits of EMG Guidance for BoNT Injections**

| Limitations | Advantages |
|---|---|
| Anatomic variations or rearrangements | Provides auditory feedback on muscle activity |
| Involuntary movements or impaired selective motor control | May provide information on location of motor point and motor endplates |
| Co-contraction, impaired relaxation<br>• EMG signal may falsely attribute to target muscle when needle is in another muscle which is co-contracting | Most physicians are familiar with EMG |

*(continued)*

**TABLE 4.3 Limitations and Benefits of EMG Guidance for BoNT Injections (*continued*)**

| Limitations | Advantages |
|---|---|
| Contracture or deformity | Equipment is accessible to most physicians and is relatively inexpensive |
| Muscle atrophy | |
| Difficult to estimate muscle depth in obese patients or small patients | |
| Obesity | |
| Impaired selective motor control | |
| Cooperation | |
| Pain | |
| Children may require sedation | |

*Abbreviations:* BoNT, botulinum neurotoxin; EMG, electromyography; e-stim, electrical stimulation.

of EMG guidance is that it may be difficult or impossible to determine whether the needle is in the target muscle in patients with synergy patterns and co-contraction. Yet in focal dystonia, EMG is often useful for isolation of individual muscle fascicles. In patients with CD, EMG can also assist identification of muscles that may contribute to complex movement patterns (102, 104). There is limited evidence on the superiority of EMG compared to other techniques. One study reported superiority of EMG compared to anatomic guidance for focal hand dystonia (105). Speelman and Brans commented that EMG guidance for CD may reduce the number and severity of side effects (627). In a methodological study comparing EMG with e-stim for patients with focal hand dystonia, there was no significant difference in outcome measures between the two techniques (106). Additional studies comparing the various techniques are reviewed in the sections that follow.

## Electrical Stimulation Guidance

E-stim is only useful for BoNT injections in which a muscle is the target structure. Equipment required for e-stim-guided procedures include a small portable stimulator (or combined EMG/stimulator) or the nerve stimulator function from an electrodiagnostic machine. An insulated injecting needle electrode is required, as described earlier for EMG-guided procedures. When using e-stim, the procedure starts with inspection and ARG/SA/P. The physician then inserts the needle electrode through the skin advancing the needle to the target. The stimulator is turned on as the physician nears the target muscle and muscle contraction/joint movement is observed. If the needle is in the target muscle, relatively low-current stimulation is required to generate a muscle twitch. Upon stimulation, if contraction occurs in several muscles or muscles other than the target, the clinician should advance or adjust the position of the needle to isolate the target muscle.

The advantage of e-stim over EMG is that it provides direct visual feedback (i.e., muscle contraction) when the needle is appropriately located in the target muscle. Disadvantages are listed in Tables 4.1 and 4.4. When using e-stim to guide BoNT procedures, physicians must avoid excessive stimulation current. Overstimulation (excessive current) may lead to volume conduction in the target muscle when the needle is located elsewhere. In addition, if a motor branch is stimulated before it imbeds into the targeted muscle, injected BoNT may end up outside the target. The use of e-stim for children requiring BoNT injections requires general sedation, a distinct disadvantage of e-stim as it increases the risk of the procedure. Furthermore, even adults may find continuous probing with stimulation very uncomfortable (18, 91, 92, 99, 102). Studies have shown that e-stim is more accurate than manual needle placement (99, 107).

**TABLE 4.4 Limitations of e-stim Guidance for BoNT Injections**

| Limitations | Advantages |
|---|---|
| Anatomic variations or rearrangements | Produces visible contraction when needle is in target muscle (see Limitations column)<br>• Useful when co-contraction limits isolation of a muscle with anatomic guidance/palpation or EMG |
| Difficult to isolate deep or overlapping muscles | May be more accurate than EMG |
| Many physicians are not familiar with this technique | Equipment is accessible to most physicians |
| Volume conduction<br>• High-stimulation intensity may lead to contraction in target muscle when stimulating needle electrode is in another muscle or outside the targeted muscle | Equipment is relatively inexpensive |
| Unlike EMG, does not provide information about muscle activity level | Can be used to isolate motor point and or motor endplate |
| Contractures or deformity may make it difficult to visualize muscle twitch | |
| Muscle atrophy | |
| Difficult to estimate muscle depth in very large or small patients or patients who are obese | |
| Time consuming to localize muscles, motor points | |
| Pain from stimulation or needle electrode | |
| Cooperation | |
| Children require sedation, analgesia | |

*Abbreviations:* BoNT, botulinum neurotoxin; EMG, electromyography.

## B-Mode Ultrasound

B-mode US is widely used to guide a range of musculoskeletal procedures and is increasingly used for BoNT procedures (17, 22, 90, 100–103, 108, 109). Unlike EMG or e-stim, US can be used for both muscle and nonmuscle targets, including the salivary glands (90, 110). High-frequency transducers provide exquisitely detailed images with a resolution similar to magnetic resonance imaging (MRI) (111).

US has many advantages when compared to other guidance techniques, including real-time imaging of the intended target, adjacent structures (e.g., nerves, vessels, viscera), and other structures to be avoided. US can provide real-time visualization of the needle as it is advanced to the target, as well as the injectate, confirming the correct location within the muscle and avoiding nearby spread of toxin. Structures are identified by pattern recognition, contour lines, and adjacent structures. This is useful when contractures, deformity, or involuntary movements prevent optimal patient positioning. Muscles or muscle fascicles can be identified by passive joint range of motion when a patient cannot isolate movement due to limited motor control or co-contraction. Over time, some patients with spasticity from upper motor neuron syndrome have fibrotic replacement of muscle tissue. US can be used to identify this change based on an increase in echo intensity of the muscle (i.e., the muscle appears hyperechoic). This information may alter dosing of BoNT. In addition, muscles that receive repeated injection of BoNT have smaller cross-sectional diameter, and US can assist in keeping the injectate within fascial borders (22).

Limitations of US include cost, access to equipment, and training specific for BoNT procedures. A list of advantages and disadvantages of US for BoNT procedures is provided in Table 4.5. US guidance has also been shown to be equivalent to fluoroscopy when performing BoNT injections for thoracic outlet syndrome (93) and when compared to cystoscopy for some urologic procedures (112).

When comparing accuracy of needle placement, every study published to date has reported superior accuracy with US compared to manual placement, EMG, and e-stim. Some studies have also found higher efficacy and fewer adverse events when US was used to guide BoNT procedures (22, 100–103).

**TABLE 4.5 Advantages/Disadvantages of US and Other Guidance**

| | Anatomic/ Palpation | EMG | Stimulation | US |
|---|---|---|---|---|
| Accuracy | – | ± | ✓ | ✓✓✓ |
| Provides information on muscle activity | ± | ✓✓ | – | ✓ |
| Isolation of motor endplate | – | ± | ✓ | – |

*(continued)*

**TABLE 4.5 Advantages/Disadvantages of US and Other Guidance (*continued*)**

| | Anatomic/ Palpation | EMG | Stimulation | US |
|---|---|---|---|---|
| Clinical practicability | ✓ | ± | ± | ✓✓ |
| Availability | ✓ | + | ± | ± |
| Pain | ✓ | ± | ± | ✓✓✓ |
| Speed | ✓ | ± | – | ✓✓✓✓ |
| Cost of equipment | ✓✓✓ | ✓✓ | ✓✓ | ± |
| Procedure cost | ✓✓✓ | ✓✓ | ✓✓ | ± |
| Acceptability to patients | ✓ | ± | – | ✓✓✓✓ |
| Future research | – | – | ✓ | ✓✓✓✓ |

*Abbreviations:* EMG, electromyography; US, ultrasound.

## Combinations of Techniques

Each guidance technique has a role when performing BoNT injections. Two or more of the aforementioned techniques can also be combined, which may provide added benefit compared to the use of any of the techniques alone. The authors and other experienced clinicians frequently combine US and EMG to guide BoNT procedures for patients with CD and limb spasticity. US is used to guide the depth and location of the target muscle, whereas EMG provides information about the level of muscle activity, which can help dosing and/or may aid selection of other, more active, muscles.

US and e-stim are frequently combined for other chemodenervation procedures, such as diagnostic or therapeutic nerve blocks using aqueous phenol. This combined approach increases the accuracy of needle placement in near-nerve locations. This prevents inadvertent injection of potentially caustic agents (e.g., phenol, 30% alcohol) into nontargeted structures, such as muscles, viscera, or blood vessels. In many institutions and for many practitioners, US combined with e-stim are always used when performing nerve blocks (113–115). US and e-stim are less commonly combined for BoNT injections.

## Other Guidance Techniques for BoNT Injections

Although CT and fluoroscopy have been used for BoNT procedures in several case reports, they are used much less frequently than other guidance techniques. This is due to the exposure to ionizing radiation, cost, and inconvenience of traveling to a radiology suite for the procedure. Unless there is a very deep, hard-to-find target, other modalities, such as US, are equally effective (116).

Cystoscopy is widely used to guide BoNT injections for urologic indications. As noted earlier, some clinicians are also using US to guide these procedures.

## Summary

When performing BoNT procedures, the primary goals are to accurately inject only the target, enhance efficacy, and reduce the risk of adverse events, such as puncture of nearby nerves or vessels. To achieve these goals, clinicians should be familiar with several of the available guidance techniques, as each has inherent advantages and disadvantages. When performing BoNT and other chemodenervation procedures, clinicians should choose the technique, or combinations of techniques, that are competent to perform and that provide the most accuracy. The current evidence suggests that additional guidance (e.g., EMG, e-stim, US) is superior to the use of ARG/SA/P alone. However, head-to-head studies are required to determine which of the techniques are best suited to each indication.

# 5

# Phenol Nerve Blocks

*Zachary Bohart, MD, MS*
*Stephen Koelbel, MD*
*Katharine E. Alter, MD*

For many physicians, phenol nerve blocks are in many ways a "lost art," with this form of chemodenervation having been largely or completely replaced by botulinum neurotoxin (BoNT) injections. However, phenol nerve or motor point blocks continue to have a role in the treatment of patients who have problematic muscle hypertonia (117–118). Physicians who treat patients with hypertonia should be familiar with this agent, its mechanism of action, safety profile, and mode of administration. This chapter provides a review of phenol and its use for chemoneurolysis.

## Why Consider Phenol Neurolysis?

Although BoNTs are very effective in reducing spasticity and other forms of hypertonia, clinicians who manage spasticity are frequently left in the position of suboptimally treating the patient's hypertonia when only BoNTs are used for chemoneurolysis. For many patients with severe spasticity, particularly those in whom lower limb muscles are affected, the total dose of BoNT required to address their hypertonia may exceed either the maximum safe dosage range or the dosage range reimbursable by third-party payers (17, 119). The use of phenol nerve blocks and intrathecal baclofen pumps may be used in conjunction with BoNT, enabling the physician to more effectively use BoNT in a targeted and efficacious manner (17, 117). Phenol is also significantly less expensive than BoNT, which may be useful when patients have limited insurance coverage for BoNT. In addition, phenol injections have a longer duration of action than BoNT, frequently lasting up to a year or more (120). Phenol, as a neurolytic agent, has advantages and disadvantages when compared to BoNT injections (Table 5.1) and physicians who treat patients with spasticity should be familiar with these factors when considering the optimal agent for chemoneurolysis procedures in their patients.

**TABLE 5.1 Chemodenervation Procedures for Muscle Hypertonia: Phenol Versus BoNT Injections**

| Advantages of Phenol | Disadvantages of Phenol |
|---|---|
| • Immediate onset of action (vs. delayed onset for BoNT)<br>• Longer duration of action (6–18 months vs. 3–4 months for BoNT)<br>• More robust reduction in tone<br>• Lower cost | • Procedures are technically more challenging<br>• Phenol injections are more painful<br>• Risk of paresthesias with phenol injections if mixed sensory nerves are targeted<br>• Limited clinical applications (relatively few nerves can be blocked with phenol)<br>• Some adult and all pediatric patients require general anesthesia for phenol injections, increasing the risk and cost of phenol procedures<br>• "All or nothing" effect of phenol (i.e., phenol is not titratable)<br>• Toxicity of phenol |

*Abbreviation:* BoNT, botulinum neurotoxin.

## Phenol Mechanism of Action

Phenol, in concentrations of 5% to 7%, when injected immediately adjacent to a nerve, diffuses into the axons causing protein denaturation and resulting in chemical neurolysis of the nerve (117, 121, 122). Concentrations of phenol greater than 5% result in protein coagulation, demyelination, and orthograde axontomesis, followed by Wallerian degeneration (123). Phenol's onset of action is immediate and the duration of action reportedly ranges from 2 months to 2 years (124). In the authors' experience, the duration of reduced spasticity following phenol neurolysis ranges from 6 to 12 months. This is clearly longer than the typical 3- to 4-month duration of action following injection of BoNT. Following phenol neurolysis, nerve regeneration occurs at a rate of approximately 1 to 3 mm/day (123). The suggested maximum dose of phenol for adults is 1 g/day and for children is 30 mg/kg with a maximum of 1 g/day (115, 117). The reported lethal dose of phenol is 8.5 g in adults, with an extrapolated fatal dose in children of 0.1 to 0.2 g/kg (117, 120).

## Muscle Hypertonia

Muscle hypertonia is one of the most commonly observed motor impairments in patients with upper motor neuron syndromes (17). Muscle hypertonia may have a wide-ranging impact on passive and active function as well as quality of life. When considering phenol injections to reduce tone, the most frequently blocked nerves are the musculocutaneous nerve for elbow flexor tone, the obturator nerve for hip adductor tone, and motor branches of the tibial nerve for ankle plantar flexion and equinus tone. The neurolytic effects of phenol are not selective; both sensory and motor nerves are affected by the injection of phenol. Phenol neurolysis of mixed nerves with a significant sensory component carries a risk of dysesthesia reported up to 23% when concentrations of 2% to 5% phenol are used (124). Therefore, the authors generally avoid phenol neurolysis in such nerves. Although both the musculocutaneous and obturator nerves have sensory distributions, the sensory component of these nerves is minor, and in the authors' experience, dysethesias are not a significant consideration for phenol neurolysis in these nerves.

## Pattern of Involvement

Increased elbow flexor tone can result in a wide array of impairments, such as difficulty with caregiving, the ability to get dressed, perform hygiene in the elbow crease, skin breakdown, and, of course, increases the risk of elbow flexion contracture (125, 126). Please note that in our clinics, we restrict the use of phenol to the musculocutaneous nerve for patients who lack significant functional elbow flexion, because the results are longer lasting than BoNT and phenol blockade cannot be titrated with the same degree of efficacy as BoNT. Phenol neurolysis is associated with more of an "all or nothing" effect than BoNT injection.

Hip adductor tone can lead to scissoring, which may destabilize gait, limit transfers, impair groin hygiene and catheterization in a more dependent patient, interfere with positioning in a wheelchair or bed, and may pose a challenge to sexual intercourse (18, 125, 126). Phenol neurolysis of the obturator nerve is particularly useful in nonambulatory patients, as there is minimal risk that decreased adductor tone will further limit the patient's function. Although the hip adductors are often considered less critical than the other hip-girdle muscle groups for standing and ambulation, caution is urged when considering phenol obturator nerve blocks in functional ambulators, as patients may use spasticity functionally to stand, transfer, and walk (18). For this reason, the authors more often recommend or prescribe BoNT for adductor muscle spasticity in patients who are functional ambulators, as BoNT will produce a more graded reduction in muscle tone and because the results, if deleterious, will be of shorter duration than the phenol blockade.

Ankle plantar flexion hypertonia may also impair the proper biomechanics of gait, make it more difficult to tolerate an ankle-foot orthosis (AFO), increase the risk of skin breakdown due to inappropriate pressure against the sole of the shoe or AFO, impair proper wheelchair positioning, and, if left untreated, greatly increase the risk of developing contracture (17, 125, 126). As with the musculocutaneous nerve, we reserve this procedure for patients with upper motor neuron lesions that have little-to-no ability to actively plantarflex the ankle.

## Injection Technique and Dosing

Electrical nerve stimulation (e-stim) is typically used to localize the nerve (117, 127). The procedure is as follows: the stimulating/injecting needle is inserted through the skin into the target muscle near the expected location of the distal nerve trunk.

The authors perform initial localization of the nerve while stimulating at 3 to 5 mA. Once muscle contraction is visualized or palpated using this stimulation intensity, the needle is advanced or repositioned while the stimulation intensity is reduced, continuing to observe for muscle contraction in the distribution of the target nerve. A near-nerve location is confirmed when muscle contraction persists with the stimulator intensity at 0.5 to 1.0 mA. At that point, a 0.5 to 1.0 mL aliquot of 5% to 7% phenol in aqueous solution is injected into the nerve. Prior to injecting phenol, the physician must always aspirate to reduce the risk of intravascular injection, which can result in cardiac arrhythmias, tremors, convulsions, hypotension, and respiratory depression (120). Following this procedure, the needle is then repositioned, the process repeated, and additional aliquots of phenol are injected until the desired effect is obtained and/or there is no more significant muscle contraction with nerve stimulation at 3.0 mA (118, 120, 127). Although many clinicians rely solely on e-stim to localize nerves, others use a combination of B-mode ultrasound and e-stim for phenol chemoneurolysis procedures (90, 127).

Some clinicians advocate performing a diagnostic nerve block using a short-acting local anesthetic agent, such as lidocaine, prior to performing a neurolysis procedure with phenol (17, 18, 115, 127). The purpose of this diagnostic/short duration nerve block is to temporarily reduce the patient's spasticity. This allows the physician, patient, therapists, and caregivers to assess the impact of reduced tone (and possibly sensation) on the patient's function. This is basically a "test run" of the phenol procedure; if the effects are not as desired, then the block will quickly wear off and the phenol injections are canceled. A temporary block will assist in differentiating between severe spasticity versus contracture in patients where this may be difficult to determine on clinical examination. If there is no effect following a diagnostic nerve block (i.e., no reduction in tone or improved range of motion), then phenol injections are unlikely to be helpful and other treatment options should be considered.

## Musculocutaneous Nerve

The musculocutaneous nerve arises from the lateral cord of the brachial plexus and innervates the coracobrachialis muscle, the biceps brachii, the brachialis muscle, and provides sensory distribution to the lateral forearm via the lateral antebrachial cutaneous nerve (note that the brachialis muscle had dual innervation from the radial nerve in >80% of cadavers studied) (128). Once the clinician is adept at performing this procedure, a phenol block of the musculocutaneous nerve is a relatively straightforward procedure and is not time consuming to perform.

To localize the musculocutaneous nerve, the authors inject just distal to the pectoralis major tendon and perpendicular to the coracobrachialis, while watching for elbow flexion and/or supination (129). Although some authors use ultrasound in addition to e-stim, the authors generally use only e-stim, as the superficial nature of the nerve allows precise localization with e-stim alone (130). During e-stim, care must be taken to not inject the median or radial nerves due to the risk of dysesthesia because both nerves have large sensory distributions. Care must also be taken to not inject into the axillary artery. As noted earlier, the neurolytic effects and resulting reduction in muscle tone following phenol injection are immediate.

## Obturator Nerve

The obturator nerve arises from the anterior divisions of L2 to L4, and it divides into anterior and posterior branches. The anterior branch innervates the adductor longus and brevis muscles, the gracilis, and sometimes the pectineus muscle. The posterior branch innervates the obturator externus, the adductor magnus, and occasionally the brevis muscles. The posterior branch also provides sensory distribution to the medial thigh (95).

The obturator nerve can be either blocked proximally as it exits the obturator foramen (thereby affecting both branches prior to the bifurcation of the nerve) or more distally by blocking each branch separately. The authors find the distal block easier to perform due to increased ease of access to this region of the limb; particularly in patients with severe hip adductor tone or contractures. Nerve stimulation is often very effective in localizing the obturator nerve or nerve branches, but in obese patients or in those with deformities caused by marked adductor tone, ultrasound may be useful as well. When using ultrasound, the anterior division of the obturator nerve is localized where it lies between the adductor longus and brevis muscles. The posterior division lies between the adductor brevis and adductor magnus muscles (131). Ultrasound is also effective in localizing the obturator nerve prior to its bifurcation into anterior and posterior branches. For the distal technique, which we customarily perform, the needle is inserted through the adductor longus, roughly 4 fingerbreadths distal to the pubic tubercle, to block the anterior branch and then advanced farther through the adductor brevis to block the posterior branch of the obturator nerve. Alternately, one could insert the needle lateral to the adductor longus, approximately 3 to 4 fingerbreadths distal to the adductor longus origin, for the anterior branch, and for the posterior branch, insert the needle medial to the adductor longus tendon. As with all phenol nerve blocks, we inject when nerve stimulation intensity is ideally at 0.5 mA and muscle contraction is visualized or palpated. Effects are immediate, and, as with all phenol blocks, it is imperative that one aspirate prior to injecting.

## Tibial Motor Nerves

When performing this procedure, care must be taken to not inject the main trunk of the tibial nerve itself, because it has a large sensory component. Rather, the targets of the injection are the muscular branches of the tibial nerve to the gastrocnemius (medial and lateral) and the soleus (132). If possible, the patient should be placed in a prone position to facilitate nerve localization and the sock and shoe should be removed. If positioning in prone is impossible, side-lying is an acceptable alternative. When in the prone position, the foot should be positioned off the end of the bed, with the toes pointed toward the floor. This position of the foot allows the physician to observe ankle plantar flexion with e-stim during nerve localization. It is of utmost importance that the physician watch for plantar flexion, signaling that the motor branches of the tibial nerve to the gastrocnemius and soleus have been isolated. If stimulation causes toe flexion and/or ankle inversion, this indicates that the needle is located near the main trunk of the tibial nerve and not in proximity to the desired motor branches to the gastrocnemius and soleus. If toe flexion or foot inversion and not plantar flexion are observed with stimulation, the needle should be repositioned while still stimulating, to isolate the desired motor branches. The skin is then prepped, and the needle is inserted two fingerbreadths distal to the posterior knee crease at midline. For the branch of the tibial nerve to the medial gastrocnemius, the needle is directed slightly medially and e-stim is gradually decreased from the initial setting of 5.0 to 0.5 mA. As with other phenol injections, aliquots of 0.5 mL are injected at a time. We customarily wait 30 to 45 seconds before subsequent injections. For the branch of the tibial nerve to the lateral gastrocnemius, the authors recommend reorienting the needle laterally (to avoid having to repenetrate the skin). For the motor branch of the tibial nerve to the soleus, the authors typically localize this motor branch by advancing the needle deeper and more inferolaterally to the motor branch to the lateral gastrocnemius. Again, the physician must carefully observe the motion of the foot during the localization procedure to ensure that the main tibial nerve is not injected. If the results of this procedure are suboptimal and plantar flexion tone (and not just contracture) remains, a second block to the distal motor nerve to the soleus can be performed. This distal branch to the soleus lies at the junction of the proximal and second quarter of the calf. The needle is inserted just lateral to the midline and carefully advanced while stimulating to localize this distal motor branch to the soleus.

## Summary

Phenol nerve blocks are a very effective arrow in the quiver of the physician who treats spasticity. Although there are limitations to use of phenol for chemodenervation procedures, this agent does have some advantages when compared to BoNT therapy (Table 5.1). In addition, by enabling the physician to treat the elbow flexors, hip adductors, and ankle plantar flexors with phenol instead of BoNT, phenol blocks allow the physician to concentrate and maximize the use of BoNT in muscles where high doses may be needed.

# Section Two

## *Clinical Applications of Botulinum Neurotoxins*

# Part I

# *Botulinum Neurotoxins for the Treatment of Muscle Overactivity Associated with Focal Dystonia Syndromes and Upper Motor Neuron Syndromes*

*Katharine E. Alter, MD*

Botulinum neurotoxin (BoNT) therapy is widely recognized as an effective treatment for muscle overactivity associated with various neurological and/or musculoskeletal disorders. This section covers the use of BoNT for the treatment of muscle overactivity associated with focal dystonia and upper motor neuron syndromes (UMNS), including dystonia and spasticity. A full discussion of the various causes of dystonic syndromes and UMNS is beyond the scope of this text and the reader is referred to several review articles and texts related to this topic (17, 176, 191, 194, 208, 616).

## Dystonia

Dystonia is a movement disorder characterized by an involuntary, sustained, or intermittent muscle contraction with limb movements and/or repeated postures that are often twisting in nature. As there are many causes of dystonia, dystonic movements and the clinical presentation of individual patients with dystonia vary considerably (176, 617).

### *Classification of Dystonia*

Traditional classification schemes for dystonia include broad categories based on the age of onset (childhood vs. adult), pattern or distribution (focal, segmental, generalized), provoking factors (action vs. rest), and cause. Classification of dystonia by its cause includes primary and secondary and idiopathic subtypes (176, 177).

Primary dystonia includes those with a clear genetic cause such as dopa-responsive dystonia (DRD), including DYT5 or Segawa's syndrome and others (176). A common cause of secondary dystonia is that associated with UMNS, for example, dystonia secondary to injury or pathology involving the brain and/or spinal cord. Depending on the location of the brain injury and the pathways involved, patients with UMNS may present with dystonia in addition to spasticity. In patients presenting with secondary dystonia, the most common cause is a focal (i.e., stroke) or traumatic brain injury. Other causes of secondary dystonia include drug-induced or metabolic issues (617). When an extensive workup fails to elicit either a genetic or secondary cause for a patient's dystonia, the patient is classified as having idiopathic dystonia. Although the causes of idiopathic dystonia are not yet established, an as-yet unidentified genetic link or genetic-environmental link is suspected as many patients report a positive family history of dystonia (194, 618).

### *BoNT for the Treatment of Dystonia*

Although BoNT therapy may be useful for treating any patient with symptomatic dystonia, it is particularly useful for patients presenting with one of the many forms of focal dystonia. Because many muscles are involved in patients with generalized dystonia, these patients are typically managed with systemic medications and/or surgical treatment. For these patients, BoNT may be useful as a supplemental treatment to address a specific issue or problem. BoNT is considered a first-line therapy or the treatment of choice for the majority of patients presenting with problematic focal dystonia (194).

## Muscle Hypertonia or Overactivity Associated with UMNS

UMNS are a collection of symptoms caused by injury or other pathology involving the central nervous system (CNS). Motor symptoms of the UMNS include positive symptoms (hyperreflexia and muscle overactivity [spasticity/dystonia/spastic dystonia]) and negative symptoms (loss of selective motor control, weakness) (207, 208). Although spasticity is well recognized in UMNS, dystonia is also common, particularly in patients with cerebral palsy (213, 619). BoNT has been found to be effective in reducing muscle overactivity associated with UMNS, but has no place in the treatment of negative UMNS symptoms (17). Chapters 6 to 8 summarize the use of BoNTs in the treatment of primary focal dystonia (blepharospasm, hemifacial spasm, oromandibular dystonia, cervical dystonia, focal limb dystonia, and dystonia of the trunk) and muscle hypertonia, including spasticity and secondary dystonia associated with UMNS.

*Craniofacial Dystonia*

# 6

# *Benign Essential Blepharospasm*

*Katharine E. Alter, MD*
*Barbara I. Karp, MD*

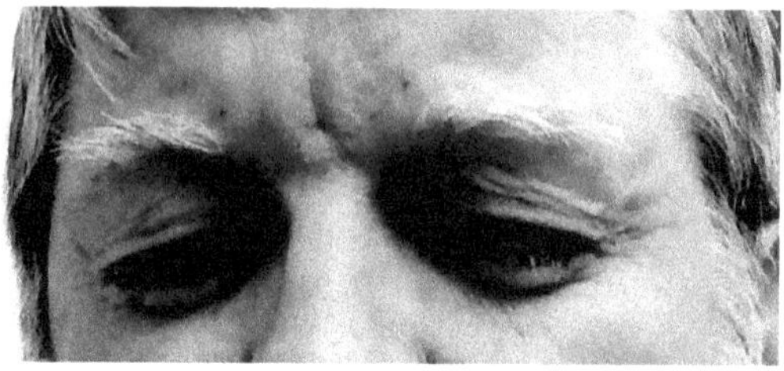

## Condition

Of the focal dystonias involving craniofacial muscles, including those of facial expression, mastication, jaw opening/closing, and the tongue, benign essential blepharospasm (blepharospasm, in this text) is the most common. Blepharospasm is an involuntary spasmodic or dystonic contraction of the eyelids and brow muscles, which causes increased blinking and forced eye closure. Although its mechanism is not well understood, many patients with blepharospasm have photosensitivity and often report a sensation of eye irritation or dry eyes, which may precede the onset of involuntary muscle activity (53, 133). Blepharospasm is more common in women and the typical age of onset is in the fifth to sixth decade. The estimated prevalence of blepharospasm is from 16 to 133 cases per million people. In the United States, 2,000 new cases are diagnosed annually with an estimated 20,000 to 50,000 individuals affected (134).

### *Clinical/Functional Impact*

Involuntary eye closure often limits a patient's function and may be so severe to cause functional blindness. Blepharospasm is often aggravated by bright light. Many clinicians recommend the use of tinted lenses or sunglasses (even indoors). Lenses with an FL-41 tint may be especially effective (135).

### *Muscle Pattern/Muscles Involved*

The pattern of abnormal movement includes eye closure and brow muscle contraction. All segments of the orbicularis oculi may be involved including orbital and palpebral (pretarsal and preseptal) portions. Corrugators and procerus muscles mediate forehead/brow movement. Blepharospasm is almost always bilateral.

### *Evaluation*

The diagnosis of blepharospasm is based entirely on clinical presentation and patient symptomatology. The differential diagnosis includes apraxia of eyelid opening, characterized by difficulty initiating eye opening. Both conditions may be treated with BoNT (136). Disease-specific rating scales include the Jankovic Rating Scale and the Blepharospasm Disability Index (BSDI) (137).

### *Treatment*

BoNT injections have been used to treat blepharospasm for over two decades and are considered the standard of care, with many patients achieving excellent clinical benefit (53, 133).

### *FDA-Approved BoNTs for Blepharospasm*

OnabotulinumtoxinA (OBTA) was approved in 1989 for the treatment of blepharospasm (34). IncobotulinumtoxinA (IBTA) is also approved for the treatment of blepharospasm in the United States (38). Outside the United States, all three marketed BoNT-A serotype toxins (OBTA, IBTA, and abobotulinumtoxinA [ABTA]) are approved for the treatment of blepharospasm.

### *Level of Evidence*

Although there are relatively few large, double-blind studies evaluating BoNT for blepharospasm, most clinicians consider BoNT to be the most effective treatment for this type of focal dystonia. Data from previously reported trials, as well as long and widespread experience, have led to acceptance of BoNT as an effective treatment for blepharospasm. Given the current recommendations, it is unlikely that additional Level I studies will be conducted. A recent evidence-based review led to a Level A (established as effective for a given condition in a given population requiring at least two Class 1 studies) recommendation for BoNT serotype A for the treatment of blepharospasm. The current level of evidence for BoNT-B for blepharospasm is U (Unproven, data inadequate or conflicting) (2, 138).

### *Treatment Goals*

The goal of BoNT treatment is to reduce involuntary movements and associated functional limitations associated with blepharospasm and to improve the patient's vision, functioning, and quality of life.

### *Injection Patterns*

Physicians use a variety of injection patterns when treating blepharospasm. The standard injection pattern for the orbicularis oculi includes four sites. Two injections are placed in the lower lid: one in the midline and the other laterally by the outer canthus. Injection of the nasal lower lid, near the inner canthus, can reduce the risk of xerophthalmia from inadvertent injection of the lacrimal gland. Two injections are placed in the upper lid. The placement in the upper lid differs from that in the lower lid in that one injection is nasal and the other is placed laterally near the lid margin. Clinicians are advised to avoid midline injections in the upper lid to reduce the risk of ptosis from inadvertent injection of the levator palpebrae. Injections may be given in the palpebral portion of the muscle; some inject the orbital portion outside the orbital rim. Injections of brow muscles, procerus or corrugator, are given bilaterally (139) (see Figure 2 following Chapter 8).

### *Dilution*

When used for blepharospasm, the toxin may be prepared at a higher dilution than used for other dystonias or when treating large muscles. The higher dilution enables clinicians to achieve the precise dosing required when treating patients with blepharospasm. OnabotulinumtoxinA and incobotulinumtoxinA are typically diluted to achieve a concentration of 1.25 units/0.1 mL or 2.5 units/0.1 mL.

To achieve a concentration of 1.25 units/0.1 mL, a 100-unit vial of OBTA or IBTA is diluted in 8 mL of preservative-free normal saline (PFNS); a 50-unit vial of IBTA is diluted in 4 mL of PFNS. To achieve a concentration of 2.5 units/0.1 mL, a 100-unit vial of OBTA or IBTA is diluted in 4 mL PFNS or a 50-unit vial of IBTA is diluted in 2 mL of PFNS. ABTA or rimabotulinumtoxinB may also be prepared at a high dilution for use in patients with blepharospasm.

### *Dosage*

A common initial recommended dose for OBTA or IBTA for blepharospasm is 1.25 units or 2.5 units (0.05–0.1 mL volume) to each site within the selected muscles. Published clinical trials have found little increased benefit from injection of >5 units per site. The dose can be titrated up, depending on the patient's response, by increasing the concentration, volume, or number of injection sites. The maximum recommended dose of OBTA for blepharospasm is a total of 200 units per treatment cycle (see Table 6.1: Benign Essential Blepharospasm BoNT Reconstitution and Dosage Table following this chapter for details).

### *Injection Technique*

Reconstituted OBTA or IBTA is injected using a sterile 27- to 30-gauge needle. For patient comfort and to avoid bruising in the delicate orbicularis oris muscle, a 30-gauge, 0.5-inch needle is often preferred. Since the orbicularis oculi is subcutaneous and the forehead muscles are superficial, injection can be guided by visual inspection alone.

Electromyographic, electrical stimulation, or ultrasound guidance is not necessary for accurate injection into these muscles.

BoNT is injected into the nasal and lateral orbicularis oculi of the upper lid (often the pretarsal portion) and into the midline and lateral pretarsal orbicularis oculi of the lower lid. As noted, avoid injection in the midline in the upper eyelid near the levator palpebrae superioris and the medial lower corner of the lower lid to avoid the lacrimal gland and inferior oblique muscle. Patient comfort may be enhanced by applying a cold pack to the eyes before injection. Ecchymosis in the eyelid soft tissues can be reduced by avoiding injection into the small veins visible under the skin around the eye and by applying gentle pressure at the injection site immediately after the injection and/or the brief application of an ice pack (see Figure 2 following Chapter 8).

## *Clinical Effect*

The initial effect of BoNT for blepharospasm is generally seen within 3 days, peaking at 1 to 2 weeks postinjection. Duration of effect is generally 12 to 14 weeks, but may last longer in some individuals. Most clinicians recommend a minimum reinjection interval of 12 weeks or longer depending on the patient's symptoms.

## *Adverse Events*

The most commonly reported adverse events when treating patients with blepharospasm are ptosis, dry eye, and lagophthalmos. Rare side effects include diplopia, ectropion, and nasal discharge (134).

**TABLE 6.1 Benign Essential Blepharospasm BoNT Reconstitution and Dosage Table (Adults ≥18 Years of Age)***

| Primary Muscles | OBTA (Botox®) | ABTA (Dysport®) | IBTA (Xeomin®) | RBTB (Myobloc®) | Notes |
|---|---|---|---|---|---|
| **Manufacturer Recommended Prescribing Information/FDA-Approved Dose** | | | | | |
| Orbicularis oculi | Initial dose: 1.25–2.5 units/site<br>Initial dose/eye: 6–12.5 units<br>Four to five injection sites<br>Volume of injectate per site: 0.05–0.1 mL | Not currently approved in the United States<br>See below for approved dosage range in other countries and published dosage range | Initial dose: 1.25–2.5 units/site (0.05–0.1 mL/site)<br>Initial dose: 25–≤35 units/eye, ≤70 units total dose, both eyes<br>No additional benefit reported with >5 units/injection site<br>Total dose ≤100 units per treatment cycle<br>Published studies:<br>Mean dose/site: 5.6 units<br>Mean dose/eye: 33.5 units | Not currently approved | Avoid injection to the midline upper lid to avoid ptosis<br>Avoid injection to the inner/medial corner, lower lid to avoid dry eye |
| Injection sites (see Figure 2 following Chapter 8) | Upper lid: medial, lateral<br>Lower lid: middle, lateral, outer | Upper lid: medial, lateral<br>Lower lid: middle, lateral, outer | Upper lid: medial, lateral<br>Lower lid: middle, lateral, outer, temporal<br>Mean number of sites: six | | Avoid midline injection to the upper lid<br>Avoid medial corner of the lower lid |

*(continued)*

**TABLE 6.1 Benign Essential Blepharospasm BoNT Reconstitution and Dosage Table (Adults ≥18 Years of Age)* (*continued*)**

| Primary Muscles | OBTA (Botox®) | ABTA (Dysport®) | IBTA (Xeomin®) | RBTB (Myobloc®) | Notes |
|---|---|---|---|---|---|
| Retreatment interval | Minimum 12 wk | Minimum 12 wk | Minimum 12 wk | | |
| Dilution | 100 units/4 mL<br>(25 units/mL, 2.5 units/0.1 mL)<br>2.5 units/0.1 mL or<br>1.25 units/0.05 mL<br>100 units/8 mL<br>(12.5 units/1 mL or<br>1.25 units/0.1 mL) | 300-unit vial diluted with 1.5 mL PFNS<br>200 units/1 mL | 50 units in 2 mL<br>(25 units/mL,<br>2.5 units/0.1 mL, or<br>1.25 units/0.05 mL)<br>or<br>50 units/4 mL<br>(12.5 units/1 mL) for<br>1.25 units/0.1mL | | |
| **Blepharospasm: Approved BoNT Dose—United Kingdom: UK MHRA-Labeled Dose** | | | | | |
| Orbicularis oculi | 1.25–2.5 units/site<br>6–12.5 units/eye<br>Four to five injection sites | Labeled dose is 120 units/eye[1]:<br>20 units (0.1 mL) medial injection sites<br>40 units (0.2 mL) lateral injection sites | 1.25–2.5 units/site<br>6–12.5 units/eye<br>Four to five sites | Not currently approved | [1]Note: Although the UK MHRA published dose is 120 units/eye, this dose exceeds that typically used in clinical practice. |

(*continued*)

**TABLE 6.1 Benign Essential Blepharospasm BoNT Reconstitution and Dosage Table (Adults ≥18 Years of Age)* (*continued*)**

| Primary Muscles | OBTA (Botox®) | ABTA (Dysport®) | IBTA (Xeomin®) | RBTB (Myobloc®) | Notes |
|---|---|---|---|---|---|
| | | Four injection sites, see standard injection site pattern (see Figure 2 following Chapter 8)<br>See Note[1] | | | In addition, doses of >50–60 units/eye of ABTA are associated with an increased incidence of weakness and ptosis<br>The authors recommend a starting dosage range of 20–50 units/eye of ABTA |
| UK MHRA published dilution | 50-unit vial diluted in 2–4 mL PFNS<br>100-unit vial diluted in 4 or 8 mL for dose/0.1 mL as described above | 300-unit vial diluted with 1.5 mL PFNS for a dilution of 200 units/1 mL or 20 unit/0.1 mL | 50 units in 2 mL PFNS or 50 units/4 mL, as described above | | |
| UK MHRA published dose increase per treatment cycle | Up to 2 times, based on response<br>Maximum dose:<br>≤5 units/site,<br>25 units/eye<br>Total dose: ≤100 units/session | Repeat injections:<br>Decreased to 80 units/eye as needed<br>0.1 mL medial<br>0.1 mL lateral<br>Further reduced to 60 units/eye, as needed | | | |

(*continued*)

**TABLE 6.1 Benign Essential Blepharospasm BoNT Reconstitution and Dosage Table (Adults ≥18 Years of Age)* (*continued*)**

| Primary Muscles | OBTA (Botox®) | ABTA (Dysport®) | IBTA (Xeomin®) | RBTB (Myobloc®) | Notes |
|---|---|---|---|---|---|
| | | NOTE: Doses of 60–80 units may be associated with an increased weakness/ adverse events. Recommended dose range is 40–50 units/ eye. | | | |
| Retreatment interval | Minimum 12 wk | Minimum 12 wk | Minimum 12 wk<br>6-wk intervals have been described | | |
| **Published Dosage Range** | | | | | |
| Orbicularis oculi | 25–50 units/eye<br>50–70 units total | 20–120 units/eye<br>Fewer adverse events reported with dose ≤80 units/eye[2] | 12–50 units/eye<br>>25 units/eye had no increased benefit | Average dosage: 3,633 units<br>Low dosage: 500–3,500 units<br>High dosage: 400–6,200 units | [2]Note: The authors recommend a starting dosage range of 20–50 units/eye of ABTA |
| **Blepharospasm: Brow Muscle Injections** | | | | | |
| Corrugator bilateral injection | 1.25–4 units/site<br>2 sites each side | 5–10 units/site<br>2 sites | 1.25–4 units at 2 injection sites, bilaterally | | |
| Procerus | 1.25–5 units<br>1 injection site | 5–10 units<br>1 site | 1.25–4 units<br>1 injection site | | |

*(continued)*

**TABLE 6.1 Benign Essential Blepharospasm BoNT Reconstitution and Dosage Table (Adults ≥18 Years of Age)* *(continued)***

| Primary Muscles | OBTA (Botox®) | ABTA (Dysport®) | IBTA (Xeomin®) | RBTB (Myobloc®) | Notes |
|---|---|---|---|---|---|
| Reported adverse events and side effects | Hematoma, pain, ptosis, weakness in injected muscle(s) or adjacent muscles, diplopia | Hematoma, pain, ptosis, weakness in injected muscle(s) or adjacent muscles, diplopia | Hematoma, pain, ptosis, weakness in injected muscle(s) or adjacent muscles, diplopia | Hematoma, pain, ptosis, weakness in injected muscle(s) or adjacent muscles, diplopia | |

*Sources:* Refs. 34–36, 38, 40, 44, 53, 68, 133, 137, 139, 149, 197, 243, 244, 300, 316, 461–464.

*Abbreviations:* ABTA, abobotulinumtoxinA; IBTA, incobotulinumtoxinA; OBTA, onabotulinumtoxinA; PFNS, preservative-free normal saline (0.9%); RBTB, rimabotulinumtoxinB.

Blepharospasm: Orbicularis oculi injection sites: Medial and lateral orbicularis oculi, upper lid; lateral orbicularis oculi lower lid. Brow muscles injected as needed: Bilateral corrugator (one to two sites/side), procerus (one site) (see Figure 2 following Chapter 8).

*UK MHRA published dose of 120 units/eye dose is higher than that typically used.

# 7

# *Botulinum Neurotoxin Therapy for Hemifacial Spasm*

*Katharine E. Alter, MD*
*Barbara I. Karp, MD*

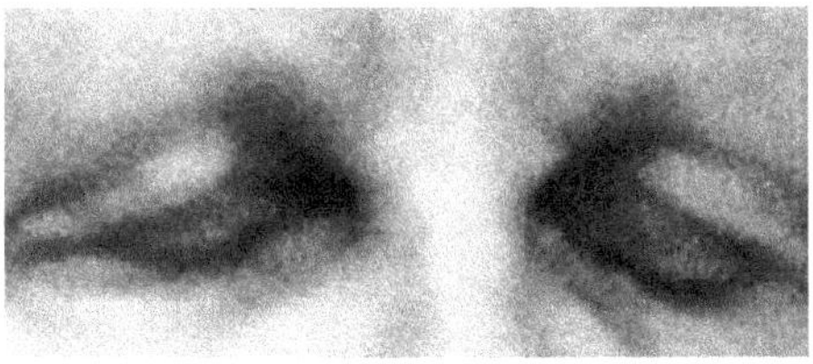
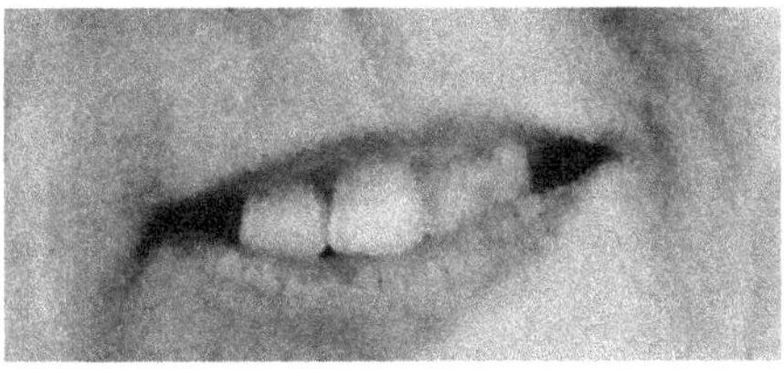

## Condition

Hemifacial spasm (HFS) is a focal movement disorder characterized by unilateral, involuntary, tonic or clonic contractions or spasms in muscles innervated by the facial nerve (cranial nerve VII [CN VII]) (140). The most common cause of HFS is mechanical compression of CN VII by an enlarged or aberrant blood vessel as it exits the brainstem. Less common causes include other compressive lesions (e.g., tumors) or damage to the peripheral facial nerve (e.g., subsequent to Bell's palsy) (141, 142). HFS is more common in women and in the Asian population, with typical onset in the fifth or sixth decade of life. In the Caucasian population, the incidence of HFS is reported to be 0.78 per 100,000, with an average prevalence of 7.4 per 100,000 people in males and 14.5 per 100,000 in females (143). Most cases are sporadic, although some patients may have a genetic predisposition to developing HFS (144). HFS is a chronic condition, and spontaneous remission is rare.

### *Clinical/Functional Impact*

Although the cause and course are typically benign and nondisabling, the intermittent involuntary movements of HFS may cause significant distress to patients, leading to a sense of facial disfigurement and social isolation. Spasms may also affect function. Involuntary eye closure, due to spasm of the orbicularis oculi muscle, may impair vision and reading. Less frequently, spasm of mouth and/or lip muscles may affect drinking, eating, or speech (140).

### *Muscle Pattern/Muscles Involved*

Any of the muscles of facial expression innervated by CN VII may be affected. Common patterns include unilateral eye closure (due to involvement of unilateral orbicularis oculi), brow muscle contraction (corrugator, procerus, and/or frontalis), mouth deviation (orbicularis oris, risorius, zygomaticus, and/or levator labii), and/or nose (nasalis) or chin (mentalis) movements (145). HFS, unlike blepharospasm, is not aggravated by sensory stimulation, such as bright light (144), but the spasms may be worsened by stress.

### *Evaluation*

The diagnosis of HFS is largely based on clinical presentation and patient symptomatology. Neuroimaging may reveal an aberrant or enlarged vessel or mass lesion overlying the facial nerve. Electrophysiologic studies of the facial nerve in HFS show ectopic excitation and ephaptic transmission (146). The differential diagnosis of HFS includes orofacial dystonia, facial myoclonus, tics, and hemimasticatory spasm (140, 147).

### *Treatment*

Treatment options for HFS include microvascular decompression, oral medications, or botulinum neurotoxin (BoNT) injections. BoNT injections have largely replaced other treatments because of the better risk/benefit ratio. Microvascular decompression entails the risk of neurosurgery, while oral medications frequently cause intolerable systemic side effects (140, 144). BoNTs have been used to treat HFS and blepharospasm for over two decades and are now considered standard of care, with many patients achieving excellent clinical benefit (53, 148). Long-term follow-up studies suggest that, over time, most patients with HFS continue to respond to BoNT treatment. Although some studies report an increase in the required dose over time, other studies report that dose escalation required to maintain clinical benefit is minimal (149).

### *BoNTs Approved for the Treatment of HFS*

Although BoNTs have been successfully used to treat HFS for many years and both onabotulinumtoxinA (OBTA) and incobotulinumtoxinA (IBTA) carry FDA approval for the treatment of blepharospasm, none of the currently approved BoNT products are specifically approved in the United States for HFS (34, 38). OBTA, IBTA, and abobotulinumtoxinA (ABTA) are approved outside the United States for the treatment of blepharospasm and OBTA and ABTA additionally have specific approval for the treatment of HFS outside the United States (35, 40, 243). RimabotulinumtoxinB (RBTB) is not currently approved in the United States or elsewhere for the treatment of blepharospasm or HFS. However, there are published reports of RBTB being used to treat both conditions, typically in patients who are unresponsive to serotype A BoNTs (150).

### *Level of Evidence*

Based on available studies of BoNTs for HFS, a 2013 evidence-based review concluded that the level of evidence for serotype A BoNTs as a class was Level B (Probably effective). Level B requires at least one Class I study or two consistent Class II studies (2, 138). Regarding individual BoNT preparations, there was Level B evidence supporting the use of OBTA and Level C (Possibly effective for the given condition/population and requires at least one Class II study or two consistent Class III studies) evidence for ABTA. The current level of evidence for IBTA and serotype B BoNTs was U (Unproven, data inadequate or conflicting data) (2, 138). A different 2013 evidence-based review found Level I evidence supporting the use of BoNTs for HFS (151).

In summary, although there are relatively few large, double-blind studies evaluating BoNTs for HFS, most clinicians consider BoNT to be the first-line treatment for this condition. Additional studies are needed to inform the optimal dose, injection interval, and indications for individual BoNT products for the treatment of both typical and atypical HFS (147).

### *Treatment Goals*

The goal of BoNT treatment is to reduce involuntary movements and associated functional limitations and/or disfigurement caused by HFS and to improve the patient's functioning and quality of life.

### *Injection Pattern*

For HFS, unilateral injections of the orbicularis oculi are performed, along with injection of other affected muscles of facial expression. When treating HFS, injections are tailored to an individual patient's pattern of dystonia. There is substantial variability in which facial muscles are affected and severity of involuntary spasm. Therefore, the injection pattern must be tailored to the individual patient's muscle pattern by observing the pattern of involuntary muscle contraction and targeting the individual muscles. Small muscles, such as the nasalis, may require only one injection site, whereas large muscles, such as the platysma, may require multiple injection sites. The dose per muscle, total dose, number of injection sites, and number of muscles injected vary widely among patients. Commonly injected muscles include the orbicularis oculi, frontalis, procerus, corrugator, orbicularis oris, zygomaticus, risorius, depressor anguli oris, buccinator, nasalis, platysma, and others. Some authors advocate injecting only upper facial muscles, especially the orbicularis oculi, at the first treatment session, as this is often sufficient to control the patient's symptoms. Patients who do not respond to the treatment of the orbicularis oculi only, or whose symptoms are limited to the lower face, should have the lower facial muscles injected. Some clinicians prefer to avoid the zygomaticus major, as weakness of that muscle visibly impairs smiling and facial expression and can result in lip biting from difficulty retracting the lip. Some clinicians also inject BoNT into muscles on the unaffected side of the face to reduce the appearance of asymmetry, which may result from unilateral injections (152).

For patients with HFS involving the eye and/or brow, the injection pattern and typical starting dose are similar to those for blepharospasm, except that the injections are unilateral. Starting dose for other affected muscles is determined by the choice of BoNT product, muscle, and severity of the problem (see Table 6.1: Benign Essential Blepharospasm BoNT Reconstitution and Dosage Table for Adults ≥ 18 Years of Age for starting dosage suggestions. For details on injection pattern and anatomy, see Figures 1 and 2 following Chapter 8. For details on dosage and dilution, see Table 7.1: Hemifacial Spasm Dosage and Dilution Table for Adults ≥18 Years of Age following this chapter.)

### *Dilution*

As when treating blepharospasm, the neurotoxin may be prepared at a higher dilution than used for dystonia involving large muscles to enable more precision in delivering small doses. For example, OBTA or IBTA may be diluted to achieve a concentration of 1.25 units/0.1 mL or 2.5 units/0.1 mL. To achieve a concentration of 1.25 units/0.1 mL, a 100-unit vial of OBTA or IBTA can be diluted in 8 mL of preservative-free normal saline (PFNS) or a 50-unit vial of IBTA can be diluted in 4 mL of PFNS. To achieve a concentration of 2.5 units/0.1 mL, a 100-unit vial of OBTA or IBTA can be diluted with 4 mL PFNS or a 50-unit vial of IBTA can be diluted in 2 mL of PFNS. A 300-unit vial of ABTA is typically diluted in 1.5 mL of PFNS for a concentration of 200 units/1 mL or 20 units/0.1 mL. RBTB is provided in solution from the manufacturer and does not require reconstitution. If a higher dilution is desired this can be achieved by adding PFNS to the vial.

### *Dosage*

Although considered the first-line treatment of HFS, none of the U.S. FDA-approved BoNT products are approved for the treatment of HFS. Dosing information is based on the literature and the serotype A BoNT approval for OBTA and ABTA in other countries (see Table 7.1: Hemifacial Spasm Dosage and Dilution Table for Adults ≥18 Years of Age for recommended starting dose, injection pattern, and dosage ranges).

### *Injection Technique*

Reconstituted OBTA or IBTA is injected using a sterile 27- to 30-gauge needle. For patient comfort and to avoid bruising, a 30-gauge, 0.5-inch needle may be preferred. While not used uniformly, electromyography, electrical stimulation, or ultrasound guidance may be helpful in locating particular muscles, such as the risorius or zygomaticus major (see Figures 2 and 3 following Chapter 8).

Pain from the injections or ecchymosis can be reduced by applying pressure at the injection site immediately after the injection and/or the brief application of an ice pack.

## *Clinical Effect*

As with blepharospasm, the initial effect of BoNT is generally seen within 3 days, peaking at 1 to 2 weeks postinjection. Duration of effect is generally 12 to 14 weeks. Most clinicians recommend a minimum reinjection interval of 12 weeks or longer depending on the patient's symptoms.

## *Adverse Events/Side Effects*

Adverse events when treating HFS include bruising and injection site pain. Other side effects include ptosis, dysphagia, xerostomia, xerophthalmia, facial asymmetry, and weakness in the injected muscles or those nearby.

**TABLE 7.1 Hemifacial Spasm Dosage and Dilution Table (Adults ≥18 Years of Age)***

| BoNT preparation | OBTA (Botox®) | ABTA (Dysport®) | IBTA (Xeomin®) | RBTB (Myobloc®) | Notes |
|---|---|---|---|---|---|
| U.S. FDA approval | Currently not FDA approved | Currently not FDA approved | Currently not FDA approved | Currently not FDA approved | |
| **Orbicularis Oculi** | | | | | |
| UK MHRA: Note: For orbicularis oculi, treat as unilateral blepharospasm | 1.2–2.5 units/site Maximum dose: ≤5 units/site, 25 units/eye | 120 units/affected eye[1] (20 units [0.1 mL] medial injection sites) (40 units [0.2 mL] lateral injection sites) See Note[1] | Currently not FDA approved | Currently not FDA approved | [1]Note: Although the UK MHRA published dose is 120 units, this dose exceeds that typically used in clinical practice. In addition, doses of >50–60 units of ABTA are associated with an increased incidence of weakness and ptosis. The authors recommend a starting dosage range of 20–50 units/eye of ABTA. |
| Orbicularis oculi injection sites | Four injection sites; see standard injection site pattern | Four injection sites; see standard injection site pattern | | | |

(*continued*)

**TABLE 7.1 Hemifacial Spasm Dosage and Dilution Table (Adults ≥18 Years of Age)* (*continued*)**

| BoNT preparation | OBTA (Botox®) | ABTA (Dysport®) | IBTA (Xeomin®) | RBTB (Myobloc®) | Notes |
|---|---|---|---|---|---|
| **Obicularis Oculi Published Dosage Range** | | | | | |
| Published dosage range | 1–50 units/eye | 20–60 units/eye | 12–43 units/eye | 100, 200, 400, and 800 units reported[3] | [2]Note: Doses >50–60 units of ABTA are associated with a higher incidence of weakness. Consider a starting dose of 20–50 units/eye.<br>[3]Clinical improvement reported at doses >200 units. Sustained improvement reported with 400 and 800 unit doses.<br>[4]Reported total per treatment session is for bilateral injections in patients with blepharospasm. Injections for hemifacial spasm are performed unilaterally. The total dose will be ½ that reported for blepharospasm. |
| Mean, total dose range | 10–46 units/eye | 20–100 units/eye[2] | 12–70 units/eye | | |
| Dose/treatment cycle | 15–80 units[4] | 28–220 units[4] | 15–80 units[4] | 1,250–9,000 units | |

(*continued*)

**TABLE 7.1 Hemifacial Spasm Dosage and Dilution Table (Adults ≥18 Years of Age)* (*continued*)**

| BoNT preparation | OBTA (Botox®) | ABTA (Dysport®) | IBTA (Xeomin®) | RBTB (Myobloc®) | Notes |
|---|---|---|---|---|---|
| **Muscles of Facial Expression** | | | | | |
| Depressor anguli oris, levator anguli oris, levator labii, nasalis, mentalis, orbicularis oris, risorius, zygomaticus | 1.25–2.5 units/muscle<br>May be increased slowly based on the patient's response | 5–10 units/muscle<br>May be increased slowly based on the patient's response | 1.25–2.5 units/muscle<br>May be increased slowly based on the patient's response | 1,200–2,500 units[5]<br>Increase to 5,000 units as needed[5] | [5]Dose divided between obicularis oculi and facial muscles (238). |
| Dilution | 100-unit vial diluted in 4 mL PFNS: 25 units/1 mL, 2.5 units/0.1 mL<br>8 mL PFNS: 12.5 units/1 mL, 1.25 units/0.1 mL<br>In UK/Europe: 50-unit vial diluted in 2–4 mL PFNS; see IBTA column | 300-unit vial diluted with 1.5 mL PFNS 200 units/1 mL or 20 unit/0.1 mL | 50 units in 2 mL: 25 units/1 mL, 2.5 units/0.1 mL<br>or<br>50 units/4 mL: 12.5 units/1 mL, 1.25 units/0.1 mL | Not required but can be further diluted; see note below† | |

*(continued)*

**TABLE 7.1 Hemifacial Spasm Dosage and Dilution Table (Adults ≥18 Years of Age)* (*continued*)**

| BoNT preparation | OBTA (Botox®) | ABTA (Dysport®) | IBTA (Xeomin®) | RBTB (Myobloc®) | Notes |
|---|---|---|---|---|---|
| Reported adverse events and side effects | Hematoma, pain, ptosis, weakness in injected muscle(s) or adjacent muscles, diplopia | Hematoma, pain, ptosis, weakness in injected muscle(s) or adjacent muscles, diplopia | Hematoma, pain, ptosis, weakness in injected muscle(s) or adjacent muscles, diplopia | Hematoma, pain, ptosis, weakness in injected muscle(s) or adjacent muscles, diplopia | |

*Note: When treating hemifacial spasm, injections are generally performed unilaterally. Some authors advocate for a low dose in contralateral muscles for facial symmetry. Any muscle innervated may be affected. Commonly affected/injected muscles include orbicularis oculi, orbicularis oris, risorius, zygomaticus, levator labii, nasalis, and mentalis.

†Note: RBTB is provided from the manufacturer in a 5,000 units/mL solution. Higher dilutions can be achieved by the addition of PFNS to the vial. For a dilution of 2,500 units/mL, 0.5 mL PFNS is added to a 2,500 unit vial or 1 mL is added to a 5,000 unit vial. For a dilution of 1,250 units per vial 1.5 mL PFNS is added to a 2,500 unit vial or 3 mL PFNS is added to a 5,000 unit vial.

*Abbreviations:* ABTA, abobotulinumtoxinA; IBTA, incobotulinumtoxinA; OBTA, onabotulinumtoxinA; PFNS, preservative-free normal saline (0.9%); RBTB, rimabotulinumtoxinB.

*Sources:* Refs. 34–36, 38, 40, 44, 96, 139, 143, 149, 152, 197, 238, 243, 461, 465–472.

# 8

# *Botulinum Neurotoxin Injections for Oromandibular Dystonias*

*Katharine E. Alter, MD*
*Barbara I. Karp, MD*

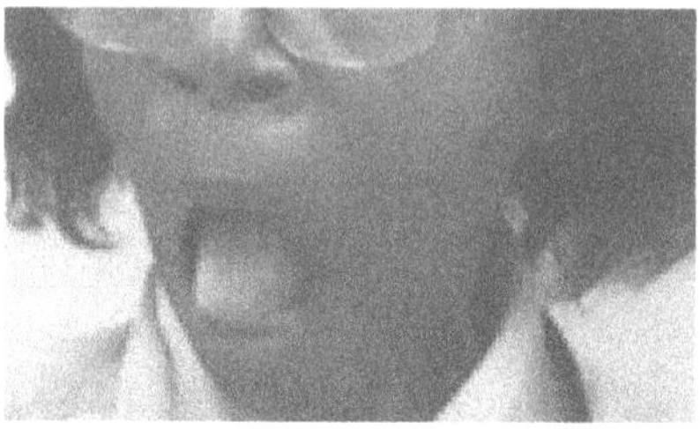

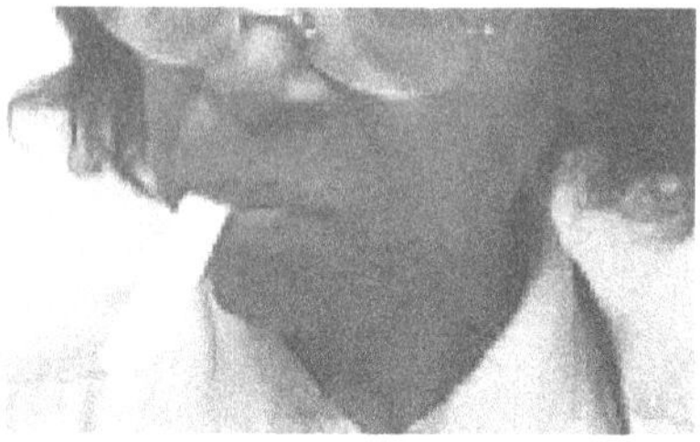

## Condition

Oromandibular dystonia (OMD) is a form of dystonia that involves the face, jaw, and oropharyngeal muscles. When occurring in isolation, it is a form of focal dystonia. OMD may also occur in combination with blepharospasm (Meige syndrome) or in patients with generalized dystonia (53, 153, 154). OMD is characterized by various combinations of intermittent or sustained movements in muscles of the face, mastication, pharynx, or the tongue. Common patterns of dystonia include jaw opening, jaw closing, and lateral deviation. Grinding or clenching of the teeth (similar to that seen in bruxism) may be present in patients with jaw closing dystonia and may also be seen in patients with secondary dystonia, such as that seen in patients with cerebral palsy or traumatic brain injury. OMD is more common in women and the mean age of onset is in the sixth decade, with a reported prevalence of 3.3 to 6.9 per million in the United States (153).

### *Clinical/Functional Impact*

OMD may affect a variety of functions including speaking, drinking, chewing, and swallowing. Patients frequently report that involuntary movements lead to repeated injury to the lips, tongue, or inside of the cheek, and/or to abnormal wear or breakage of teeth. They also often report jaw or temporomandibular pain and headache. The involuntary movements are often visible and may provoke significant emotional distress, interfere with communication, and lead to dysphagia with subsequent weight loss and social isolation (142). If associated with blepharospasm, vision may also be compromised.

### *Pattern of Involvement*

The common patterns of OMD noted previously include jaw opening, which implicates the lateral pterygoid muscles and anterior belly of the digastric muscle, jaw closing or trismus (masseters, temporalis, and medial pterygoids), bruxism (masseter, temporalis, and/or medial pterygoid), jaw deviation (asymmetric involvement of the muscles listed previously). Other patterns include lip pursing (orbicularis oris) or lip retraction, grimacing (muscles of facial expression), and abnormal movements in the chin or neck (mentalis and/or platysma). Abnormal tongue movements include tongue protrusion, deviation, and complex writhing movements due to involvement of genioglossus and other tongue musculature (142).

### *Evaluation*

The diagnosis of OMD is largely based on clinical presentation and patient symptomatology. A detailed medication history, specifically for neuroleptics, should be taken in patients with OMD to rule out tardive dyskinesia, which often involves orofacial muscles (154).

### *Treatment*

Oral medications such as anticholinergics or benzodiazepines may be helpful in some patients with OMD, but their benefit is often outweighed by their side effects. Many patients with OMD report that their dystonic movements are temporarily improved with a "sensory trick," such as placing a toothpick between the teeth, using a mouth guard, or chewing gum. Sensory tricks should be sought in people with OMD and a prescriptive occlusal device or mouth guard should also be considered. A nighttime mouth guard or relaxation and/or behavioral therapy may be helpful for some patients, but is often less helpful in patients with OMD than in those with bruxism. Due to the complexity of the movements, botulinum neurotoxin (BoNT) therapy is not as effective for OMD as it is for blepharospasm or hemifacial spasm. However, BoNT therapy can be considered and may reduce the severity of OMD symptoms and improve quality of life. There are limited data on the starting dose, dose titration, and dosage range of BoNT when treating OMD. Clinicians should begin therapy at the lower end of the dosage range for each toxin product and adjust the dose based on the patient's response (53).

### *BoNTs Approved for the Treatment of OMD*

None of the BoNT products currently approved by the FDA carry a specific approval for the treatment of OMD.

### *Approvals Outside the United States*

None of the BoNT products currently available carry specific approval for the treatment of OMD.

### *Level of Evidence*

In a 2013 evidence-based review using the American Academy of Neurology (AAN) clinical practice guidelines, the current evidence supports a Level C (Possibly effective, ineffective or harmful for the given condition in the specified population; Level C requires one Class II study or two consistent Class III studies) recommendation for serotype A BoNTs for the treatment of OMD (2, 138). A different 2013 evidence-based review reported Level 1 evidence supporting the use of BoNTs for the treatment of OMD (151).

### *Injection Pattern*

Muscle selection is based on the dominant pattern of the dystonic movement. Since the most common pattern is jaw-closing dystonia, the most common muscles injected are the bilateral masseters, temporalis, and medial pterygoids (see Figures 3 and 4 located at the end of this chapter). This pattern is also reportedly more amenable to treatment with BoNT therapy than other forms of OMD. Jaw-opening dystonia is less common and may be more difficult to treat (53). Muscles typically injected for jaw-opening dystonia include the lateral pterygoids and anterior belly of the digastric muscle, all injected bilaterally. The genioglossus or other tongue muscles can be targeted for lingual involvement.

### *BoNT Dilution*

For precise dosing of small muscles, a higher dilution of BoNT is required. A 100-U vial of onabotulinumtoxinA (OBTA) is generally diluted with 2 mL preservative-free normal saline (PFNS), resulting in a concentration of 50 units/1 mL or 5 units/0.1 mL. For abobotulinumtoxinA (ABTA), 300 units are diluted into 1.5 mL PFNS for a concentration of 200 units/1 mL or 20 unit/0.1 mL. A 50-unit vial of incobotulinumtoxinA (IBTA) is diluted with 1 mL PFNS or a 100-unit vial with 2 mL PFNS for a concentration of 50 units/1 mL or 5 units/0.1 mL. RimabotulinumtoxinB (RBTB) is supplied in solution (5,000 units/mL) and does not require reconstitution. If desired, PFNS can be added to the vial to further dilute the product; 0.5 mL PFNS added to a 2,500-unit vial will result in a concentration of 1,250 units/mL or 125 units/0.1 mL. A 5,000-unit vial can be further diluted with 1 mL for a resulting concentration of 2,500 units/mL, 250 units/0.1 mL. Alternately, a 5,000 unit vial can be diluted with 3 mL for a concentration of 1,250 units/mL or 125 units/0.1 mL.

### *Dosage*

When treating patients with OMD, the dose per muscle and the total dose should be based on the severity of the dystonic movement and the size of the muscle. There are limited data to guide the dose for these muscles or the total dose. The available data on published dose and dose range/muscle are provided in Table 8.1: Oromandibular Dystonia Dosage/Dilution Table for Adults ≥18 years of Age (53, 151, 154, 155).

### *Injection Technique*

Most studies recommend the use of electromyography (EMG) guidance for many of the muscles injected when treating OMD, as palpation is often not possible and the muscles are near structures (such as the facial nerve or blood vessels), which should be avoided. Such guidance can also ensure that the injection is delivered into the correct muscle. B-mode ultrasound, which provides direct visualization of the muscles, vessels, and nerves, may also be used either alone or in combination with EMG to guide these injections (156, 157).

### *Clinical Effect*

Many patients report significant benefit from BoNT injections, with reduced involuntary movements, improved speech, chewing, and reduced emotional distress. As noted, those with jaw-closing dystonia often respond better than those with jaw-opening dystonia. Complex OMD with involvement of the tongue, oropharynx, or multiple muscles are particularly difficult to treat with BoNT.

### *Adverse Events*

Dysphagia and dry mouth are common adverse events in those treated for OMD and are largely due to excessive weakness and spread to adjacent muscles or unintended targets like the salivary glands. Dysphagia is a common side effect with lingual injections (53).

**TABLE 8.1 Oromandibular Dystonia Dosage/Dilution Table (Adults ≥18 Years of Age)**

| BoNT Preparation | OBTA (Botox®) | ABTA (Dysport®) | IBTA (Xeomin®) | RBTB (Myobloc®) | Notes |
|---|---|---|---|---|---|
| U.S. FDA approval | Currently not FDA approved | Currently not FDA approved | Currently not FDA approved | Currently not FDA approved | |
| UK MHRA | Currently not an approved indication | Currently not an approved indication | Currently not an approved indication | Currently not an approved indication | |
| **Published Dosage Ranges** | | | | | |
| **Jaw-Opening Dystonia** | | | | | |
| Digastric, anterior belly | 1.5–5 units | No data available | No data available | No data available | Assists jaw opening<br>Elevates hyoid, also pulls tongue/jaw back, down, and open |
| Mylohyoid<br>Per injection site<br>Total dose | 1.25–5 units<br>10–20 units | 4–20 units<br>30 units | 1.25–5 units<br>10–20 units | No data available | Assists jaw opening<br>Elevates hyoid, pushes tongue up or out (protrusion) |
| Platysma | 20 units | 60 units | No data available | 100–1,000 units | Assists jaw opening |
| Pterygoid, lateral<br>dose<br>Dosage range | 5–15 units<br>7.5–40 units | 40–60 units<br>Dose increase >60 units as needed | 5–15 units<br>5–25 units | 500–1,000 units | Primary muscle responsible for jaw opening (along with gravity)<br>For localization, consider US or US and EMG. Ask patient to open jaw and deviate side to side |

*(continued)*

**TABLE 8.1 Oromandibular Dystonia Dosage/Dilution Table (Adults ≥18 Years of Age) (*continued*)**

| BoNT Preparation | OBTA (Botox®) | ABTA (Dysport®) | IBTA (Xeomin®) | RBTB (Myobloc®) | Notes |
|---|---|---|---|---|---|
| Mentalis – Submentalis complex<br>Starting dose | 5–20 units | 30–50 units | 5–20 units | 250–500 units | Assists in initial jaw opening |
| Dosage range | 20–50 units (up to 200 units reported) | 50–90 units | 5–50 units | 500–1,000 units | |
| **Jaw-Closing Dystonia** | | | | | |
| Masseter<br>Starting dose | 25–50 units | 50–100 units | 15–50 units | 1,500–2,500 units | Consider US or US and EMG to avoid the parotid gland |
| Dosage range | 15–75 units | 50–300 units | 15–75 units | | |
| Pterygoid, medial | 10–20 units | 30–50 units | 10–20 units | 500–1,000 units | |
| Temporalis | 10–30 units | 50–100 units | 5–20 units | No data available | Multiple injection sites for this fan-shaped muscle |
| Meige syndrome (blepharospasm + OMD): Treat as blepharospasm with other oromandibular muscles, as above. | | | | | |
| **Lingual Muscle Dystonia** | | | | | |
| Lingual/tongue muscles<br>Starting dose | 2.5–5 units | 10–30 units | 2.5–5 units | 200–500 units | Treat with caution due to reported high incidence of dysphagia; consider treating unilaterally |
| Dosage range | 2.5–10 units | | | | |

(*continued*)

**TABLE 8.1 Oromandibular Dystonia Dosage/Dilution Table (Adults ≥18 Years of Age) (*continued*)**

| BoNT Preparation | OBTA (Botox®) | ABTA (Dysport®) | IBTA (Xeomin®) | RBTB (Myobloc®) | Notes |
|---|---|---|---|---|---|
| **Dilution** | | | | | |
| Dilution | 100 units with 2 mL PFNS, for a concentration of 50 units/mL | 300 units with 1.5 mL PFNS for a concentration of 200 units/mL | 50 units with 0.5 mL or 100 units with 1 mL for a concentration of 100 units/mL, 10 units/ 0.1 mL | Provided in solution (5,000 units/mL), reconstitution is not required. If desired RBTB can be further diluted, see Notes column | Dilution of RBTB: Add 0.5 mL or 1.5 mL PFNS to a 2,500 unit vial (0.5 mL) for a concentration of 2,500 units/mL or 1,250 units/mL RBTB, respectively. To a 5,000 unit vial add 1 mL or 3 mL for a concentration of 2,500 units/1 mL or 1,250 units/mL, respectively. |
| Adverse events/ side effects | Xerostomia, dysphagia, weakness | Xerostomia, dysphagia, weakness | Limited data for OMD | Limited data for OMD | |

*Abbreviations:* ABTA, AbobotulinumtoxinA; EMG, Electromyography; IBTA, IncobotulinumtoxinA; OBTA, OnabotulinumtoxinA; OMD, Oromandibular Dystonia; PFNS, Preservative-Free Normal Saline (0.9%); RBTB, RimabotulinumtoxinB; US, Ultrasound.

*Sources:* Refs. 34–36, 38, 40, 44, 53, 96, 151, 153, 154–156, 197, 243, 473.

# Illustrations for Craniofacial Dystonia—Chapters 6–8

*FIGURE 1* *Technique for intradermal botulinum neurotoxin injections.*

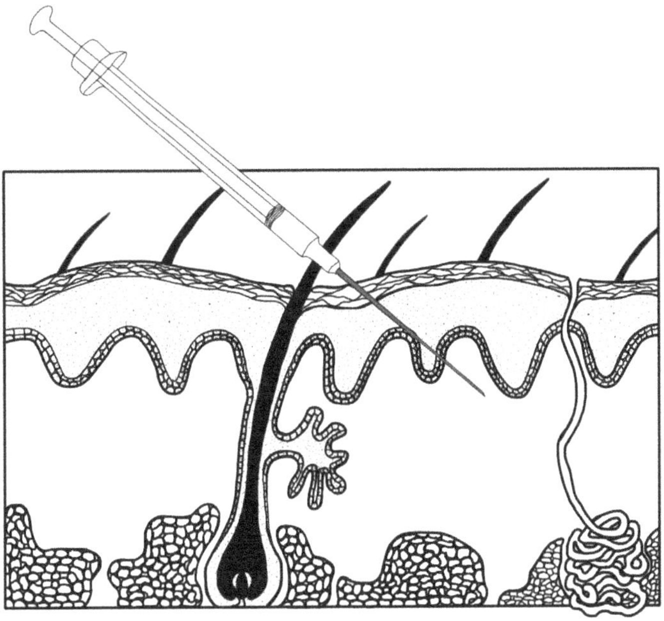

*FIGURE 2* *Injection patterns for blepharospasm.*

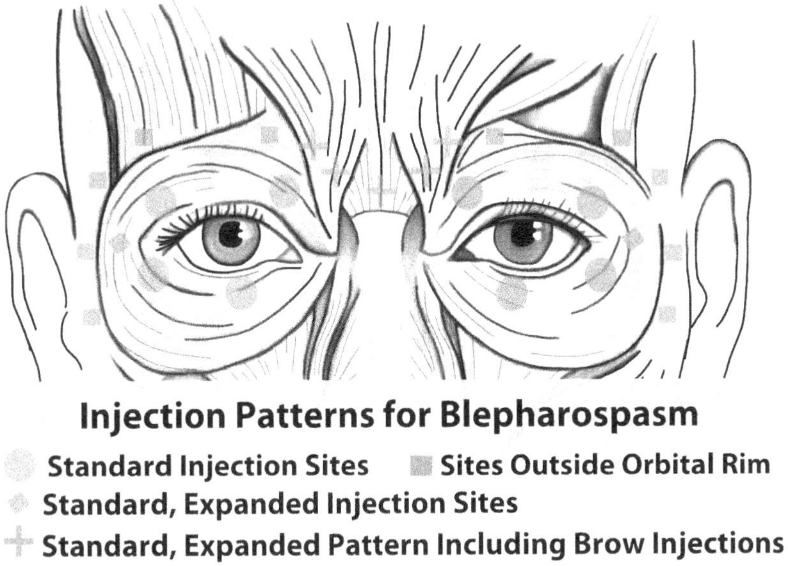

*FIGURE 3* *Muscles of facial expression, hemifacial spasm.*

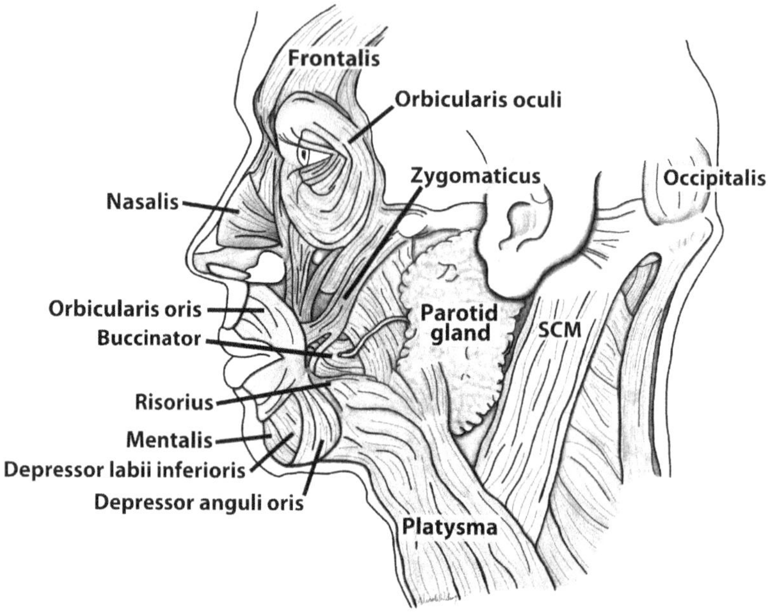


*FIGURE 4* *Temporalis muscle, oromandibular dystonia.*

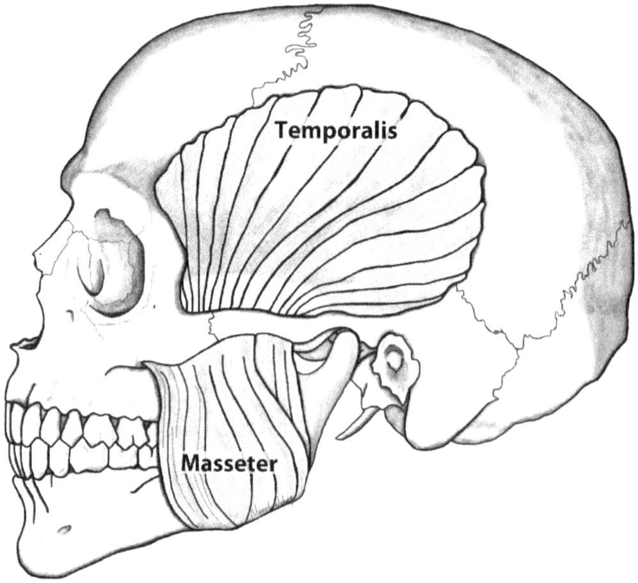

*FIGURE 5* *Medial and lateral pterygoid muscles, oromandibular dystonia.*

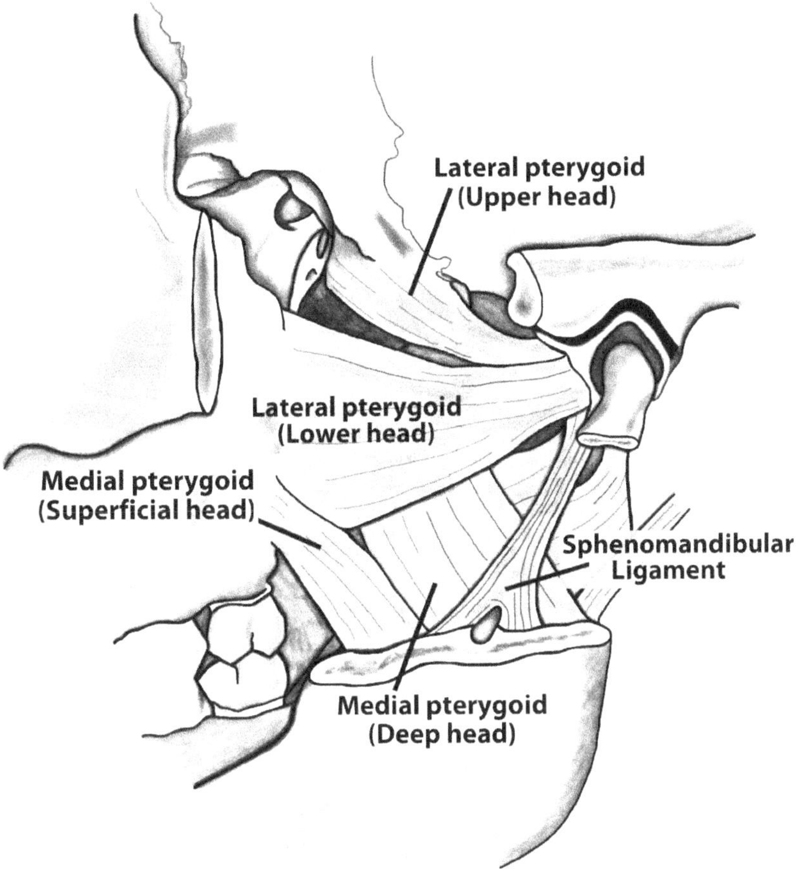

*Cervical Dystonia*

# 9

# *Botulinum Neurotoxin Injections for Cervical Dystonia*

*Katharine E. Alter, MD*
*Michael C. Munin, MD, FAAPMR*
*Sherry A. Downie, PhD*

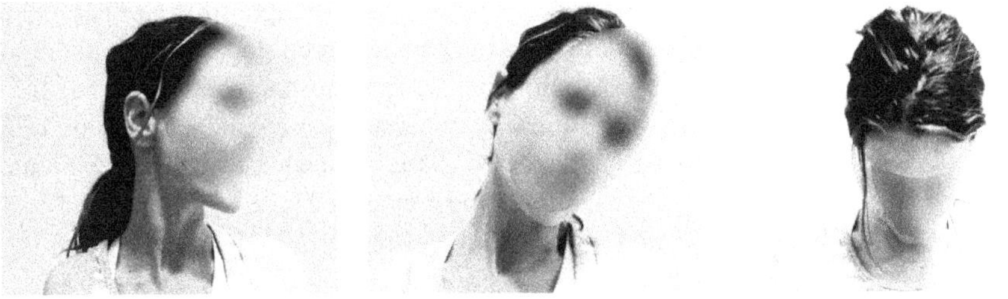

## Condition

### *Clinical Presentation/Functional Impact*

Cervical dystonia (CD or spasmodic torticollis) is a focal movement disorder characterized by co-contraction of agonist and antagonist muscles leading to involuntary movements or postures of the head and/or neck. The disorder places the head away from its customary central position. CD is classified by the movement pattern or presenting posture and includes several subtypes (i.e., torticollis [lateral rotation], laterocollis [lateral tilt], retrocollis [extension], anterocollis [flexion], sagittal shift, lateral shift, and frequently, combinations of these patterns). Patients often report improvement in their symptoms with some type of tactile stimulus (called a "sensory trick" or *geste antagoniste*), such as touching the chin (85, 158, 159). Abnormal movements, postures, and pain frequently impede functional tasks at home and work, like reading, watching television, viewing a computer screen, and/or driving. These impairments reduce quality of life, may result in social isolation, and may affect mood or cause depression.

### *Muscle Pattern*

When evaluating patients with CD, one of the most critical principles for clinicians to recognize is that a muscle can only move a bone or a structure to which it is attached. Although the aforementioned classification system of CD refers to "collis" (from *collum*, Latin referring to the neck), patients may present with an abnormal position of the "caput," that is, the head or both the head and neck. Therefore, clinicians should record the position of both the head and the neck, as this distinction is important when considering which muscles should be injected (85, 158). For example, torticaput (lateral rotation of the head) may be caused by dystonic movements in the ipsilateral obliquus capitis inferioris (OCI) and/or the splenius capitis. Torticollis (lateral rotation of the neck) may be caused by dystonic contraction in the ipsilateral splenius cervicis or levator scapulae, the contralateral sternocleidomastoid (SCM), or other muscles (Table 9.1). Combined torticollis and torticaput may be caused by co-contraction of the combined muscles listed previously (Table 9.1).

Abnormal movements associated with CD may include sustained postures, dystonic tremor, jerky movements, spasms, or combinations of these movements. In addition to abnormal movements, the majority of patients with CD also report pain that may be more disabling than the abnormal head posture (143, 160, 161). The vast majority of patients with CD are categorized as having a primary dystonia restricted to the head and neck region. CD may also present as one symptom of a generalized primary dystonia or a secondary dystonia, caused by another etiology, such as cerebral palsy. The diagnosis of secondary posttraumatic CD remains controversial (159, 162, 163). CD is the most common form of focal dystonia and psychogenic cases are rare (143, 159, 160). Although the true incidence of CD is somewhat difficult to estimate due to variability in establishing the diagnosis, the prevalence is reported to be 0.4% of the population with women affected twice as often as men (159, 164, 165).

### *Evaluation*

The diagnosis of CD is largely based on clinical evaluation. Radiologic studies may be helpful in some patients with atypical presentations or when a boney abnormality is suspected. Clinical evaluation of CD is based on one or more of the available semiquantitative clinical rating scales. These scales include the Burke–Fahn–Marsden (BFM) Scale and the Unified Dystonia Rating Scale (UDRS) (166, 167). Rating scales specific for CD include the Toronto Western Spasmodic Torticollis Rating Scale (TWSTRS), the Tsui Scale, and the Dystonia Discomfort Scale (DDS) (167–171). The TWSTRS is the most widely used scale in clinical practice for evaluation of CD. It includes several sections, specifically a severity section based on examination, and both disability and pain sections informed by historical information provided by the patient. The TWSTRS also queries for the presence or absence of a *geste antagoniste* and whether sensory stimulation improves abnormal postures. The DDS evaluates the patient's report of pain or discomfort associated with CD. Patients are asked to keep a daily diary and to rate their symptoms in multiples of 5%, ranging from no pain (0%) to maximum pain (100%). This scale has been reported to be valid and sensitive (see also www.dds.iabnetz.de) (171).

**TABLE 9.1 Cervical Dystonia: Head, Neck, and/or Shoulder Postures and Muscles Contributing to the Observed Patterns**

**Pattern explanations:** Muscles can only move structures to which they are attached (e.g., head, neck, shoulder). To determine which muscles may be involved, carefully observe the patient's abnormal posture or movement to determine whether the abnormal posture or movement involves the head, the neck, or both the head and neck. This requires that the patient's abnormal postures or movements be observed from the front, back, and both sides.

| Possible Muscle Involvement | Torticollis (Neck Rotation) or Torticaput (Head Rotation) | Laterocollis (Neck Tilt) and/or Laterocaput (Head Tilt)[1] | Torticollis (Neck Rotation) + Laterocollis (Neck Tilt) | Sagittal Shift (Anterior Head Shift With Neck Maintained in Neutral or Flexion)[2a] | Lateral Shift (Head Is Shifted Laterally, Away From the Midline, Toward the Shoulder)[2b] | Anterocollis (Neck Flexion) and/or Anterocaput (Head Flexion)[3,4a] | Anterocollis (Neck Flexion) + Retrocaput (Head Extension)[3,4a,4b] | Retrocollis (Neck Extension) and/or Retrocaput (Head Extension) | Shoulder Elevation (With Upward or Downward Rotation of Glenohumeral (GH) joint) |
|---|---|---|---|---|---|---|---|---|---|
| Levator scapulae | Ipsilateral neck | Ipsilateral neck | Ipsilateral (T, L) | Bilateral, holds neck in neutral or flexion | | | | Bilateral neck | Ipsilateral (D) |
| Longissimus capitis | Ipsilateral head | Ipsilateral head | | | | | Bilateral head | Bilateral head | |
| Longissimus cervicis | Ipsilateral neck | Ipsilateral neck | Ipsilateral (T, L) | Bilateral, holds neck in neutral or flexion | | | | Bilateral neck | |
| Longus capitis | | | | | | Bilateral head | | | |
| Longus colli | Contralateral neck (2°) | | | | | Bilateral neck | | | |

(continued)

**TABLE 9.1 Cervical Dystonia: Head, Neck, and/or Shoulder Postures and Muscles Contributing to the Observed Patterns (*continued*)**

**Pattern explanations:** Muscles can only move structures to which they are attached (e.g., head, neck, shoulder). To determine which muscles may be involved, carefully observe the patient's abnormal posture or movement to determine whether the abnormal posture or movement involves the head, the neck, or both the head and neck. This requires that the patient's abnormal postures or movements be observed from the front, back, and both sides.

| Possible Muscle Involvement | Torticollis (Neck Rotation) or Torticaput (Head Rotation) | Laterocollis (Neck Tilt) and/or Laterocaput (Head Tilt)[1] | Torticollis (Neck Rotation) + Laterocollis (Neck Tilt) | Sagittal Shift (Anterior Head Shift With Neck Maintained in Neutral or Flexion)[2a] | Lateral Shift (Head Is Shifted Laterally, Away From the Midline, Toward the Shoulder)[2b] | Anterocollis (Neck Flexion) and/or Anterocaput (Head Flexion)[3,4a] | Anterocollis (Neck Flexion) + Retrocaput (Head Extension)[3,4a,4b] | Retrocollis (Neck Extension) and/or Retrocaput (Head Extension) | Shoulder Elevation (With Upward or Downward Rotation of Glenohumeral (GH) joint) |
|---|---|---|---|---|---|---|---|---|---|
| Multifidus | Contralateral neck | Ipsilateral neck | Contralateral (T) Ipsilateral (L) | Bilateral, holds neck in neutral or flexion | | | | Bilateral neck | |
| Scalene, anterior | Contralateral neck | Ipsilateral neck | Contralateral (T) Ipsilateral (L) | | Contralateral, holds neck in neutral or tilt | Bilateral neck | Bilateral neck | | |
| Scalene, middle | | Ipsilateral neck | Ipsilateral (L) | | Contralateral, holds neck in neutral or tilt | Bilateral neck | Bilateral neck | | |
| Scalene, posterior | Ipsilateral neck (2°) | Ipsilateral neck | Ipsilateral (T, L) | Bilateral, holds neck in neutral or flexion | Contralateral, holds neck in neutral or tilt | | | Bilateral neck (2°) | |
| Semispinalis capitis | | Ipsilateral head | | | | | Bilateral head | Bilateral head | |

(*continued*)

**TABLE 9.1 Cervical Dystonia: Head, Neck, and/or Shoulder Postures and Muscles Contributing to the Observed Patterns (*continued*)**

**Pattern explanations:** Muscles can only move structures to which they are attached (e.g., head, neck, shoulder). To determine which muscles may be involved, carefully observe the patient's abnormal posture or movement to determine whether the abnormal posture or movement involves the head, the neck, or both the head and neck. This requires that the patient's abnormal postures or movements be observed from the front, back, and both sides.

| Possible Muscle Involvement | Torticollis (Neck Rotation) or Torticaput (Head Rotation) | Laterocollis (Neck Tilt) and/or Laterocaput (Head Tilt)[1] | Torticollis (Neck Rotation) + Laterocollis (Neck Tilt) | Sagittal Shift (Anterior Head Shift With Neck Maintained in Neutral or Flexion)[2a] | Lateral Shift (Head Is Shifted Laterally, Away From the Midline, Toward the Shoulder)[2b] | Anterocollis (Neck Flexion) and/or Anterocaput (Head Flexion)[3,4a] | Anterocollis (Neck Flexion) + Retrocaput (Head Extension)[3,4a,4b] | Retrocollis (Neck Extension) and/or Retrocaput (Head Extension) | Shoulder Elevation (With Upward or Downward Rotation of Glenohumeral (GH) joint) |
|---|---|---|---|---|---|---|---|---|---|
| Semispinalis cervicis | Contralateral neck | Ipsilateral neck | Contralateral (T) Ipsilateral (L) | Bilateral, holds neck in neutral or flexion | | | | Bilateral neck | |
| Splenius capitis | Ipsilateral head | Ipsilateral head | | | Contralateral, pulls head away from midline | | | Bilateral head | |
| Splenius cervicis | Ipsilateral neck | Ipsilateral neck | Ipsilateral (T, L) | Bilateral, holds neck in neutral or flexion | | | | Bilateral neck | |
| SCM | Contralateral head | Contralateral head | | Bilateral, extends head and/or shifts head forward | Contralateral, pulls head away from midline | | Bilateral head and neck | Bilateral head extension (then flexes neck) | |
| Trapezius, upper | Contralateral head | Ipsilateral head | Contralateral (T) Ipsilateral (L) | | | | Bilateral head | Bilateral head | Ipsilateral (U) |

(*continued*)

**TABLE 9.1 Cervical Dystonia: Head, Neck, and/or Shoulder Postures and Muscles Contributing to the Observed Patterns (*continued*)**

**Pattern explanations:** Muscles can only move structures to which they are attached (e.g., head, neck, shoulder). To determine which muscles may be involved, carefully observe the patient's abnormal posture or movement to determine whether the abnormal posture or movement involves the head, the neck, or both the head and neck. This requires that the patient's abnormal postures or movements be observed from the front, back, and both sides.

| Possible Muscle Involvement | Torticollis (Neck Rotation) or Torticaput (Head Rotation) | Laterocollis (Neck Tilt) and/or Laterocaput (Head Tilt)[1] | Torticollis (Neck Rotation) + Laterocollis (Neck Tilt) | Sagittal Shift (Anterior Head Shift With Neck Maintained in Neutral or Flexion)[2a] | Lateral Shift (Head Is Shifted Laterally, Away From the Midline, Toward the Shoulder)[2b] | Anterocollis (Neck Flexion) and/or Anterocaput (Head Flexion)[3,4a] | Anterocollis (Neck Flexion) + Retrocaput (Head Extension)[3,4a,4b] | Retrocollis (Neck Extension) and/or Retrocaput (Head Extension) | Shoulder Elevation (With Upward or Downward Rotation of Glenohumeral (GH) joint) |
|---|---|---|---|---|---|---|---|---|---|
| **Suboccipital Group: Cross Only Occipital C1, Occipital C2, or C1–C2[5]** | | | | | | | | | |
| OCI | Ipsilateral (C1–head)[6] | | | | Contralateral, pulls head away from midline | | | | |
| OCS | | | | Bilateral, extends head and/or shifts head forward | | | Bilateral head (OCC–C1) | Bilateral head (OCC–C1) | |
| Rectus capitis anterior | | Ipsilateral head (2° muscle) | | | | Bilateral head (OCC–C1) | Bilateral head (OCC-C1) | | |
| Rectus capitis posterior major | Ipsilateral head (OCC–C2) | Ipsilateral head (OCC–C2) | | | | | Bilateral head (OCC–C2) | Bilateral head (OCC–C2) | |
| Rectus capitis posterior minor | Ipsilateral head (OCC–C1) | Ipsilateral head (OCC–C1) | | | | | Bilateral head (OCC–C1) | Bilateral head (OCC–C1) | |

(*continued*)

**TABLE 9.1 Cervical Dystonia: Head, Neck, and/or Shoulder Postures and Muscles Contributing to the Observed Patterns (*continued*)**

[1]Clinicians should carefully observe the position of both the head and the neck. This evaluation will guide in determining which muscles may be contributing to the abnormal posture or movement. When a patient presents with lateral deviation or tilt, remember that either the head or the neck or both may be affected. If a patient presents with *laterocollis* (neck tilt), then the splenius cervicis may be involved; if a patient presents with *laterocaput* (head tilt), then the splenius capitis may be contributing to the abnormal posture. If both the neck and the head are tilted, then both the splenius capitis and the cervicis may be contributing to the posture/movement.

[2a]Sagittal shift: In anterior sagittal shift, the head is shifted or moved anteriorly, while the neck is maintained in neural or flexion. This shift occurs due to the combined effect of contraction of muscles that shift the head in an anterior direction and the action of neck extensor muscles.

[2b]Lateral shift: In lateral shift, the head is deviated or shifted away from its normal midline position, toward the shoulder, whereas the neck remains in a midline position or is deviated toward the opposite shoulder. For example, in *left* lateral shift, the head is shifted away from midline toward the left shoulder. The neck remains in midline or is shifted to the right by the right cervical muscles. Muscles that may be involved in a left shift include the right SCM pulling the head toward the left shoulder, the right splenius capitis, and right OCI resist the head rotation force from the SCM and contribute force shifting the head away from midline toward the left shoulder. The right scalenes may act to keep the neck in the midline or tilt it to the right.

[3]In the literature, the term anterocollis is often used to refer to a flexed posture of the neck and/or head. However, although some patients present with both head and neck flexion, others may present with neck flexion and head extension. To be biomechanically correct, clinicians should observe and record the position of the head (caput) and neck (collis) separately. Neck flexion may be caused by the bilateral longus colli and/or the bilateral scalenes. Head flexion may be caused by the longus capitis.

[4a]Clinical pearl: To correctly identify the subtype of anterocollis, observe the position of the patient's head and neck. If the neck is flexed but the chin is pointed up or out, then the head is in extension. If the neck is flexed and the chin is pointed toward the chest, then the head is also in flexion. These two clinical patterns are distinctly different with different muscles involved; see Table 9.1.

[4b]Neck flexion with head extension: When evaluating patients with anterocollis, carefully observe the position of the patient's neck and head. Some patients will present with retrocaput or head extension superimposed on a flexed neck posture. This posture is generally caused by bilateral SCM involvement. Although the SCM, when acting bilaterally, may flex the neck, this muscle first extends the head. It does so because its superior attachment on the mastoid and superior nuchal line is posterior to the axis of head flexion/extension. Once the head reaches full range of motion in extension, continued force from the SCM will pull the neck (and extended head) forward.

[5]The suboccipital muscles cross only the occipital C1 and occipital C2 joints. Contraction of these muscles produces only a small range of motion. Although the excursion is small, these muscles exert significant force and are quite powerful. When evaluating a patient with a dystonic contraction of the suboccipital muscle(s), the head may feel "stuck." This is due to the combined action of dystonic muscle contraction, the small arc of motion at these joints, and the tight ligaments that span the involved joints at occipital C1.

[6]The OCI rotates C1 on C2. C1 and the skull base are held together by dense membranes, the anterior and posterior atlantooccipital membranes. Thus, when C1 is rotated, the head also rotates. Although the OCI does not directly attach to the head, it is considered a rotator of the head.

*Abbreviations:* D, downward; GH, glenohumeral; L, laterocollis; OCC, occipital; OCI, obliquus capitis inferioris; OCS, obliquus capitis superioris; SCM, sternocleidomastoid; T, torticollis; U, upward; 2°, secondary.

### *Treatment*

Botulinum neurotoxin (BoNT) injections are considered the standard of care (preferred treatment) for CD. BoNT injections are well tolerated and provide symptomatic relief of the pulling, abnormal postures, and pain associated with CD. Patients may also benefit from physical therapy and/or the intermittent use of cervical collars. Various oral medications (e.g., anticholinergics, antidopaminergics, dopamine depletors, benzodiazepines) may be prescribed for some patients with CD, but none have been proven as effective as BoNT injections (143, 160, 164, 172).

### *BoNTs Approved for the Treatment of CD*

Currently, several BoNT products are approved by the Food and Drug Administration (FDA) for the treatment of CD: onabotulinumtoxinA (OBTA), abobotulinumtoxinA (ABTA), incobotulinumtoxinA (IBTA), and rimabotulinumtoxinB (RBTB) (34, 36, 38, 44).

### *Level of Evidence*

There is high-quality Level A evidence to support the efficacy of OBTA, ABTA, IBTA, and RBTB in the treatment of CD (2, 138).

### *Treatment Goals*

The goal of BoNT treatment is to decrease pain, improve abnormal postures, increase function, and improve quality of life in patients with CD.

### *Treatment of Various Patterns of CD*

Muscle selection is based on the pattern of dystonic movements involving the head, neck and/or shoulder, tremor and/or dystonic movements, and pain. Physicians must be well versed in the regional anatomy and kinesiology of the individual muscles responsible for the abnormal head movements, which can be located either ipsilateral or contralateral to the movement (Table 9.1). When injecting BoNT for CD, the most commonly targeted muscles include the SCM, splenius capitis, splenius cervicis, levator scapulae, scalenes (anterior and middle), longissimus capitis, semispinalis capitis, and trapezius. Other muscles that may be targeted by experienced clinicians include the OCI, longus colli, and longus capitis. When targeting the longus colli and longus capitis, most clinicians recommend the use of real-time imaging to guide the injections, since these muscles are surrounded by large vessels and nerves and lie immediately adjacent to the pharynx (90).

### *Dosage*

In neurotoxin-naïve patients, clinicians are advised to initiate treatment with the lowest recommended published dose listed in the full prescribing information for each BoNT product. (See Tables 9.1–9.3 for additional information.) When switching within or between BoNT serotypes, most manufacturers recommend starting with the lowest recommended starting dose for their product (34, 36, 38, 44). Although there are published data on dosage conversion ratios, these data are not fully reliable, since each medication has its own biologic formulation. Thus, unlike drugs such as opioids, these drugs cannot be directly converted between serotypes. Currently, all the manufacturers and the FDA recommend against the use of conversion ratios (55, 59, 63, 173–175). Until there is agreement on whether conversion ratios can be used safely, physicians should convert between serotypes with caution and use the lowest possible dose ratio.

### *Muscle Localization*

The majority of physicians who perform BoNT injections for CD and the manufactures of BoNT products recommend the use of a supplementary guidance technique (in addition to palpation) to localize involved muscles. Commonly used localization techniques include electromyography, electrical stimulation, B-mode ultrasound, and/or combinations of these techniques (90). Each of these guidance techniques has advantages and disadvantages, and this topic is covered in detail in Chapter 4.

### *Adverse Events*

The most common side effect from injections with BoNT is dysphagia, with an incidence varying between 10% and 30% in randomized trials, regardless of serotype. Other adverse events include injection-site pain, dry mouth, flu-like symptoms, and any of the adverse events listed in the full prescribing information included with each vial of BoNT.

**TABLE 9.2 BoNT for Cervical Dystonia: Manufacturer's Recommended Dosage Range (Adults ≥18 Years of Age)**

| BoNT Preparation | OBTA (Botox®) | ABTA (Dysport®) | IBTA (Xeomin®) | RBTB (Myobloc®) | Notes |
|---|---|---|---|---|---|
| **Manufacturer's Recommended Dose, Dosage Range from Package Insert/Prescribing Information (PI)** | | | | | |
| Dose | 236 units[1] | 500 units[2] | 120 units[2] | 2,500-5,000 units | [1]Mean dosage<br>[2]Initial dose<br>[3]No added benefit, and increased AE reported with a 10,000-unit dose in registration trials<br>[4]Increased AE reported with dosages ≥1000 units<br>[5]In registration trials, no meaningful difference in efficacy with 240 units, compared to 120 units |
| Dosage range | 198–300 units (25th–75th percentile) | — | — | 2,500–5,000 units | |
| **Published Total Dosage Ranges (from Published Studies)** | | | | | |
| Dosage range | 50–500 units | 125–1,200 units[4] (500 units, most commonly reported maximum dose) | Toxin-naïve patients: ≤120 units<br>Dosage range: 50–180 units, in most studies<br>Previously treated patients:<br>Mean dose: 245 units<br>Dosage range: 120–300 units[5] | 579–25,000[3] | |
| Recommended or reported dose increase per session: | 5%–20% | 250 units/session | 5%–20% | Not reported | |

*(continued)*

**TABLE 9.2 BoNT for Cervical Dystonia: Manufacturer's Recommended Dosage Range (Adults ≥18 Years of Age) (*continued*)**

| BoNT Preparation | OBTA (Botox®) | ABTA (Dysport®) | IBTA (Xeomin®) | RBTB (Myobloc®) | Notes |
|---|---|---|---|---|---|
| Dose modifiers | Consider lower initial total dose for milder symptoms, smaller muscles, or history of dysphagia with other BoNT products | Consider lower initial total dose for milder symptoms, smaller muscles, or history of dysphagia with other BoNT products | Consider lower initial total dose for milder symptoms, smaller muscles, or history of dysphagia with other BoNT products | Consider lower initial total dose for milder symptoms, smaller muscles, or history of dysphagia with other BoNT products | |
| Mean duration of effect | 94 days<br>No significant differences among other BoNT products | 84 days<br>No significant differences among other BoNT products | 95.9 days<br>No significant differences among other BoNT products | 93.4 days<br>No significant differences among other BoNT products | |
| Retreatment interval | 12–16 weeks or longer, based on return of symptoms | 12–16 weeks or longer, based on return of symptoms | 12–16 weeks or longer, based on return of symptoms<br>Published range: 6–16 weeks | 12–16 weeks or longer, based on return of symptoms | |

(*continued*)

**TABLE 9.2 BoNT for Cervical Dystonia: Manufacturer's Recommended Dosage Range (Adults ≥18 Years of Age) (*continued*)**

| BoNT Preparation | OBTA (Botox®) | ABTA (Dysport®) | IBTA (Xeomin®) | RBTB (Myobloc®) | Notes |
|---|---|---|---|---|---|
| Dilution and resultant concentration | 100-unit vial with 1-mL PFNS<br>100 units/1 mL<br>10 units/0.1 mL | 300-unit vial with 0.6-mL PFNS<br>250 units/1 mL<br>25 units/0.1 mL | 50-unit vial with 0.5-mL PFNS<br>100 units/1 mL<br>10 units/0.1 mL | N/A, product is provided in solution, 5,000 units/1 mL<br>500 units/0.1 mL | All dilutions using PFNS for injection |
| | 100-unit vial with 2-mL PFNS<br>50 units/1 mL<br>5 units/0.1 mL | 500-unit vial with 1-mL PFNS<br>500 units/1 mL<br>50 units/0.1 mL | | | |
| | 200-unit vial with 2-mL PFNS<br>100 units/1 mL<br>10 units/0.1 mL | | 100-unit vial with 1-mL PFNS<br>100 units/1 mL<br>10 units/0.1 mL | | |
| | 200-unit vial with 4-mL PFNS<br>50 units/1 mL<br>5 units/0.1 mL | | | | |
| **AEs** | | | | | |
| Dysphagia | 3.4%–19% | 19.4%–26.8% | 13%–18% | 15.6%–25% | See manufacturer's full PI for a full list of AEs |
| Xerostomia | 0.8%–41% | 2.9%–36.7% | Incidence not reported in PI | 3.2%–90% | |

*Abbreviations:* ABTA, abobotulinumtoxinA; AE, adverse events; BoNT, botulinum neurotoxin; IBTA, incobotulinumtoxinA; OBTA, onabotulinumtoxinA; PFNS, preservative-free normal saline (0.9%); PI, prescribing information; RBTB, rimabotulinumtoxinB; SCM, sternocleidomastoid.

*Sources:* Refs. 34, 36, 38, 41, 44, 59, 85, 96, 133, 151, 172, 173, 195, 197, 198, 474–486.

**TABLE 9.3 BoNT for Cervical Dystonia: Published Dosage Range per Muscle (Adults ≥18 Years of Age)**

This table provides information on the published dosage range per muscle and maximum dose from clinical trials for the four FDA-approved BoNT products.

The dose per muscle and total dose per treatment session for toxin-naïve patients or patients with prior exposure to BoNT is determined by the severity of symptoms, size of the target muscle, response to prior injections, adverse events with prior injections, number of muscles to be injected, and medical comorbidities.

| BoNT Preparation | OBTA (Botox®) | ABTA (Dysport®) | IBTA (Xeomin®) | RBTB (Myobloc®) | Notes |
|---|---|---|---|---|---|
| Levator scapulae | 20–100 units* | Median: 105.3 units*<br>Range: 50–200 units* | 23–32 units* | 325–750 units* | |
| | 5–100 units** | 20–200 units** | 5–60 units** | 325–750 units** | |
| Longissimus capitis | Not reported* | Median: 150 units*<br>Range: 100–200 units* | 20–47.3 units mean dose* | 500–1,000 units* | |
| | Not reported** | 100–200 units | Not reported** | Not reported** | |
| | 20–50 units[1] | 100–200 units[1] | 20–50 units[1] | 250–500 units[1] | [1]First author's dosage range |
| Longus colli, longus capitis | Not reported* | Not reported* | Not reported* | Not reported* | |
| | 30–33 units[3] | 20–60 units[2] | Not reported** | Not reported** | [2]Flowers et al. (479)<br>[3]Herting et al. (482) |
| | 15–25 units[1] | 25–75 units[1] | 15–25 units[1] | 150–250 units[1] | [1]First author's dosage range |
| Obliquus capitis inferioris | Not reported* | Not reported* | Not reported* | Not reported* | |
| | Not reported** | Not reported** | Toxin-naïve patients: 12 units mean dosage**<br>All patients: 23 units mean dosage** | Not reported** | |

*(continued)*

**TABLE 9.3 BoNT for Cervical Dystonia: Published Dosage Range per Muscle (Adults ≥18 Years of Age) (*continued*)**

| BoNT Preparation | OBTA (Botox®) | ABTA (Dysport®) | IBTA (Xeomin®) | RBTB (Myobloc®) | Notes |
|---|---|---|---|---|---|
| Obliquus capitis inferioris (*continued*) | 10–25 units[1] | 25–60 units[1] | 10–25 units[1] | 100–150 units[1] | [1]First author's dosage range |
| Scalenes, middle/anterior | 15–50 units, divided* | Median: 115.5 units*<br>Range: 50–300 units* | Median: 20 units*<br>75th percentile: 25 units* | 150–250 units, divided* | |
| | 5–25 units/muscle** | 20–300 units/muscle** | Toxin-naïve patients: 10 units/muscle mean dose**<br>All patients: 17 units/muscle mean dose**<br>Dosage range: 5–25 units/muscle** | 150–500 units** | |
| Semispinalis capitis | 30–100 units* | Median: 131 units*<br>Range: 50–250 units* | Range: 20–100 units* | 500–1,800 units* | |
| | 20–100 units** | 80–400 units** | Toxin-naïve patients: 18 units mean dosage**<br>All patients: 33 units mean dosage** | 500–2,500 units** | |
| Splenius capitis | 30–100 units* | Median: 131.6 units*<br>Range: 50–300 units* | Median: 48 units*<br>75th percentile: 63 units* | 500–1,250 units* | |
| | 10–100 units** | 40–450 units** | Range: 10–100 units<br>Toxin-naïve patients: 34.4 units mean dosage<br>All patients: 43.6 units mean dosage | 500–1,500 units** | |
| Splenius cervicis | 20–60 units* | Not reported separately | Not reported separately by manufacturer | Not reported separately* | |

(*continued*)

**TABLE 9.3 BoNT for Cervical Dystonia: Published Dosage Range per Muscle (Adults ≥18 Years of Age) (*continued*)**

| BoNT Preparation | OBTA (Botox®) | ABTA (Dysport®) | IBTA (Xeomin®) | RBTB (Myobloc®) | Notes |
|---|---|---|---|---|---|
| Splenius cervicis (*continued*) | 20–100 units, divided between splenius capitis and cervicis** | 40–400 units, divided between splenius capitis and cervicis** | Toxin-naïve patients: 14.5 units mean dosage**<br>All patients: 28.9 units mean dosage**<br>Range: 10–100 units** | 500–2,500 units, divided between splenius capitis and cervicis** | |
| SCM | 15–100 units*,[4] | Median: 125 units*<br>Range: 50–350 units* | Median: 25 units*<br>75th percentile: 35 units*<br>Range: 5–50 units* | 250–1,500 units | [4]Limiting dose in SCM to <100 units may decrease the incidence of dysphagia |
| | 5–150 units**,[4] | 20–300 units**<br>Note: Unilateral dose >150 units associated with increased incidence of dysphagia | Toxin-naïve patients: 37.2 units mean dosage**<br>All patients: 47.3 units mean dosage** | 250–1,500 units** | |
| Trapezius | 20–100 units* | Median: 150 units*<br>Range: 50–350 units* | Median: 25 units*<br>75th percentile: 25 units* | 250–1,750 units | |
| Trapezius, upper | 5–50 units** | 20–300 units** | Toxin-naïve patients: 45 units mean dosage**<br>All patients: 47.3 units mean dosage**<br>Range: 5–50 units** | 250–2,500 units** | |

*Reported dosage in manufacturer's prescribing information.

**Published dosage range from published studies.

*Abbreviations:* ABTA, abobotulinumtoxinA; AE, adverse events; BoNT, botulinum neurotoxin; FDA, Food and Drug Administration; IBTA, incobotulinumtoxinA; OBTA, onabotulinumtoxinA; RBTB, rimabotulinumtoxinB; SCM, sternocleidomastoid.

*Sources:* Refs. 34, 36, 38, 41, 44, 59, 85, 96, 133, 151, 172, 173, 195, 197, 198, 474–486.

# Illustrations for Cervical Dystonia—Chapter 9

*FIGURE 1* *Cervical muscles, anterolateral view, superficial and intermediate muscle layers.*

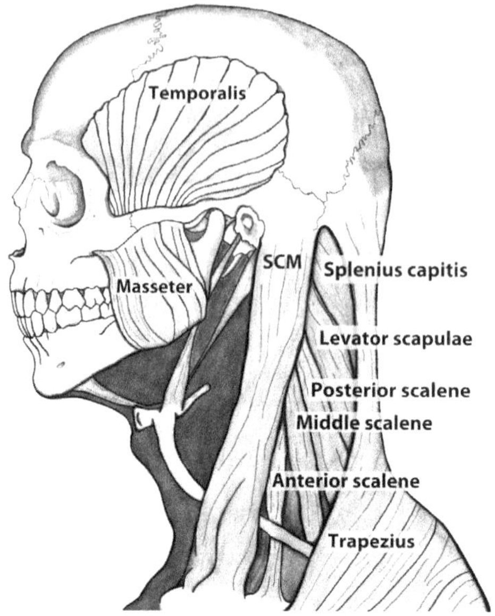


*FIGURE 2* *Cervical muscles, anterior view, intermediate and deep muscle layers.*

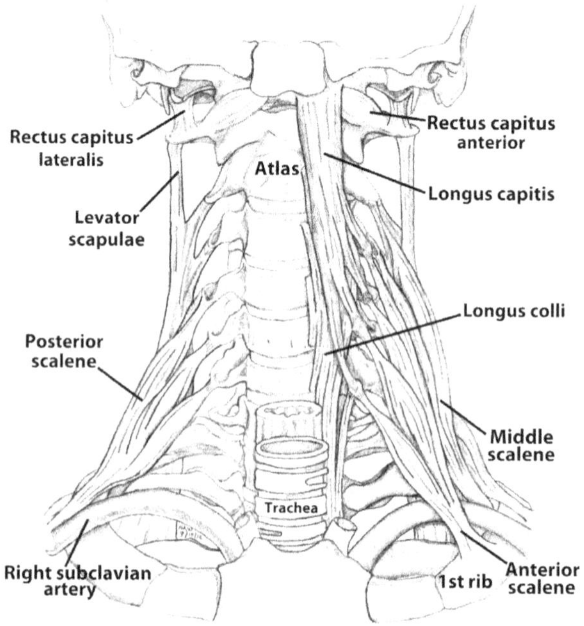

*FIGURE 3* Cervical muscles, posterior view, intermediate and deep muscle layers.

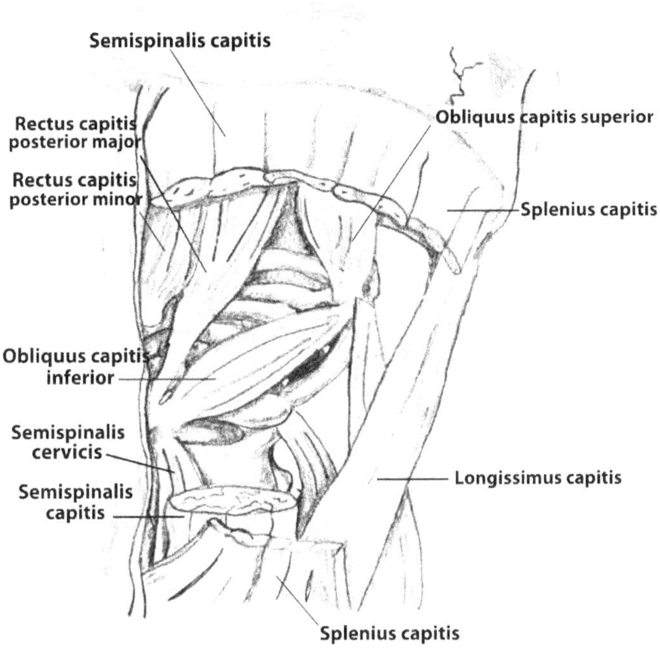

# *Upper Limb, Lower Limb, and Trunk Dystonia*

# 10

# Botulinum Neurotoxin for the Treatment of Idiopathic Primary Focal Limb Dystonia

Katharine E. Alter, MD
David Simpson, MD, FAAN
Elie Elovic, MD

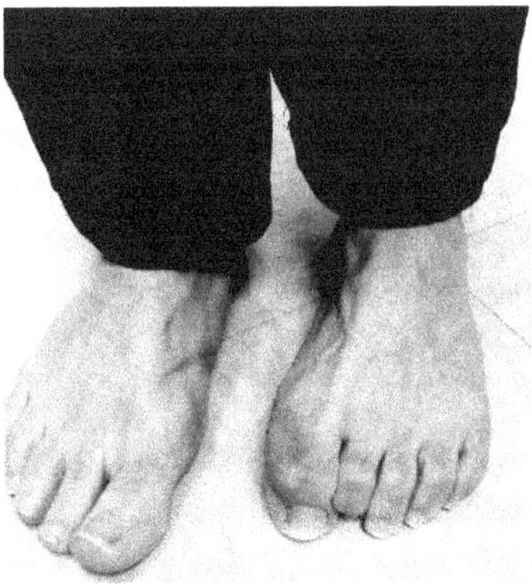

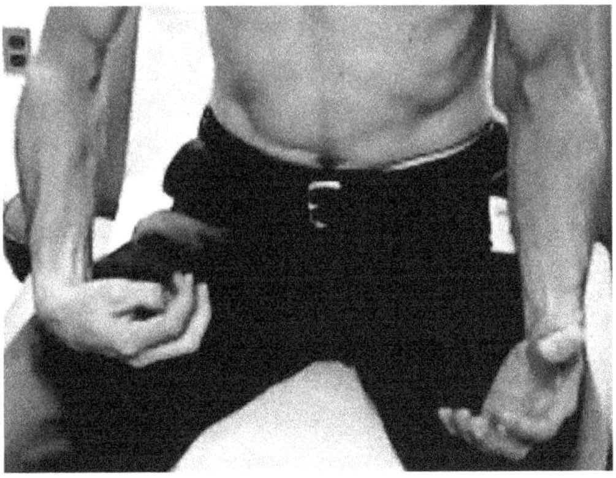

## Condition

Dystonia is a movement disorder characterized by involuntary movements or repetitive postures. These postures and movements are often, but not always, twisting in nature, may be hyperkinetic or hypokinetic, and may be accompanied by a dystonic tremor. Dystonia is classified using several subtypes based on patterns or regions of the body involved. Subtypes include focal dystonia, where a limited portion of the limb is affected; segmental dystonia, where the entire limb is affected; or generalized dystonia (176, 177). Botulinum neurotoxin (BoNT) therapy may be useful in treating any form of symptomatic dystonia. This chapter focuses on the treatment of idiopathic primary focal limb dystonia (IPFLD), one form of idiopathic focal dystonia. Other types of primary idiopathic focal dystonia including blepharospasm, hemifacial spasm, cervical, oromandibular, cervical, and trunk dystonia are covered elsewhere in this text.

Although patients with IPFLD may present with dystonia involving the upper or lower limbs, the upper limbs are much more commonly affected (178, 179). Focal dystonia involving the lower limb is rare, and additional care should be taken during the workup of these patients to rule out other potential causes for the patients' symptoms, including a variety of neurological conditions (spasticity, stiff person syndrome, Parkinson disease, and others) (178, 180).

Focal dystonia is often task specific, such as that seen in patients with writer's cramp, musician's cramp, and task-specific lower limb disorders including "runner's dystonia" (177, 178). Task specificity implies that the involuntary movement is induced by performing a specific task, such as holding a pen or playing the piano, but not by other tasks involving the same muscle or muscle groups, for example, holding a toothbrush or typing. Task specificity may be lost over time, and involuntary movements may generalize or spread to other muscles or may be provoked by other tasks. Examples include writer's cramp, where dystonia initially involves only thumb muscles, but eventually spreads to affect the finger, wrist, or forearm muscles. Another example of the loss of task specificity is in patients with lower limb dystonia where symptoms are initially present only with running but eventually may be present with walking (177, 179, 180). IPFLD, like other forms of idiopathic focal dystonia, typically begins in middle age and affects both males and females. Unlike most other forms of idiopathic primary dystonia (e.g., blepharospasm and cervical dystonia), IPFLD is more common in men than in women (157). The prevalence of primary dystonia varies somewhat by country/ethnicity and increases with age. In the general population, the prevalence of IPFLD is estimated to be 10 to 16.4/100,000 with an overall prevalence of primary focal dystonia (PFD) estimated to be 15.6/100,000. Of the PFDs, cervical dystonia is the most common with a reported prevalence of 4.98/100,000. The reported prevalence of primary focal limb dystonia (PFLD) is 1.24/100,000 and that of writer's cramp is 1.65/100,000 (181).

### *Clinical/Functional Impact*

The involuntary movements and postures associated with IPFLD interfere with activities of daily living (ADLs), occupational tasks, writing, walking, running, sports, avocational interests, and with quality of life (182). As noted, the dystonic postures and involuntary movements are frequently task specific; examples include focal hand dystonia (writer's cramp, musician's cramp, and others) or patients with involuntary movements when dancing or running (157, 183, 184). As a form of compensation or an attempt to improve function, patients often adapt their pen/pencil grip; modify techniques when writing or typing; use their nondominant hand; or change their gait. Involuntary movements and compensations may lead to other postural problems, abnormal joint biomechanics, pain, or discomfort. The dystonic movements or postures may severely limit the patient's function including ADLs, hand use, and/or mobility.

### *Pattern of Involvement*

While the presenting posture or abnormal movements vary among patients, there are some commonalities.

## *Upper Limb IPFLD*

In IPFLD involving the upper limbs, forearm and hand muscles are affected more often than proximal muscles (185, 186). When proximal muscles are involved, a flexed elbow pattern is more common than extension. Shoulder elevation often accompanies elbow flexion. In the forearm, pronation and flexion of the wrist are more common than extension. Finger flexion is also more common than extension. In patients presenting with musician's cramp (focal, task-specific hand dystonia), different patterns of involvement are noted with different instruments. In pianists, flexion of the fourth and fifth fingers is common; in guitarists, flexion of the third finger is common; and in clarinet players extension of the third finger is common (187). Although the aforementioned patterns are more common, virtually any muscle and/or groups of muscles may be involved in an individual patient. Because each patient may present with a unique pattern, the patient should be observed performing the task or function that provokes the abnormal movement (188). In a 10-year review of BoNT therapy for focal hand dystonia, Lungu et al. reported that the average number of muscles treated in musicians was 1.7 (± 0.08) and in nonmusicians was 3.1 (± 0.08) (189).

## *Lower Limb IPFLD*

As with upper limb IPFLD, the abnormal movement patterns involving the lower limb are quite variable and distal muscles are affected more commonly than proximal muscles. At the ankle, plantar flexion, foot inversion, and toe flexion are more common than dorsiflexion, eversion, and toe extension. At the knee, involuntary knee flexion and/or extension patterns are common (179). Involvement of hip girdle muscles (flexion, extension, and adduction) is less common, but is occasionally seen.

## *Evaluation*

The evaluation of a patient presenting with IPFLD starts with a detailed history, including history of the present problem, and medical and family history, inquiring specifically about involuntary movements or neurological problems in other family members. The patient should be questioned about onset/duration of his or her involuntary movements or symptoms, pattern of involvement, factors that worsen or improve the involuntary movements, as well as practice history for musicians. The patient should also be asked if the involuntary movements have spread or generalized to affect other areas or tasks and for the presence of a sensory trick (*geste antagoniste*). A detailed physical examination is imperative. Physical examination should include detailed neurological and musculoskeletal examinations. The patient should be observed while performing tasks that provoke the symptoms (writing, playing an instrument, walking, running, etc.). All patients with focal hand dystonia should undergo a thorough examination to rule out a peripheral neuropathy or entrapment neuropathy (188). Patients with a neuropathy will present with weakness and/or sensory loss that is not typical for a patient with IPFLD. Imaging and/or metabolic workup should be considered, particularly in patients with atypical presentation or symptoms, and in all who present with IPFLD involving the lower limb(s), which is exceedingly rare.

### *Treatment*

Although there are other treatment options for IPFLD (rehabilitation therapies, splinting, oral medications, BoNT injections, and surgery), BoNT is the treatment of choice for the vast majority of patients. Many patients may benefit from physical or occupational therapy, adaptive aids, splinting, or orthotic devices. Not all therapists are familiar with the evaluation or treatment of dystonia and physicians should establish a therapist's level of expertise prior to referring patients.

### *Oral Medications*

Side effects of oral medications are fairly common and these agents (baclofen, L-dopa, tetrabenazine, trihexyphenidyl, benzodiazepines, and others) are generally reserved for patients who fail BoNT therapy (190, 191).

### *Other Interventions*

Transcranial magnetic stimulation has also been used for the treatment of focal dystonia (192). Surgical interventions, such as intrathecal or intraventricular baclofen and/or deep brain stimulation, may also be considered for patients who fail medical therapy but these interventions are rarely recommended (176, 191, 193).

### *BoNT Injections*

BoNT is widely accepted as the treatment of choice and standard of care for the treatment of IPFLD, including writer's cramp, musician's cramp, and other occupational or focal limb dystonia (157, 188, 190, 194, 195). Many patients report significant symptomatic and functional benefits from BoNT injections and the majority continue the treatment, often for many years (189, 196). The most commonly reported reason for discontinuing the treatment is insufficient benefit (189, 196). Evaluation of benefit is made difficult by the lack of validated, standardized scales for the various forms of IPFLD (186, 196).

## Regulatory Approval Status for the Treatment of IPFLD

Although none of the currently approved BoNT products are approved by the Food and Drug Administration (FDA) or international regulatory authorities for the treatment of IPFLD, BoNT therapy is considered the treatment of choice by most expert clinicians.

### *Level of Evidence*

In their review of evidence for IPFLD, Hallett et al. (2003) concluded that the current level of evidence supports a Level B (Probably effective, ineffective or harmful for the given condition in the specified population (197). Level B requires one Class II study or two consistent Class II studies) recommendation for onabotulinumtoxinA (OBTA) and abobotulinumtoxinA (ABTA) for the treatment of IPFLD (Levels of Evidence, see [138]). Due to lack of evidence, the same authors reported Level U (Unproven, data inadequate or conflicting; given current knowledge, treatment is unproven) evidence for incobotulinumtoxinA (IBTA) and rimabotulinumtoxinB (RBTB) for the treatment of IPFLD. Simpson et al. (2008) reviewed the evidence for BoNT for the treatment of movement disorders including focal dystonia and concluded that there was Level B evidence for the treatment of focal hand dystonia (198).

### *Injection Pattern and Technique*

Prior to injection, patients should be observed performing the task or function, such as writing, typing, playing an instrument, or running/walking, that provokes their symptoms. This close observation is the key to establishing which muscles are responsible for dystonic movements and which may be compensatory. For a neurotoxin-naïve patient, in the first treatment session, injection of a few key muscles may be considered (188). This may help establish whether a few muscles are triggering other muscles and/or contracting as a form of compensation for the dystonia.

Muscles and muscle fascicles are localized using surface anatomy, anatomic reference guides, palpation, and with active and passive ranges of motion. When treating patients with IPFLD, in which muscle involvement is very localized, precise targeting of a muscle and/or muscle fascicle is required. Many expert clinicians recommend the use of an adjunctive localization technique in addition to the aforementioned techniques. Supplementary techniques include electromyography (EMG), electrical stimulation (e-stim), and B-mode ultrasound (US). Each of these techniques has advantages and disadvantages (90) (see Chapter 4). However, there is limited evidence related to the use of supplementary targeting techniques and whether these techniques improve outcome or reduce adverse events. Evidence is also limited regarding the superiority or inferiority of one technique over another. In their review, Hallett et al. (2013) reported evidence from two Class II studies (138), one of which supported enhanced accuracy of needle placement using EMG (105, 106, 197, 198). While many, if not most, clinicians recommend a supplementary localization technique when performing BoNT injections, additional studies are needed to establish which technique(s) is superior (92). Charles and Gill reported potential benefits of more accurate localization, including reduction in the required effective dose of BoNT and reduced antibody formation (187). Additional studies are required to determine the most effective, most accurate localization technique for BoNT injections, including those for IPFLD.

### *Retreatment Interval*

Most clinicians recommend a minimum treatment interval of 12 weeks between injections. The reinjection interval should be determined by the return of symptoms. In a 10-year follow-up of patients with focal hand dystonia, Lungu et al. reported that musicians tended to wait longer between treatment sessions than patients with focal hand dystonia due to other causes (189). The same authors reported a trend toward greater efficacy with shorter injection intervals. While the practice of booster dosing has been reported, at the time of publication of this text this practice is discouraged by many clinicians and researchers (199). Clinical research into the safety of booster dosing is ongoing.

## *Toxin Dilution*

When precise dosing with a small number of units is required for small muscles, a higher dilution of BoNT is required. There is limited data from clinical trials related to dilution of BoNT for IPFLD and additional studies are required to determine the optimal dilution of the various BoNT products for this and other conditions.

OBTA

For a dosage of higher than 5 units per muscle or fascicle, most clinicians recommend using a dilution of 100 units with 1 mL of preservative-free normal (0.9%) saline (PFNS) (concentration: 100 units/mL, 10 units/0.1 mL). When a dosage of less than 5 units per muscle or muscle fascicle is required, clinicians may consider a higher dilution, for example, 100 units diluted with 2-mL PFNS (concentration: 50 units/mL, 5 units/0.1 mL).

ABTA

For ABTA, the published dilution from clinical trials is 20 units/0.1 mL. To achieve this dilution, 300 units of ABTA are diluted in 1.5-mL PFNS for a concentration of 200 units/mL (20 unit/0.1 mL). A 500-unit vial is required if the treatment dosage is of 500 or higher units. To achieve a dilution of 200 units/mL (20 units/0.1 mL), a 500-unit vial is reconstituted with 2.5-mL PFNS.

IBTA

A 50-unit vial is used when the total treatment dosage is less than 50 units, and a 100-unit vial is required for a dosage of 50 or higher units. For a dosage per muscle or muscle fascicle of less than 5 units, most clinicians recommend using a concentration of 100 units/mL (10 units/0.1 mL). To achieve this dilution, a 50-unit vial is reconstituted with 0.5-mL PFNS or a 100-unit vial is reconstituted with 1-mL PFNS (concentration: 100 units/mL, 10 units/0.1 mL). When the recommended treatment dosage is less than 5 units per muscle or muscle fascicle, clinicians may consider a higher dilution, for example, reconstituting a 50-unit vial with 1-mL PFNS or a 100-unit vial of IBTA with 2-mL PFNS. This results in a concentration of 50 units/mL or 5 units/0.1 mL.

RBTB

RBTB is supplied in solution (5,000 units/mL), does not require reconstitution, and is available in 2,500-, 5,000-, or 10,000-unit vials. If desired, PFNS can be added to the vial to further dilute the product. For example, 0.5-mL or 1.5 mL PFNS can be added to a 2,500-unit vial for dilutions of 2,500 units/mL or 250 units/0.1mL and 1,250 units/mL or 125 units/0.1mL, respectively. Alternately, a 5,000-unit vial can be further diluted with 1 mL or 3 mL PFNS, for resulting dilutions of 2,500 units/mL (250 units/0.1mL) or 1,250 units/mL (125 units/0.1/mL).

See Table 10.1 for BoNT dosage.

# TABLE 10.1 BoNT for Focal Hand Dystonia; Injection Patterns (Adults ≥18 Years of Age)

| BoNT Preparation | OBTA (Botox®) | ABTA (Dysport®) | | IBTA (Xeomin®) | RBTB (Myobloc®) | Notes |
|---|---|---|---|---|---|---|
| U.S. FDA approval | Currently not FDA approved | Currently not FDA approved | | Currently not FDA approved | Currently not FDA approved | |
| Approvals, other countries | Currently not an approved indication | Currently not an approved indication | | Currently not an approved indication | Currently not an approved indication | |
| **Published Dosage Range: Adults (≥18 Years of Age)** | | | | | | |
| **Writer's Cramp** | | | | | | |
| Average number of muscles injected | 3.1 | | | No published information on dose/dosage range | No published information on dose/dosage range | (189) |
| Mean dose, first treatment session | 24.9 units | 82 units (range: 20–178 units) | | | | |
| Mean dose, repeat treatment session | 49.9 units | 142 units (range: 0–280 units) | | | | |
| Dosage range | 2.5–120 units | 30–240 units | | | | |
| **Musician's Cramp** | | | | | | |
| Average number of muscles injected | 1.7 | | | | | (189) |
| Mean dose (dose range): | | First Tx (units) | Repeat Tx (units) | | | (196) |
| Shoulder muscles | | 55 (40–70) | 55 (40–70) | | | |
| Forearm flexors | | 56 (10–60) | 47.4 (5–250) | | | |
| Forearm extensors | | 34.6 (4–100) | 31.5 (4–100) | | | |
| Hand | | 22.4 (4–100) | 17.7 (1.5–100) | | | |
| Mean total dosage (range) | | 126.9 (5–420) | 112.2 (3–1,000) | | | |

*Abbreviation*: Tx, treatment.

## General Principles

When treating patients with IPFLD:

- None of the available BoNT products is approved by regulatory agencies for the treatment of IPFLD and there are no published manufacturer data on the optimal starting dose per muscle or muscle fascicle or maximum dose when treating patients with IPFLD.
- There are a limited number of studies published on the topic of BoNT dosage as a class and for individual BoNT products. Therefore, the optimal starting dose, minimal effective dose, and maximum dose for individual BoNT products are unknown.
- The optimal starting, effective, and maximum dose of a given BoNT product when treating patients with IPFLD are likely patient-specific. This is due to variation in the pattern of dystonic movements, patient/muscle size, number of muscles/muscle fascicles involved, and severity of the problem.
- Because of individual patient differences, recommendations for a specific starting and/or maximum dose must be interpreted with caution. Because of patient differences, a starting/maximum dose range may be more appropriate.
- When treating a neurotoxin-naïve patient for IPFLD, most expert clinicians recommend starting with a lower dose and "underdosing" in most patients, particularly musicians or others presenting with focal hand dystonia.
- The dose per muscle and the total dose of BoNT are much lower than those typically used when treating patients with generalized or segmental dystonia or patients with spasticity or secondary dystonia associated with upper motor neuron syndromes.
- A lower dose per muscle and per fascicle is typically used when treating upper limb muscles compared with the dose used in lower limb muscles. This dosing difference may be due to the larger size of lower limb muscles or because the precise movements and control required for hand movements require exquisite accuracy in dosing.
- A lower dose per muscle and per fascicle is reported when treating patients with musician's cramp/dystonia than those with writer's cramp.

### *OnabotulinumtoxinA (OBTA, Botox)*

The published dose range of OBTA for IPFLD is 2.5 to 120 units (14, 106, 189, 200–202). For patients presenting with focal hand dystonia, higher doses are generally reported in writer's cramp than in musician's cramp. For more detailed dosing information, see the dosage tables in this chapter.

### *AbobotulinumtoxinA (ABTA, Dysport)*

The published dose range for the treatment of writer's cramp is 20 to 280 units (186, 203). Kruisdijk et al. reported a mean starting dose of 82 units and a mean dose of

142 units at the second treatment session (186). For more detailed dosing information, see the dosage tables in this chapter.

### *IncobotulinumtoxinA (IBTA, Xeomin)*

There are no published studies on dose or dose range for IBTA for the treatment of IPFLD. For more detailed dosing information, see the dosage tables in this chapter.

### *RimabotulinumtoxinB (RBTB, Myobloc/NeuroBloc)*

There are no published studies on dose or dose range for RBTB for the treatment of IPFLD. For more detailed dosing information, see the dosage tables in this chapter.

### *Clinical Effect*

The onset and duration of action of OBTA and IBTA, serotype A BoNTs are similar with the reported onset of effect at 3 to 7 days, peak effect at 4 to 6 weeks, and duration of effect approximately 12 weeks or 3 months for IBTA and 3 to 6 months for OBTA. The onset of action of ABTA is reported to be evident within 2 weeks of injection, with peak effect at 4 to 8 weeks, and duration of efficacy 10 to 16 weeks (194).

### *Adverse Events/Side Effects*

The most common side effects or adverse events following BoNT injections for IPFLD are pain at injection site and weakness in the target muscle. Additional risks include xerostomia, dysphagia, and/or the risks listed in the manufacturer's full prescribing information and the FDA-mandated boxed warning for all FDA-approved BoNT products.

**TABLE 10.2 BoNT for Focal Dystonia, Upper Limb Muscles: Shoulder/Elbow (Adults ≥18 Years of Age)**

| BoNT Preparation | OBTA (Botox®) | ABTA (Dysport®) | IBTA (Xeomin®) | RBTB (Myobloc®) | Notes |
|---|---|---|---|---|---|
| USA FDA approval | Currently not FDA approved | Currently not FDA approved | Currently not FDA approved | Currently not FDA approved | |
| UK MHRA | Currently not an approved indication | Currently not an approved indication | Currently not an approved indication | Currently not an approved indication | |
| **Published Dosage Range, Dilution** | | | | | |
| **Shoulder Girdle Muscles** | | | | | |
| Deltoid:<br>Starting dosage<br>Published dosage range<br>Injection sites | <br>5–50 units<br>5–200 units<br>1–3 | <br>40–100 units<br><br>1–2 | <br>5–50 units<br><br>1–2 | <br>150–1,000 units[a]<br><br>1–2 | [a]No published information on dosage. These ranges represent the dosage ranges used by the first author.<br>[b]Published dosage range includes treatment of spasticity and focal dystonia. Consider lower dosage range for focal dystonia. |
| Latissimus dorsi:<br>Dosage range<br>Injection sites | <br>20–100 units<br>1–3 | <br>80–400 units<br>1–3 | <br>20–100 units<br>1–3 | <br>150–1,000 units[a]<br>1–3 | |
| Infraspinatus:<br>Starting dosage<br>Dosage range<br>Injection sites | <br>5–40 units<br>5–100 units<br>1–3 | <br>20–80 units<br>20–150 units<br>1–3 | <br>5–20 units<br><br>1–3 | <br>1,000–3,000 units[b]<br><br>1–3 | |
| Pectoralis major:<br>Starting dosage<br>Dosage range<br>Injection sites | <br>10–40 units<br>10–200 units<br>1–2 | <br>40–100 units<br><br>1–2 | <br>10–40 units<br><br>1–2 | <br>150–1,000 units[a]<br><br>1–2 | |
| Pectoralis minor:<br>Dosage range<br>Injection sites | <br>10–40 units<br>1–2 | <br>40–100 units<br>1–2 | <br>10–40 units<br>1–2 | <br>150–1,000 units[a]<br>1–2 | |

*(continued)*

**TABLE 10.2 BoNT for Focal Dystonia, Upper Limb Muscles: Shoulder/Elbow (Adults ≥18 Years of Age) (*continued*)**

| BoNT Preparation | OBTA (Botox®) | ABTA (Dysport®) | IBTA (Xeomin®) | RBTB (Myobloc®) | Notes |
|---|---|---|---|---|---|
| Rhomboids, major/minor: | | | | | |
| Dosage range | 25–20 units | 20–80 units | 5–20 units | 150–500 units[a] | |
| Injection sites | 1 | 1 | 1 | 1 | |
| Serratus anterior: | | | | | |
| Dosage range | 5–10 units | 20–80 units | 5–10 units | 100–500 units[a] | |
| Injection sites | 1–6 | 1–6 | 1–6 | 1–6 | |
| Subscapularis: | | | | | |
| Dosage range | 25–100 units | 50–200 units[a] | 25–100 units[a] | 1,000–3,000 units[b] | |
| Injection sites | 1–3 | 1–3 | 1–3 | 1–3 | |
| Supraspinatus: | | | | | |
| Dosage range | 5–20 units | 20–80 units | 5–20 units | 1,000–3,000 units[b] | |
| Injection sites | 1–2 | 1–2 | 1–2 | 1–2 | |
| Teres major: | | | | | |
| Dosage range | 5–100 units | 20–150 units | 5–40 units | 1,000–3,000 units | |
| Injection sites | 1–2 | 1–2 | 1–2 | 1–2 | |
| Teres minor: | | | | | |
| Dosage range | 5–100 units | 20–80 units | 5–40 units | 1,000–3,000 units[b] | |
| Injection sites | 1–2 | 1–2 | 1–2 | 1–2 | |
| Trapezius: | | | | | |
| Starting dose | 5–20 units | 20–80 units | 5–20 units | 50–1,000 units | |
| Published dosage range | 40–100 units | — | — | — | |
| Injection sites | 2–4 | 2–4 | 2–4 | 2–4 | |

(*continued*)

**TABLE 10.2 BoNT for Focal Dystonia, Upper Limb Muscles: Shoulder/Elbow (Adults ≥18 Years of Age) (*continued*)**

| BoNT Preparation | OBTA (Botox®) | ABTA (Dysport®) | IBTA (Xeomin®) | RBTB (Myobloc®) | Notes |
|---|---|---|---|---|---|
| **Elbow Muscles** | | | | | |
| Biceps brachii:<br>Starting dose<br>Dosage range<br>Injection sites | <br>20–40 units<br>20–150 units<br>2–4 | <br>60–100 units<br>60–400 units<br>2–4 | <br>20–40 units<br>20–100 units<br>2–4 | <br>—<br>1,000–3,000 units[a]<br>2–4 | [a]Published dosage range includes treatment of spasticity and focal dystonia. Consider lower dosage range for focal dystonia.<br>[b]No published information on dosage. These ranges represent the dosage ranges used by the first author. |
| Brachialis:<br>Starting dose<br>Dosage range<br>Injection sites | <br>10–30 units<br>20–60 units<br>1–2 | <br>50–75 units<br>50–200 units<br>1–2 | <br>10–30 units<br>20–60 units<br>1–2 | <br>100–1,000 units[b]<br>—<br>1–2 | |
| Brachioradialis:<br>Starting dose<br>Dosage range<br>Injection sites | <br>15–40 units<br>15–100 units<br>1–3 | <br><br><br>1–3 | <br>20–40 units<br>20–100 units<br>1–3 | <br>—<br>500–3,750 units[a]<br>1–3 | |
| Triceps brachii:<br>Starting dose<br>Dosage range<br>Injection sites | <br>25–50 units<br>25–120 units<br>2–3 | <br>75–100 units<br>75–500 units<br>2–3 | <br>—<br>20–120 units<br>2–3 | <br>—<br>500–5,000 units[a]<br>2–3 | |

(*continued*)

**TABLE 10.2 BoNT for Focal Dystonia, Upper Limb Muscles: Shoulder/Elbow (Adults ≥18 Years of Age) (*continued*)**

| BoNT Preparation | OBTA (Botox®) | ABTA (Dysport®) | IBTA (Xeomin®) | RBTB (Myobloc®) | Notes |
|---|---|---|---|---|---|
| Dilution Reconstitute with (PFNS) (0.9%) | 100-unit vial with 1-mL PFNS (concentration: 10 units/0.1 mL) or with 2-mL PFNS (5 units/0.1 mL) | 300-unit vial with 1.5-mL PFNS, or 500 units with 2.5-mL PFNS for a concentration of 20 units/0.1 mL | 50-unit vial with 0.5-mL PFNS (10 units/0.1 mL) or with 1 mL (5 units/0.1 mL)<br>100-unit vial with 1 mL (10 units/0.1 mL) or with 2 mL (5 units/0.1 mL) | Comes in solution 5,000 units/mL (no dilution required)[c] | [c]If desired, PFNS can be added for additional dilution. See Chapter 3. |
| Adverse events | Weakness, pain at injection site (see boxed warning for others) | Weakness, pain at injection site (see boxed warning for others) | Weakness, pain at injection site (see boxed warning for others) | Weakness, pain at injection site (see boxed warning for others) | |

*Abbreviations:* ABTA, abobotulinumtoxinA; IBTA, incobotulinumtoxinA; OBTA, onabotulinumtoxinA; PFNS, preservative-free normal saline (0.9%); RBTB, rimabotulinumtoxinB.

*Sources:* Refs. 185, 199, 487.

**TABLE 10.3 BoNT for Focal Dystonia, Upper Limb Muscles: Forearm/Wrist (Adults ≥18 Years of Age)**

| BoNT Preparation | OBTA (Botox®) | ABTA (Dysport®) | IBTA (Xeomin®) | RBTB (Myobloc®) | Notes |
|---|---|---|---|---|---|
| U.S. FDA approval | Currently not FDA approved | Currently not FDA approved | Currently not FDA approved | Currently not FDA approved | |
| UK MHRA | Currently not an approved indication | Currently not an approved indication | Currently not an approved indication | Currently not an approved indication | |
| **Published Dosage Range/Dilution: Adults (≥18 Years of Age)** | | | | | |
| **Forearm/Wrist Muscles** | | | | | |
| AbP longus:<br>Starting dosage<br>Dosage range<br>Injection sites | <br>2.5–5 units<br>2.5–20 units<br>1 | <br>10–20 units<br>20–80 units<br>1 | <br>2.5–5 units<br>5–20 units<br>1 | <br>50–30 units[a]<br>— | [a]No published information on dosage. These ranges represent the dosage ranges used by the first author.<br>[b]Published dose range includes treatment of spasticity and focal dystonia. Consider lower dose ranges for focal dystonia. |
| FDS:<br>Dosage<br>Total dosage<br>Injection sites | <br>2.5–10 units/fascicle<br>2.5–10 units/fascicle<br>1–4 | <br>40–60 units/fascicle<br>60–200 units<br>1–4 | <br>2.5–10 units/fascicle<br>20–60 units<br>1–4 | <br>75–150 units/fascicle<br>75–1,000 units[b]<br>1–4 | |
| FPL:<br>Starting dosage<br>Dosage range<br>Injection sites | <br>2.5–5 units<br>2.5–70 units<br>1 | <br>20–40 units<br>20–80 units<br>1 | <br>2.5–5 units<br>2.5–20 units<br>1 | <br>75–150 units<br>75–1,000 units[b]<br>1 | |
| Palmaris longus:<br>Starting dosage<br>Dosage range<br>Injection sites | <br>5–20 units<br>5–60 units<br>1–2 | <br>20–40 units<br>20–60 units<br>1–2 | <br>5–20 units<br>5–60 units<br>1–2 | <br>100–500 units[a]<br>— | |

*(continued)*

**TABLE 10.3 BoNT for Focal Dystonia, Upper Limb Muscles: Forearm/Wrist (Adults ≥18 Years of Age) (*continued*)**

| BoNT Preparation | OBTA (Botox®) | ABTA (Dysport®) | IBTA (Xeomin®) | RBTB (Myobloc®) | Notes |
|---|---|---|---|---|---|
| Pronator teres:<br>Starting dosage<br>Dosage range<br>Injection sites | <br>10–15 units<br>10–70 units<br>1–2 | <br>40 units<br>40–100 units<br>1–2 | <br>10–15 units<br>10–30 units<br>1–2 | <br>150–500[a]<br>150–2,500[b]<br>1–2 | |
| Pronator quadratus:<br>Starting dosage<br>Dosage range<br>Injection sites | <br>5–10 units<br>5–30 units<br>1–2 | <br>20–40 units<br>20–80 units<br>1–2 | <br>10–15 units<br>5–20 units<br>1–2 | <br>100–250 units<br>150–2,500 units[b]<br>1–2 | |
| Supinator:<br>Starting dosage<br>Dosage range<br>Injection sites | <br>5–10 units<br>5–60 units<br>1–2 | <br>10–50 units<br>20–100 units<br>1–2 | <br>5–10 units<br>5–30 units<br>1–2 | <br>50–300 units[b]<br>—<br>1–2 | |
| Dilution | 100-unit vial with 1-mL PFNS (10 units/0.1 mL) or with 2-mL PFNS (5 units/0.1 mL) | 300-unit vial with 1.5-mL PFNS or 500 units with 2.5-mL PFNS for a concentration of 20 units/0.1 mL | 50-unit vial with 0.5-mL PFNS (concentration: 10 units/0.1 mL) or with 1-mL PFNS (5 units/0.1 mL)<br>100-unit vial with 1-mL PFNS (concentration: 10 units/0.1 mL) or with 2-mL PFNS (5 units/0.1 mL) | Comes in solution 5,000 units/mL (no dilution required)[c] | [c]If desired, PFNS can be added for additional dilution. See Chapter 3. |
| Adverse events | Weakness, pain at injection site (see boxed warning for others) | | Weakness, pain at injection site (see boxed warning for others) | Weakness, pain at injection site (see boxed warning for others) | |

*Abbreviations:* AbP, abductor pollicis; ABTA, abobotulinumtoxinA; IBTA, incobotulinumtoxinA; FDS, flexor digitorum superficialis; FPL, flexor pollicis longus; OBTA, onabotulinumtoxinA; PFNS, preservative-free normal saline (0.9%); RBTB, rimabotulinumtoxinB.

*Sources:* Refs. 14, 96, 185–187, 189, 196, 199, 200, 201, 203.

**TABLE 10.4 BoNT for Focal Dystonia, Upper Limb: Intrinsic Hand Muscles (Adults ≥18 Years of Age)**

| BoNT Preparation | OBTA (Botox®) | ABTA (Dysport®) | IBTA (Xeomin®) | RBTB (Myobloc®) | Notes |
|---|---|---|---|---|---|
| U.S. FDA approval | Currently not FDA approved | Currently not FDA approved | Currently not FDA approved | Currently not FDA approved | |
| UK MHRA | Currently not an approved indication | Currently not an approved indication | Currently not an approved indication | Currently not an approved indication | |
| **Published Dosage Range: Adults (≥18 Years of Age)** | | | | | |
| AbPB, AbDM, AdPB:<br>Starting dosage<br>Dosage range<br>Injection sites | <br><br>2.5 units<br>2.5–10 units<br>1 | <br><br>10–20 units<br>10–40 units<br>1 | <br><br>2.5 units<br>2.5–10 units<br>1 | <br><br>20–50 units[a]<br><br>1 | [a]No published information on dosage. These ranges represent the dosage ranges used by the first author. |
| Interossei (dorsal and palmar):<br>Dosage<br>Dosage range | <br><br>2.5–5 units/fascicle<br>10–50 units | <br><br>10–20 units/fascicle<br>— | <br><br>2.5–5 units/fascicle<br>— | <br><br>10–50 units/fascicle<br>— | |
| FPB:<br>Starting dosage | <br>1.25–5 units | <br>10–20 units | <br>1.2–5 units | <br>25–50 units | |
| Lumbricals:<br>Dosage<br>Injection sites | <br>2.5–5 units/fascicle<br>One per fascicle | <br>10–20 units/fascicle<br>One per fascicle | <br>2.5–5 units/fascicle<br>One per fascicle | <br>10–50 units/fascicle<br>One per fascicle | |
| ODM:<br>Dosage range<br>Injection sites | <br>2.5–5 units<br>1 | <br>10–20 units<br>1 | <br>2.5–5 units<br>1 | <br>20–50 units[a]<br>1 | |

*(continued)*

**TABLE 10.4 BoNT for Focal Dystonia, Upper Limb: Intrinsic Hand Muscles (Adults ≥18 Years of Age) (*continued*)**

| BoNT Preparation | OBTA (Botox®) | ABTA (Dysport®) | IBTA (Xeomin®) | RBTB (Myobloc®) | Notes |
|---|---|---|---|---|---|
| Opponens pollicis:<br>Dosage range<br>Injection sites | 2.5–10 units<br>1 | 10–40 units<br>1 | 2.5–10 units<br>1 | 10–50 units[a]<br>1 | |
| Palmaris brevis:<br>Dosage range<br>Injection sites | 2.5 units<br>1–3 | 10 units<br>1–3 | 5–20 units<br>1–3 | 20–50 units[a]<br>1–3 | |
| Dilution | 100-unit vial with 1-mL PFNS (concentration: 10 units/0.1 mL)<br>100 units with 2-mL PFNS (5 units/0.1 mL) | 300-unit vial with 1.5-mL PFNS or 500 units with 2.5-mL PFNS for concentration of 20 units/0.1 mL | 50-unit vial with 0.5-mL PFNS (concentration: 10 units/0.1 mL) or with 1-mL PFNS (5 units/0.1 mL)<br>100-unit vial with 1-mL PFNS (concentration 10: units/0.1 mL) or with 2-mL PFNS (5 units/0.1 mL) | Comes in solution 5,000 units/mL (no dilution required)[b] | [b]May be diluted with PFNS if desired. |
| Adverse events | Weakness, pain at injection site (see boxed warning for others) | Weakness, pain at injection site (see boxed warning for others) | Weakness, pain at injection site (see boxed warning for others) | Weakness, pain at injection site (see boxed warning for others) | |

*Abbreviations:* AbDM, abductor digiti minimi; AbPB, abductor pollicis brevis; ABTA, abobotulinumtoxinA; AdPB, adductor pollicis brevis; AbPL, abductor pollicis longus; FPB, flexor pollicis brevis; IBTA, incobotulinumtoxinA; OBTA, onabotulinumtoxinA; ODM, opponens digiti minimi; PFNS, preservative-free normal saline (0.9%); RBTB, rimabotulinumtoxinB.

*Sources:* Refs. 14, 96, 105, 106, 185–187, 189, 195, 196, 199, 200–203, 238.

**TABLE 10.5 BoNT for Focal Dystonia, Lower Limb: Hip/Thigh Muscles (Adults ≥18 Years of Age)**

| BoNT Preparation | OBTA (Botox®) | ABTA (Dysport®) | IBTA (Xeomin®) | RBTB (Myobloc®) | Notes |
|---|---|---|---|---|---|
| U.S. FDA approval | Currently not FDA approved | Currently not FDA approved | Currently not FDA approved | Currently not FDA approved | |
| UK MHRA | Currently not an approved indication | Currently not an approved indication | Currently not an approved indication | Currently not an approved indication | |
| **Published Dosage Range: Adults (≥18 Years of Age)** | | | | | |
| Adductor brevis:<br>Dosage range<br>Injection sites | <br>20–80 units<br>1–2 | <br>50–300 units<br>1–2 | <br>20–80 units<br>1–2 | <br>100–1,000 units[a] | [a]No published information on dosage. These ranges represent the dosage ranges used by the first author.<br>[b]Published dose range includes treatment of spasticity and focal dystonia. Consider lower dose range for focal dystonia. |
| Adductor longus:<br>Dosage range<br>Injection sites | <br>20–100 units<br>1–3 | <br>50–400 units<br>1–3 | <br>20–100 units<br>1–3 | <br>100–1,000 units[a] | |
| Adductor magnus:<br>Dosage range<br>Injection sites | <br>30–150 units<br>1–3 | <br>100–500 units<br>1–3 | <br>30–150 units<br>1–3 | <br>100–1,500 units[a] | |
| Gluteus maximus:<br>Dosage range<br>Injection sites | <br>40–100 units<br>1–2 | <br>140–400 units<br>1–3 | <br>40–100 units<br>1–3 | <br>100–1,500 units[a] | |
| Gluteus medius and minimus:<br>Dosage range<br>Injection sites | <br>20–60 units<br>1–2 | <br>70–200 units<br>1–2 | <br>20–60 units<br>1–2 | <br>100–1,000 units[a] | |
| Gracilis:<br>Dosage range<br>Injection sites | <br>20–60 units<br>1–3 | <br>50–200 units<br>1–3 | <br>20–50 units<br>1–3 | <br>100–750 units[a] | |

(continued)

**TABLE 10.5 BoNT for Focal Dystonia, Lower Limb: Hip/Thigh Muscles (Adults ≥18 Years of Age) (*continued*)**

| BoNT Preparation | OBTA (Botox®) | ABTA (Dysport®) | IBTA (Xeomin®) | RBTB (Myobloc®) | Notes |
|---|---|---|---|---|---|
| Iliacus:<br>Dosage range<br>Injection sites | 50–150 units[a]<br>1–2 | 75–300 units[a]<br>1–2 | 50–100 units[a]<br>1–2 | 100–1,000 units[a] | |
| Iliopsoas:<br>Dosage range<br>Injection sites | 25–200 units<br>1–3 | 100–700 units<br>1–3 | 25–200 units<br>1–3 | 100–1,500 units[a]<br>1–3 | |
| Pectineus:<br>Dosage range<br>Injection sites | 20–50 units<br>1 | 80–180 units<br>1 | 20–50 units<br>1 | 100–750 units[a]<br>1 | |
| Sartorius:<br>Dosage range<br>Injection sites | 10–40 units<br>1–2 | 40–140 units<br>1–2 | 10–40 units<br>1–2 | 100–500 units[a]<br>1–2 | |
| Tensor fasciae latae:<br>Dosage range<br>Injection sites | 20–40 units<br>1–2 | 80–300 units<br>1–2 | 20–40 units<br>1–2 | 100–750 units[a]<br>1–2 | |
| **Thigh Muscles** | | | | | |
| Hamstrings:<br>Biceps femoris<br>Semimembranosus<br>Semitendinosus<br>Injection sites | 40–140 units<br>20–100 units<br>20–80 units<br>1–3 per muscle | 100–500 units<br>80–400 units<br>60–300 units<br>1–3 per muscle | 40–140 units<br>20–100 units<br>20–80 units<br>1–3 per muscle | Medial hamstrings:<br>2,500–7,500 units[b]<br>Lateral hamstrings:<br>2,500–7,500 units[b]<br>1–3 per muscle | |

(*continued*)

**TABLE 10.5 BoNT for Focal Dystonia, Lower Limb: Hip/Thigh Muscles (Adults ≥18 Years of Age) (*continued*)**

| BoNT Preparation | OBTA (Botox®) | ABTA (Dysport®) | IBTA (Xeomin®) | RBTB (Myobloc®) | Notes |
|---|---|---|---|---|---|
| Quadriceps femoris components: | | | | 1,000–5,000 units, divided among all four muscles[b] | |
| Rectus femoris | 20–100 units | 50–400 units | 50–100 units | | |
| Vastus intermedius | 20–80 units | 50–300 units | 20–80 units | | |
| Vastus lateralis | 20–80 units | 50–300 units | 20–80 units | | |
| Vastus medialis | 20–80 units | 50–300 units | 20–80 units | | |
| Injection sites | 1–3 per muscle | 1–3 per muscle | 1–3 per muscle | 1–3 per muscle | |
| Dilution | 100-unit vial with 1-mL PFNS (concentration: 10 units/0.1 mL) or with 2-mL PFNS (5 units/0.1 mL) | 300-unit vial with 1.5-mL PFNS or 500 units with 2.5-mL PFNS for concentration of 20 units/0.1 mL | 50-unit vial with 0.5-mL PFNS (concentration: 10 units/0.1 mL) or with 1-mL PFNS (5 units/0.1 mL)<br>100-unit vial with 1-mL PFNS (concentration: 10 units/0.1 mL) or with 2-mL PFNS (5 units/0.1 mL) | Comes in solution 5,000 units/mL (no dilution required)[c] | [c]May be diluted with PFNS if desired. |
| Adverse events | Weakness, pain at injection site (see boxed warning for others) | Weakness, pain at injection site (see boxed warning for others) | Weakness, pain at injection site (see boxed warning for others) | Weakness, pain at injection site (see boxed warning for others) | |

*Abbreviations:* ABTA, abobotulinumtoxinA; IBTA, incobotulinumtoxinA; OBTA, onabotulinumtoxinA; PFNS, preservative-free normal saline (0.9%); RBTB, rimabotulinumtoxinB.

*Sources:* Refs. 96, 178, 199, 488.

**TABLE 10.6 BoNT for Focal Dystonia, Lower Limb Muscles: Calf/Foot Intrinsic Muscles (Adults ≥18 Years of Age)**

| BoNT Preparation | OBTA (Botox®) | ABTA (Dysport®) | IBTA (Xeomin®) | RBTB (Myobloc®) | Notes |
|---|---|---|---|---|---|
| U.S. FDA approval | Currently not FDA approved | Currently not FDA approved | Currently not FDA approved | Currently not FDA approved | |
| UK MHRA | Currently not an approved indication | Currently not an approved indication | Currently not an approved indication | Currently not an approved indication | |
| **Published Dosage Range: Adults (≥18 Years of Age)** | | | | | |
| EDL:<br>Dosage range<br>Injection sites | <br>5–30 units<br>1–2 | <br>20–140 units<br>1–2 | <br>5–30 units<br>1–2 | <br>100–500 units[a]<br>1–2 | [a]No published information on dosage. These ranges represent the dosage ranges used by the first author.<br>[b]Published dose range includes treatment of spasticity and focal dystonia. Consider lower dose range for focal dystonia. |
| EHL:<br>Starting dosage<br>Dosage range<br>Injection sites | <br>20–40 units<br>20–60 units<br>1–2 | <br>—<br>80–140 units<br>1–2 | <br>—<br>20–40 units<br>1–2 | <br>—<br>100–1,500 units[b]<br>1–2 | |
| Fibularis brevis:<br>Starting dosage range[a]<br>Injection sites | <br>5–20 units[a]<br>1 | <br>20–40 units[a]<br>1 | <br>5–20 units[a]<br>1 | <br>50–500 units[a]<br>1 | |
| Fibularis longus:<br>Dosage range<br>Injection sites | <br>5–40 units<br>1–2 | <br>20–100 units<br>1–2 | <br>5–40 units<br>1–2 | <br>100–1,000 units[a]<br>1–2 | |
| FDL:<br>Starting dosage<br>Dosage range<br>Injection sites | <br>10–40 units<br>10–125 units<br>1–2 | <br>—<br>80–200 units<br>1–2 | <br>—<br>10–40 units<br>1–2 | <br>—<br>500–3,000 units<br>1–2 | |

*(continued)*

**TABLE 10.6 BoNT for Focal Dystonia, Lower Limb Muscles: Calf/Foot Intrinsic Muscles (Adults ≥18 Years of Age) (*continued*)**

| BoNT Preparation | OBTA (Botox®) | ABTA (Dysport®) | IBTA (Xeomin®) | RBTB (Myobloc®) | Notes |
|---|---|---|---|---|---|
| FHL:<br>Dosage range<br>Injection sites | <br>20–125 units<br>1–2 | <br>80–200 units<br>1–2 | <br>20–40 units<br>1–2 | <br>100–1,000 units[a]<br>1–2 | |
| Gastrocnemius:<br>Dosage range<br>Injection sites | <br>20–100 units<br>1–3 per head | <br>80–200 units<br>1–3 per head | <br>20–100 units<br>1–3 per head | <br>1,000–3,000 units<br>1–3 per head | Consider higher doses in the medial gastrocnemius, which is generally larger. |
| Soleus:<br>Starting dosage<br>Dosage range<br>Injection sites | <br>20–50 units<br>20–200 units<br>2–4 | <br><br>80–300 units<br>2–4 | <br><br>20–80 units<br>2–4 | <br><br>1,000–2,500 units[a]<br>2–4 | [a]Published dose range includes treatment of spasticity and focal dystonia. Consider lower dose ranges for focal dystonia.<br>[b]No published information on dosage. These ranges represent the dosage ranges used by the first author. |
| Tibialis anterior:<br>Starting dosage<br>Dosage range<br>Injection sites | <br>20–80 units<br>20–150 units<br>1–3 | <br>80–100 units<br>80–300 units<br>1–3 | <br>20–40 units<br>20–80 units<br>1–3 | <br><br>1,000–5,000 units[a]<br>1–3 | |
| Tibialis posterior:<br>Starting dosage<br>Dosage range<br>Injection sites | <br>20–50 units<br>20–350 units<br>1–3 | <br>50–75 units<br>50–200 units<br>1–3 | <br><br>20–80 units<br>1–3 | <br><br>1,000–7,500 units[a]<br>1–3 | |

(*continued*)

**TABLE 10.6 BoNT for Focal Dystonia, Lower Limb Muscles: Calf/Foot Intrinsic Muscles (Adults ≥18 Years of Age) (*continued*)**

| BoNT Preparation | OBTA (Botox®) | ABTA (Dysport®) | IBTA (Xeomin®) | RBTB (Myobloc®) | Notes |
|---|---|---|---|---|---|
| **Intrinsic Foot Muscles** | | | | | |
| AbH, AdH:<br>Starting dosage<br>Dosage range<br>Injection sites | <br>5–20 units<br>5–80 units<br>1 | <br>20–80 units<br>—<br>1 | <br>5–20 units<br>—<br>1 | <br>100–500 units[b]<br>—<br>1–2 | [a]Published dose range includes treatment of spasticity and focal dystonia. Consider lower dose range for focal dystonia.<br>[b]No published information on dosage. These ranges represent the dosage ranges used by the first author. |
| EDB, FHB:<br>Dosage range<br>Injection sites | <br>5–30 units<br>1–2 | <br>20–100 units<br>1–2 | <br>5–30 units<br>1–2 | <br>100–500 units[b]<br>1–2 | |
| FDB:<br>Starting dosage<br>Dosage range<br>Injection sites | <br>10–50 units<br>10–120 units<br>1–3 | <br>—<br>40–400 units<br>1–3 | <br>—<br>10–100 units<br>1–3 | <br>—<br>150–750 units[b]<br>1–3 | |
| FDMP:<br>Dosage range<br>Injection sites | <br>5–20 units<br>1–2 | <br>20–80 units<br>1–2 | <br>5–20 units<br>1–2 | <br>100–500 units[b]<br>1–2 | |
| Interossei/ lumbricals:<br>Dosage range<br>Injection sites | <br>5–10 units/muscle belly<br>1 per muscle belly<br>1–3 for interossei<br>2–4 for lumbricals | <br>20–40 units/muscle belly<br>1 per muscle belly<br>1–3 for interossei<br>2–4 for lumbricals | <br>5–10 units/muscle belly<br>1 per muscle belly<br>1–3 for interossei<br>2–4 for lumbricals | <br>75–100 units/ muscle belly[b]<br>1 per muscle belly<br>1–3 for interossei<br>2–4 for lumbricals | |

(*continued*)

**TABLE 10.6 BoNT for Focal Dystonia, Lower Limb Muscles: Calf/Foot Intrinsic Muscles (Adults ≥18 Years of Age) (*continued*)**

| BoNT Preparation | OBTA (Botox®) | ABTA (Dysport®) | IBTA (Xeomin®) | RBTB (Myobloc®) | Notes |
|---|---|---|---|---|---|
| Quadratus plantae:<br>Dosage range<br>Injection sites | 5–20 units<br>1–2 | 20–80 units<br>1–2 | 5–20 units<br>1–2 | 100–500 units[b]<br>1–2 | |
| Dilution | 100-unit vial with 1-mL PFNS (concentration: 10 units/0.1 mL) or with 2-mL PFNS (5 units/0.1 mL) | 300-unit vial with 1.5-mL PFNS or 500 units with 2.5-mL PFNS for concentration of 20 units/0.1 mL | 50-unit vial with 0.5-mL PFNS (concentration: 10 units/0.1 mL) or with 1-mL PFNS (5 units/0.1 mL)<br><br>100-unit vial with 1-mL PFNS (concentration: 10 units/0.1 mL) or with 2-mL PFNS (5 units/0.1 mL) | Comes in solution 5,000 units/mL (no dilution required)[c] | [c]May be diluted with PFNS if desired. |
| Adverse events | Weakness, pain at injection site (see boxed warning for others) | Weakness, pain at injection site (see boxed warning for others) | Weakness, pain at injection site (see boxed warning for others) | Weakness, pain at injection site (see boxed warning for others) | |

*Abbreviations:* AbH, abductor halluces; ABTA, abobotulinumtoxinA; AdH, adductor halluces; EDB, extensor digitorum brevis; EDL, extensor digitorum longus; EHL, extensor hallucis longus; FDB, flexor digitorum brevis; FDL, flexor digitorum longus; FDMP, flexor digiti minimi pedis; FHB, flexor hallucis brevis; FHL, flexor hallucis longus; IBTA, incobotulinumtoxinA; OBTA, onabotulinumtoxinA; PFNS, preservative-free normal saline (0.9%); RBTB, rimabotulinumtoxinB.

*Sources:* Refs. 96, 178, 195, 199, 238, 489, 490.

# 11

# *Botulinum Neurotoxin for Treatment of Muscle Overactivity Associated with Upper Motor Neuron Syndromes*

*Katharine E. Alter, MD*
*John McGuire, MD*
*Stephen Nichols, MD*

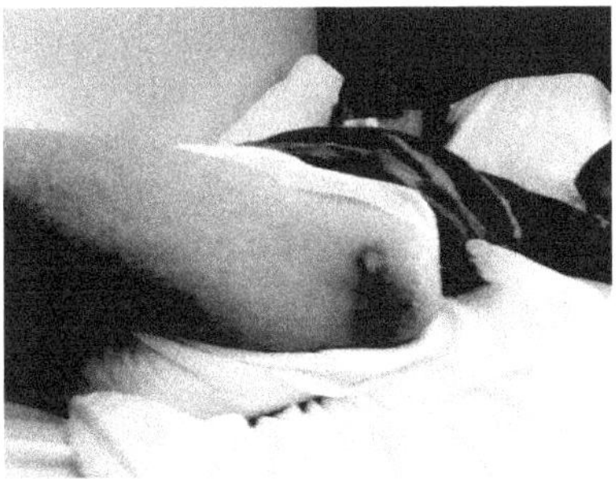

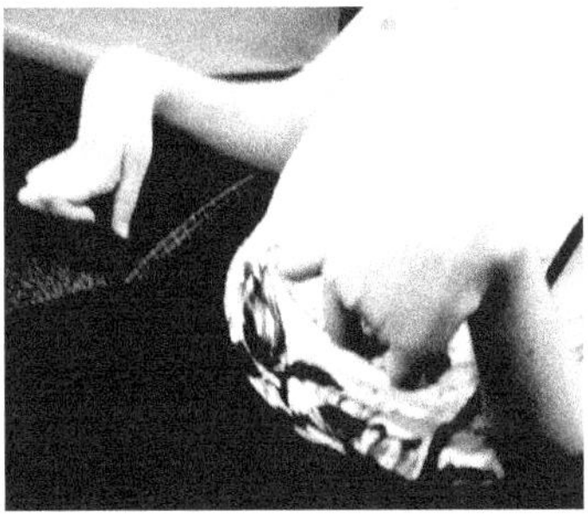

## Condition

A wide range of conditions or injuries affecting the central nervous system (CNS) can lead to muscle overactivity as part of a constellation of sensorimotor signs or symptoms collectively referred to as the upper motor neuron syndrome (UMNS). Lance described the positive and negative signs associated with UMNS. Negative signs associated with UMNS include weakness, loss of selective motor control or dexterity, and impaired sensory perception (204, 205). Positive signs include hyperreflexia, pathological reflexes, spasms, and muscle hypertonia (e.g., spasticity, dystonia, rigidity) (204–206).

UMNS-related muscle overactivity or hypertonia is one of the most common problems leading to a referral for chemodenervation procedures, including botulinum neurotoxin (BoNT) injections. In adult patients, the most common causes of UMNS are stroke, traumatic brain injury (TBI), cerebral palsy (CP), spinal cord injury (SCI), and multiple sclerosis (MS). In the pediatric population, CP, resulting from injury to or a lesion in the developing brain, is the most common cause of UMNS. Hypertonia is also seen in pediatric patients following SCI, TBI, stroke, and in association with myelodysplasia, hereditary spastic paraplegia, inherited/genetic metabolic/neurologic disorders, and other conditions (207, 208).

Hypertonia is the net result of complex changes in reflex activity in upper motor neuron (UMN) lesions, the effects of which are not fully understood. It is known that changes occur in the CNS in monosynaptic and polysynaptic pathways at both the segmental level and in descending inhibitory input from higher cortical centers (208–210). The resulting loss of inhibition leads to a net increase in alpha motor neuron excitability and resulting muscle hypertonia (211).

As noted previously, the signs and symptoms of UMNS include both positive (hypertonia, hyperreflexia) and negative symptoms (weakness, loss of selective motor control) (125, 207). The full impact of UMNS is due to a combination of these positive and negative symptoms, as well as rheological changes such as contracture, fibrosis, and atrophy (212). Types of muscle hypertonia include spasticity, spastic dystonia, dystonia, spasms, and stiffness.

The most common forms of muscle overactivity seen in patients with UMNS are spasticity and dystonia and many patients present with a combination of spasticity and dystonia. Spasticity is defined as a velocity-dependent increase in tonic stretch reflexes (204–206, 213). During assessment on physical exam, spasticity will be perceived as increased resistance to stretch as the velocity of stretch increases. Typically, during rapid stretch, a "spastic catch" will be felt by the clinician, but may be obscured if the patient has combined spasticity/dystonia. Dystonia is a movement disorder characterized by involuntary postures or sustained movements that often have a twisting quality. Dystonia may be associated with hypertonia and be either hyperkinetic or hypokinetic (213).

### *Clinical Pearl*

Spasticity will be "felt" on the physical exam (as a spastic catch), whereas dystonia may be "seen" when the patient is observed as he or she attempts to move or at times when the patient is apparently "at rest." In addition to increasing with voluntary movement attempts, dystonia often increases if a patient talks, is in pain, or is excited or agitated.

### *Clinical/Functional Impact*

Any or all the preceding forms of hypertonia may cause discomfort/pain, joint deformity, lead to contractures, contribute to skin breakdown, and affect quality of life, activities of daily living (ADLs), mobility, and other function in patients with UMNS.

However, these impairments are only one aspect of the UMNS and may change over time (125, 126).

In pediatric patients, the symptoms caused by a static UMN lesion combined with ongoing linear growth and disuse often lead to progressive musculoskeletal consequences (muscle shortening, contractures, limb/joint deformity) (207, 214).

## *Pattern of Involvement*

Although each patient presents with a unique combination of UMNS motor impairments, there are some commonalities and pattern of muscle overactivity. For example:

1. Poststroke upper limb spasticity (ULS)/dystonia: The most common upper limb pattern/posture is shoulder adduction/internal rotation, elbow flexion, forearm pronation, and wrist and/or finger flexion. Muscles typically involved include the pectoralis major, latissimus dorsi, teres major, subscapularis, biceps, brachialis, brachioradialis, pronators teres/quadratus, flexor carpi radialis (FCR), flexor carpi ulnaris (FCU), flexor digitorum profundus (FDP), flexor digitorum superficialis (FDS), flexor pollicis longus (FPL), and the lumbricals.
2. Poststroke lower limb spasticity (LLS)/dystonia: In the lower limb, ankle plantar flexion, equinovarus foot, and toe flexion are common. A flexed hip, flexed knee, stiff knee/limited knee flexion, and thigh adduction may also be seen. Commonly affected muscles include the gastrocnemius, soleus, posterior tibialis, flexor digitorum longus (FDL), flexor hallucis longus (FHL), extensor hallucis longus (EHL), flexor digitorum brevis (FDB), flexor hallucis brevis (FHB), and possibly the hip adductors, hamstrings, and quadriceps.
3. CP, spastic diplegia: In young patients (2–4 years of age) with spastic diplegia, ankle plantar flexion with or without equinus is the most common pattern, with involvement of the plantar flexors, invertors, and toe flexors (gastrocnemius and/or soleus, FDL, tibialis posterior, tibialis anterior). In older, school-age children, in addition to the calf muscles, the hamstrings are typically involved. In patients with quadriplegia, lower limb involvement typically affects the hip flexors, adductors, and quadriceps, in addition to many of the muscles mentioned earlier.
4. CP, quadriplegia: Bilateral upper and lower limb involvement is seen and tone is often asymmetric. Adduction/internal rotation at the shoulder with elbow wrist and finger flexion is common in the upper limbs. Hip flexion, adduction, knee flexion, and ankle plantar flexion is common in the lower limbs.

## *Evaluation*

Evaluation of a patient with UMNS-related muscle overactivity starts with a history and physical examination. If the causes of the patient's symptoms/findings on physical examination are not known, the cause must be established prior to proceeding with treatment. UMNS is a clinical diagnosis that is supported by the findings (or absence of findings) from various diagnostic evaluations. Workup is determined largely by the patient's history and physical examination and may require testing including CNS imaging, electrodiagnostic testing, or other evaluations. A full discussion of the workup of UMNS is beyond the scope of this chapter and readers are referred to review articles and texts on this topic (208, 211, 215).

Prior to initiating any treatment, a detailed patient evaluation of sensorimotor impairments, including hypertonia, as well as function is required. The assessment of the impact of the patient's hypertonia on his or her active and passive function and quality of life will identify problematic muscle groups and will direct selection of the most appropriate treatment and aftercare (17, 18, 207, 216). As a part of treatment planning, the physician, patient, and/or family and caregivers should collectively identify realistic treatment goals. Patients and families frequently focus on the impact of hypertonia/muscle stiffness/pain/spasms and fail to recognize the impact of other UMNS-related impairments (sensory loss, weakness, loss of selective motor control). To avoid unrealistic expectations related to treatment, it is critical that the physician and medical team educate patients and families about all the impairments associated with UNMS.

### *Evaluation of Muscle Overactivity/Hypertonia*

Evaluation of muscle hypertonia includes a complete examination including the skin, musculoskeletal, and neurologic systems. The most commonly used hypertonia evaluation scales used for the assessment of patients with UMNS, are the Ashworth and Modified Ashworth Scales (AS and MAS, respectively) and the Tardieu or Modified Tardieu (217). Each of these scales has limitations, but their use provides some objective documentation of spasticity and the response to treatment (218). The Modified Tardieu Scale is used extensively by pediatric physicians/therapists and has the advantage of evaluating the effect of velocity on the patient's tone (219) (see Appendix 6). Other scales used for the assessment of impact of spasticity on a patient's functional status include the Barthel Index and the Functional Independence Measure (FIM) (220, 221).

The Hypertonia Assessment Tool (HAT) is a scale that discriminates among spasticity, dystonia, and rigidity. The HAT can easily be incorporated into a physical examination or performed by a therapist (222). In addition to evaluation of tone, evaluation of passive and active range of motion (ROM) and of motor control is critical. Various motor control assessment tools are available including the Selective Control Assessment of the Lower Extremity (SCALE) and the Shriner's Hospital Upper Extremity Evaluation (SHUEE) (223, 224). For reasonable goal setting related to hypertonia management, Goal Attainment Scaling is recommended by many physicians, therapists, and researchers (207, 225).

### *Treatment*

Adequate assessment of the severity, scope, and impact of hypertonia on the patient's function and quality of life will direct treatment selection. Not all patients with hypertonia require treatment of their muscle overactivity. Some patients, because of associated weakness, use spasticity functionally to assist in transfers and other tasks. Treatment of hypertonia is only necessary when it causes symptoms or problems such as pain or ROM limitations, and affects quality of life, ADLs, mobility, or other functional tasks (17, 207, 226).

## Nonpharmacologic Treatment Options

Nonpharmacologic treatment options include reducing noxious stimuli, positioning, splinting, and ROM exercises. Pharmacologic and surgical treatment options include oral medications, chemodenervation procedures, and surgery (orthopedic, baclofen pump, deep brain stimulation). During the course of their lives following an UMN injury, adult and pediatric patients may benefit from multiple treatment options, including nonpharmacologic treatment, oral medications, injectable agents (BoNT, phenol blocks), and/or surgery (17, 117, 118, 227, 228). A full discussion of all these modalities is beyond the scope of this chapter and the reader is referred to several review articles on this topic (17, 119, 208, 226, 229).

### *BoNT for Treatment of Muscle Hypertonia*

There are numerous scholarly articles, reviews, controlled trials, and case series supporting the efficacy and safety of BoNT as a therapy for adult and pediatric spasticity. BoNT therapy is widely used to treat hypertonia associated with UMNS, including stroke, TBI, SCI, and CP (86, 230, 231). BoNT has been used successfully in patients with localized and regional muscle overactivity and it may also be helpful in patients with generalized spasticity if treatment goals are correctly selected.

### *FDA-Approved BoNTs for the Treatment of Spasticity*

At the time of publication, onabotulinumtoxinA (OBTA, Botox®) is the only BoNT product available in the United States that has Food and Drug Administration (FDA) approval for the treatment of spasticity (ULS in adult patients aged 18 years or older). The approved muscles are as follows: biceps (Bi), FCR, FCU, FDP, and flexor digitorum sublimis/superficialis (FDS). Treatment of spasticity involving other upper limb muscles or LLS in adults is off-label for all the FDA-approved BoNT products.

Treatment of pediatric patients less than 18 years of age is also currently off-label in the United States for all FDA-approved BoNT products (OBTA, abobotulinumtoxinA [ABTA, Dysport®], incobotulinumtoxinA [IBTA, Xeomin®], and rimabotulinumtoxinB [RBTB, Myobloc®/NeuroBloc®]) (34, 36, 38, 44).

### *Approvals Outside of the United States*

OBTA and ABTA are approved for the treatment of spasticity in adults and pediatric patients with CP (more than 2 years of age) in many countries outside the United States, including Canada, the United Kingdom, Europe, Australia, and New Zealand. Xeomin is approved in many countries outside the United States for the treatment of spasticity associated with ULS and LLS in adults (18 years of age or older).

### *Level of Evidence for BoNT for the Treatment of UMNS Muscle Overactivity: Adults*

Esquenazi et al. (214): This is a 2013 review article using the American Academy of Neurology (AAN) Classification of Quality of Evidence for Clinical trials (138) to evaluate the evidence from published studies of BoNT for the treatment of spasticity in adults.

- ULS/adults: The authors concluded that there was sufficient evidence from Class I trials for a Level A recommendation (Established as effective) for the use of OBTA and ABTA. For IBTA, the authors concluded that there was sufficient evidence to support a Level B recommendation (Probably effective). They reported that the current evidence is insufficient (Level U, Unestablished or unproven) to support a recommendation for RBTB.
- LLS: Although there are fewer studies evaluating BoNT for LLS, the authors concluded that there was sufficient evidence to support a Level A recommendation for OBTA individually and for serotype A BoNTs in aggregate. A Level C recommendation (Possibly effective) was given for ABTA, based on the evidence from current trials, and a Level U recommendation was reported for both IBTA and RBTB due to insufficient evidence to support a higher recommendation.

Teasell et al. (527): The authors reviewed the evidence for poststroke upper and LLS (see also www.ebsr.com).

- Upper limb: There was strong Level Ia evidence that BoNT either alone or in combination with physical therapy decreases spasticity, but it was unclear whether the improvements were sustained or improved function or quality of life. There was moderate Level Ib evidence that intra-articular injections do not improve pain or passive ROM in the hemiplegic shoulder. In addition, there was conflicting Level IV evidence that BoNT injections in the subscapularis muscle reduce pain and improve passive ROM of the shoulder.
- Lower limb: There was strong Level Ia evidence that BoNT decreases spasticity, but conflicting Level IV evidence that BoNT injections improve function. In addition, there was strong Level Ia evidence that electrical stimulation (e-stim) combined with BoNT, reduces spasticity in the upper/lower limbs, but conflicting Level IV evidence that reduced tone improved function.

### *Level of Evidence for BoNT for the Treatment of Pediatric UMNS Muscle Overactivity*

Novak et al. (257): In a systematic review of evidence of treatments/interventions for children with CP, Novak et al. concluded that BoNT injections were effective at reducing muscle spasticity and should be considered for children with CP.

Esquenazi et al. (510): An international panel of experts reviewed the evidence for BoNT for the treatment of neurological impairments. In reviewing pediatric studies, the authors concluded that there was sufficient evidence to support a Level A recommendation (Established as effective) for BoNT as effective at reducing LLS and sialorrhea. The authors reported a Level B recommendation (Probably effective) for BoNT effectiveness in reducing ULS and a Level U recommendation (Unestablished or unproven) for BoNT effectiveness at reducing spasticity in neck muscles.

### *2010 Practice Parameter AAN/Child Neurology Society*

The authors concluded that there was sufficient Level I evidence to support a recommendation that serotype A BoNT is effective in reducing spasticity. Due to insufficient evidence, the authors reported a Level U recommendation for serotype B BoNT, phenol, or alcohol blocks (232).

**Note**: The majority of studies and evidence related to BoNT in pediatric UMNS spasticity is in patients with CP. The evidence from these studies may or may not be generalizable to UMNS from other causes.

### *Injection Pattern/Technique*

Injections of BoNT for spasticity require localization of the target muscle. Physicians who perform BoNT procedures must have extensive knowledge of functional, surface, and cross-sectional anatomy. Expertize with palpation and procedural skills is also required. The injection pattern and the dose/muscle are determined by the patient's clinical presentation (i.e., muscles involved, severity of the hypertonia, and functional goals).

Many, if not most, physicians who perform BoNT procedures to treat muscle overactivity use either electromyography (EMG), e-stim, B-mode ultrasound (US), or a combination of these techniques for muscle targeting (18, 156). Each localization technique has advantages and disadvantages, and for specifics, the reader is referred to the chapter comparing localization techniques in this text. Although studies suggest that EMG, US, or e-stim are superior to palpation alone, the superiority of one localization technique over another has not been established. Additional research with head-to-head comparison trials is required to establish the superiority of one technique over another.

Some clinicians also advocate injecting BoNT near the motor point of the target muscle (212, 233). Additional research is required to determine whether this technique is superior and leads to better outcomes, a lower required dose, and reduced adverse events.

### *Number of Injection Sites*

When performing BoNT injections for UMNS-related muscle overactivity, the number of injection sites is determined by the size of the muscle and the dose/volume of the injectate. A single injection site may be sufficient when a small muscle is injected. Multiple injections are typically performed for large or long muscles or when a large dose or volume is injected. Multiple injection sites are often used to reduce the potential for local spread of BoNT to nontargeted muscles or to distant sites. To avoid multiple skin penetrations, many clinicians will redirect the needle to several sites within the muscle(s) (redirecting the needle in the subcutaneous space, not in the muscle itself), such as is performed during needle EMG evaluation of muscles. This allows the BoNT to be distributed into several sites in the muscle with a single skin penetration (18, 156).

### *Dosage of BoNT for UMNS Muscle Overactivity*

The dosage of BoNT is product specific, including the starting, retreatment, and maximum recommended dose. Detailed information related to dosing is provided in the manufacturer's full prescribing information (PI) and product labels, albeit only for approved indications. There are numerous published studies on the topic of BoNT for UMNS-related spasticity. Many of these studies report only the total BoNT dose/treatment session and possibly the number of muscles injected, but unfortunately not the individual dose per muscle.

When treating patients with muscle overactivity, selecting the correct dose of BoNT depends on a number of other factors:

- The individual BoNT product to be used.
- The cause of a patient's muscle overactivity. For example, effective treatment of spasticity associated with UMNS generally requires higher doses of BoNT than that required when treating patients with focal dystonias. The dose also varies by UMNS condition (Figures 11.1 and 11.2) (207, 234).
- There is a significant variation in response to BoNT from patient to patient with some patients being more sensitive (i.e., requiring a lower dose to obtain the desired effect). Because of this variation, physicians should consider a conservative dose per muscle and total dose in toxin-naïve patients. After observing the patient's response, the dose per muscle and total dose can then be increased incrementally over a series of treatment sessions (125, 126, 207, 235, 236).
- When treating patients with spasticity, the goal is to use the lowest dose of BoNT that provides adequate muscle relaxation to achieve the goals set during treatment planning. In general, larger doses of BoNT are used in patients with severe spasticity, in large muscles, and when passive functional goals are selected (125, 126, 235, 236). Lower doses are often required for smaller muscles and milder spasticity.
- In some patients with severe spasticity or dystonia, physicians may recommend combined therapy with BoNT and phenol (or alcohol) nerve or motor-point blocks.

*FIGURE 11.1 Distribution of injected muscles. SA, shoulder adductor; D, deltoid; PM, pectoralis major; BB, biceps brachii; TB, triceps brachii; BR, brachioradialis; B, brachialis; PT, pronator teres; FDS, flexor digitorum superficialis; FDP, flexor. From Ref. 234. Phadke CP, Davidson C, Ismail F, Boulias C. The effect of neural lesion type on botulinum toxin dosage: a retrospective chart review.* PM R. *2014;6(5):406–411. Reprinted with permission from Elsevier.*

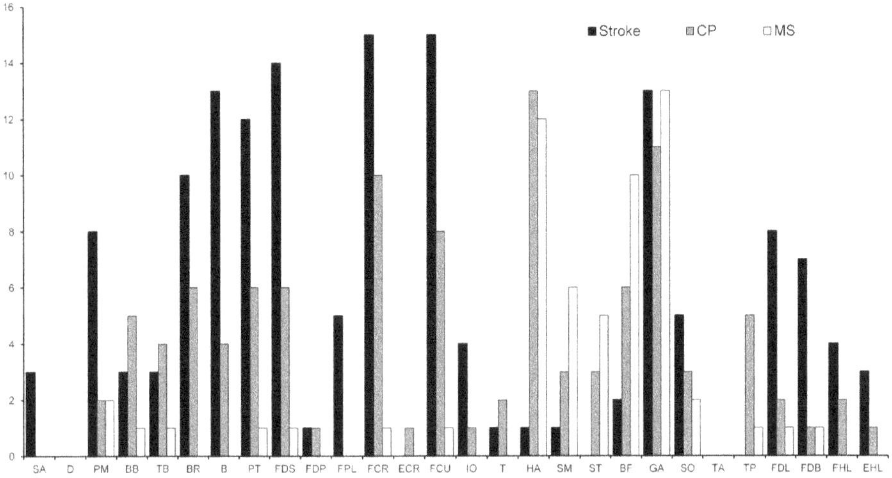


*FIGURE 11.2 Differences in toxin dosage in leg muscles between CP, MS, and stroke populations. *Significantly different (P < 0.05); kg = kilogram. From Ref. 234. Phadke CP, Davidson C, Ismail F, Boulias C. The effect of neural lesion type on botulinum toxin dosage: a retrospective chart review.* PM R. *2014;6(5):406–411. Reprinted with permission from Elsevier.*

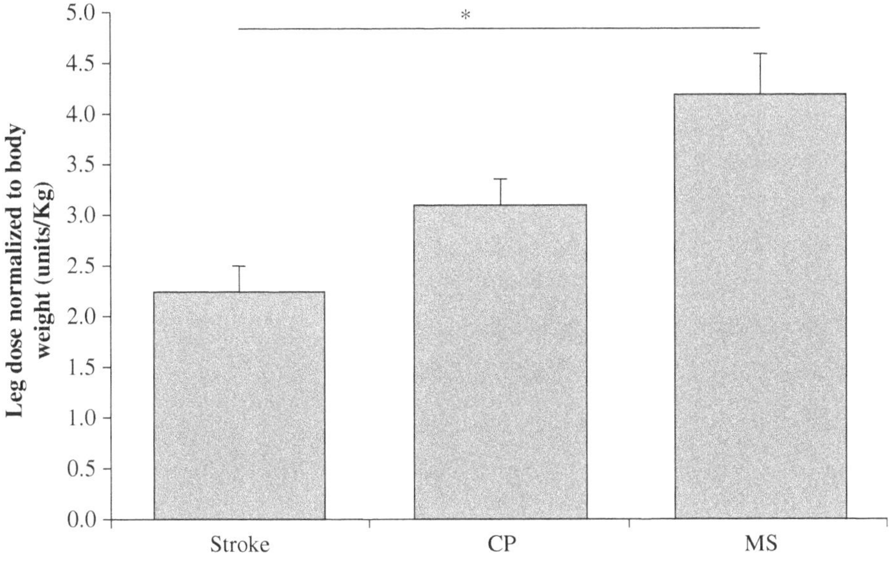

Phenol can be used as a "toxin-sparing" technique. This practice may be useful when the dose of BoNT required to treat the identified target muscles exceeds recommended dose limits. For example, in a patient with severe lower extremity spasticity, adductor tone may be addressed with phenol obturator nerve blocks, thereby "saving" toxin for other muscles (117, 118, 229, 236).

## Maximum Dose/Treatment Session

The approved/manufacturer's published dose of the various BoNT products for the treatment of UMNS-related muscle overactivity varies by individual country. There is a wide range in the published maximum dose per treatment session for each of the BoNT products from clinical trials and in clinical practice (237–239). For example, for OBTA, the manufacturer's published maximum dose for ULS is 360 units, whereas the maximum dose typically used in clinical practice is 400 to 600 units. A dose as high as 850 to 1,200 units has been reported in the literature (237, 239). These high doses (>400 units) should not be used in toxin-naïve patients and should only be used with caution and with careful dose escalation. For the published dosage ranges of the each of the BoNT products, see Tables 11.1 to 11.9.

### *OnabotulinumtoxinA: Manufacturer's Published Dosage for Hypertonia/UMNS*

- United States: Adult ULS 75 to 360 units, divided (biceps brachii, FCR, FCU, FDP, FDS) (34).
- United Kingdom/Medicines and Healthcare products Regulatory Agency (MHRA): Approved dose—240 units, divided (biceps brachii, FCR, FCU, FDP, FDS, abductor pollicis longus [AdPL], FPL) (35).
- United Kingdom/Medicines and Healthcare products Regulatory Agency (MHRA): Approved dose, pediatric spasticity (ambulatory CP)—≥4 units/kg, total dose, divided if bilateral lower limb injections are performed (gastrocnemius) (35).
- New Zealand, upper limb, adults: Dose determined by severity of spasticity, weakness, and patient response to prior treatment. Maximum dose 360 units (240).
- New Zealand, pediatric spasticity (CP, ≥2 years of age): Exact dose and number of injections dependent on size and location of muscles (240).
  - Upper limb muscles: 0.5–2 units/kg/muscle
  - Lower limb muscles: 2–4 units/kg/muscle
  - Maximum dose: 3–8 units/kg or 300 units
- Canada, upper limb, adults: Maximum dose 360 units, divided (biceps brachii, FCR, FCU, FDP, FDS, AdPL, FPL) (241).

- Canada, pediatric spasticity (CP, ≥2 years of age): Maximum dose 6 units/kg (4 units/kg, if unilateral) (241).
- EU, adult ULS: 200–240 units (FCR, FCU, FDP, FDS, adductor pollicis brevis [AdPB]) (242).
- EU, pediatric LLS (CP, ≥2 years of age): Maximum dose 6 units/kg (4 units/kg, if unilateral) (242).

### *AbobotulinumtoxinA and Dose for Hypertonia/UMNS*

- United Kingdom/MHRA: Approved dose, adult ULS—1,000 units (243).
- United Kingdom/MHRA: Approved dose, pediatric LLS (ambulatory CP, ≥2 years of age): Initial dose 10 units/kg (unilateral) and 20 units/kg (bilateral). Titrate to 30 units/kg at repeat injection (243).
- New Zealand: Approved dose for adult ULS (biceps, FCR, FCU, FDP, FDS). Maximum dose 1,000 units (244).
- New Zealand: Approved dose, pediatric spasticity (ambulatory CP, ≥2 years of age): Initial dose 10 units/kg (unilateral) and 20 units/kg (bilateral). Titrate to 30 units/kg at repeat injection. Maximum dose 1,000 units (244).
- EU: Approved for adult ULS, all countries (245).
- EU: Approved for adult LLS, most countries (245).

### *IncobotulinumtoxinA and Dose for Hypertonia/UMNS*

- United States: Not an approved indication (38).
- United Kingdom: Approved for ULS in adults ≥18 years of age—170 to 400 units (40).
- Canada: Approved for ULS, adults—FCR, FCU, FDP, FDS, AdPB, FPL (limited coverage in some providences) (246).
- European Union: Approved in some countries for ULS in adult patients (≥18 years of age) (biceps, brachialis, brachioradialis, pronator quadratus, pronator teres, FCR, FCU, FDP, FDS, AdPB, FPL, opponens pollicis [OP]): 200 to 300 units, up to 400 units in some countries (247, approved/granted a waiver for pediatric spasticity/ dystonia in some countries, www.ema.europa.eu/).
- New Zealand: Approved for upper and lower limb adult (≥18 years of age) spasticity. Maximum dose 360 units (biceps FCR, FCU, FDP, FDS, AdPB, FPL, OP) (248).

### *RimabotulinumtoxinB and Dose for Hypertonia/UMNS*

- Currently, there are no reported approvals/published dosage ranges in the United States or in countries outside the United States.

## *Published Dose Range from Clinical Trials for OBTA, ABTA, IBTA, RBTB: See Tables 11.2, 11.4, 11.7, and 11.9*

## *Toxin Dilution/Reconstitution*

The manufacturers of the three FDA-approved serotype A BoNT products recommend reconstitution with preservative-free normal saline (PFNS, 0.9%) (34, 36, 38). RBTB is provided in solution and does not require reconstitution. Studies evaluating the effect of dilution on treatment outcomes and adverse events are limited. Therefore, the optimal dilution of the various BoNT products for the treatment of spasticity and other uses is unknown. Additional high-quality trials are required to establish the optimal dilution of each of the serotype A BoNT products. Although some clinicians further dilute RBTB, studies are also required to establish the safety, efficacy, and optional postmanufacturing dilution of RBTB.

### OBTA RECONSTITUTION

The manufacturer's recommended dilution of OBTA when treating adults with spasticity, published in the PI is 50 units/1 mL (5 units/0.1 mL). To achieve this dilution, a 100-unit vial is reconstituted with 2-mL PFNS or a 200-unit vial with 4-mL PFNS (34). When injecting BoNT for UMNS-related hypertonia, experienced clinicians report using a variety of dilutions.

### ABTA RECONSTITUTION

The typical dilution for ABTA when treating spasticity is 300 units in 1.5-mL PFNS or 500 units in 2.5-mL PFNS (36). This results in a concentration of 50 units/1 mL or 5 units/0.1 mL. A lower volume of saline may be used when treating small muscles or for small children.

### IBTA RECONSTITUTION

The typical dilution used when treating patients with spasticity is a 100-unit vial reconstituted with 2-mL PFNS.

### RBTB RECONSTITUTION

RBTB is provided by the manufacturer in a 5,000 units/mL solution and therefore does not require reconstitution.

## *Clinical Effect*

The clinical effects of BoNT therapy are generally apparent within several days to 1 to 2 weeks. The peak effect is reported to occur at 4 to 6 weeks, with duration of clinical effect for at least 3 months. Some patients treated with BoNT for spasticity will report a longer duration of benefit—up to 6 months is reported. Many patients will require or benefit from repeat BoNT treatment at 3- to 6-month intervals. Re-evaluation of the patient and the extent and pattern of muscle hypertonia should be performed prior to each treatment cycle (17, 207, 208).

### *Adverse Events/Side Effects*

The most common adverse events following BoNT injections in patients with UMNS-related muscle hypertonia are local and include injection site pain or bruising and weakness in injected or adjacent muscles. Other symptoms can include flu-like symptoms, dysphagia, and weakness in sites distant to the injection. Remote risks include all the risks published in the boxed warning in the full PI for each BoNT product. High-dose protocols should be used with caution as they are associated with an increased risk of adverse events.

### *Boxed Warning and Compromised Patients*

A number of years ago, the FDA mandated the addition of a boxed warning to all BoNT products, warning of the risk of systemic side effects, aspiration, and possible death (see manufacturer PI). The risk of aspiration pneumonia and death can occur in any patient, but it has primarily been reported in compromised pediatric patients with CP. These patients had a prior history of dysphagia and/or aspiration pneumonia. Although mandating the boxed warning, the FDA did not conclude that there was a direct link between the BoNT procedure and the aspiration event/death (see Special Populations/Pediatric Patients Section). In addition to the boxed warning, the FDA mandated the addition of a Risk Evaluation Management System (REMS) to the package insert for BoNT products that includes a patient information sheet, which should be provided to the patient.

### *Special Populations/Pediatric Patients*

Pediatric patients represent a special subgroup of patients presenting with UMNS as it relates to BoNT and other chemodenervation procedures. Because of the observed clinical efficacy in reducing muscle hypertonia, chemodenervation procedures using BoNT and/or other agents (phenol or alcohol) are widely used in clinical practice (117, 118, 227–229, 249). Although none of the FDA-approved BoNT products are currently approved for use in children, they are approved in Canada, Ireland, United Kingdom, New Zealand, EU, Australia, and other countries. In 2014, BoNTs are considered the standard of care for children with UMNS-related spasticity and for other impairments (e.g., problematic sialorrhea) (227, 250). When prescribing BoNT for children, treatment goals are similar to those for adults and include improved passive/active function; brace/splint tolerance; reduced contracture/deformity; improved pain, spasms, and perioperative pain; and quality of life (17, 207, 228, 229, 250, 251). To date, the majority of CP-related studies in the use of BoNT included only ambulatory patients. Additional studies are required to determine the most effective and safe dose for patients at higher impairment levels (Gross Motor Functional Classification Scale [GMFCS] Levels IV and V) (252).

### *Pediatric Dose Calculation*

When prescribing BoNT therapy, the recommended dose is product specific. Although "dosage conversion ratio" calculations are used by some clinicians, this practice is not recommended by the manufacturers of the various BoNT products. The evidence to date on this topic is primarily in the adult population and is limited at best. To be established as safe, the practice of using "dosage conversion" requires additional research in comparison studies and head-to-head trials in both children and adults.

When treating younger children, the dose of a given BoNT product is generally calculated by body weight. This includes the dose per muscle and the total dose/kg/treatment session. If the dose per muscle or total treatment dose exceeds the recommended (or published) dose for adult patients, then a child should receive the lower (adult) dose (207, 227, 229, 250).

### *Maximum Dose per Treatment Cycle*

The recommended/published maximum dose varies from study to study and has evolved from the earliest reports of BoNT use in children in the early 1990s. Over the years, as clinicians have gained familiarity with BoNT, the dose used in clinical practice has increased significantly. There are risks associated with high-dose protocols that include generalized or local weakness and reported dysphagia. A 2006 consensus panel (253) concluded that the "safe" dosage range of OBTA was 6 to 25 units/kg (60–400 units) and dosage range of ABTA was 11 to 25 units/kg (900 units). In 2009, the same panel revised their recommendations, lowering the recommended dose range of OBTA to 1 to 20 units/kg (400 units) and ABTA 1 to 20 units/kg (500–1,000 units) (250). Therefore, when using higher doses, clinicians should weigh the risk-benefit ratio for higher doses for each patient (250, 254, 255).

### *Pediatric Dosage Modifiers*

When calculating dose, clinicians should take into account a variety of patient-related factors. When calculating dose per muscle, the first author uses a paradigm whereby the dose per muscle and total dose for a given patient is determined by the following factors:

- Age of the patient: Patients <2 years. Many physicians suggest a lower starting maximum dose for this younger age group (256).
- Size of the target muscle (small, medium, large)
- Severity of impairment (mild, moderate, severe)
- Selective motor control (mild, moderate, severe impairment)
- Functional goal (improved ease of care/passive function vs. independent function, transfers/independent mobility)

- Medical risk factors (history of aspiration, dysphagia)
- Response to prior injections

Based on the aforementioned factors, the dosage range for a patient is calculated based on a low-, moderate-, or high-dose range per muscle and for total dose. Other reported dose modifiers include the GMFCS impairment level. At higher impairment levels, disuse atrophy and muscle weakness are common. A lower dose may be effective (250). When considering BoNT treatment for a patient, there are a number of factors that must also be considered including access to care, financial burden (if the patient has no insurance or limited pharmacy benefit), access to follow-up treatment, and family/patient compliance with physical therapy/home exercise program.

### *Post-BoNT Injection Interventions*

BoNT injections in isolation may reduce tone, but may not improve function or even ROM. Therefore, following BoNT procedures, clinicians should strongly consider referring a child to physical therapy if the child is not already receiving services (257).

### *Adverse Events/Risks in Pediatric Patients*

As noted, reports of aspiration and death in pediatric patients following BoNT therapy led the FDA to add a boxed warning for all BoNTs used in the United States. Although the FDA added this warning to all BoNT products marketed in United States, the FDA did not conclude that BoNT therapy was the cause of death in these patients. A question raised by the preceeding aspiration events in pediatric patients is whether those patients who aspirated and/or died were sedated for the BoNT procedure and if so, how. All physicians who recommend sedation for BoNT procedures for patients with a history of dysphagia and poor oromotor control should be aware that sedation/anesthesia carries a higher risk than in healthy uncompromised patients (ASA [American Society of Anesthesiologists] classification and perioperative risk) (258).

**TABLE 11.1 BoNT for UMNS-Related Upper Limb Muscle Hypertonia: Manufacturer Recommended Dosage/Dilution Table (Adults ≥18 Years of Age)**

| BoNT Preparation | OBTA (Botox®) | ABTA (Dysport®) | IBTA (Xeomin®) | RBTB (Myobloc®) | Notes |
|---|---|---|---|---|---|
| U.S. FDA approval | Adult upper limb spasticity (biceps, FCR, FCU, FDP, FDS) | Currently not FDA approved | Currently not FDA approved | Currently not FDA approved | |
| Outside the United States | Adult upper limb spasticity[1–4]<br>Equinus[1–5] | Adult upper limb spasticity[1,2]<br>Equinus[1,2,5] | Adult upper limb spasticity[1–4]<br>Equinus[1,2,5] | Currently not approved | [1]United Kingdom<br>[2]New Zealand<br>[3]Canada [4]EU [5]In children with CP, <2 years of age |
| **Manufacturer Recommended Dosage Range, United States: Adults (≥18 years of Age)** | | | | | |
| Biceps brachii | 100–200 units, divided among 4 sites | Not an approved indication | Not an approved indication | Not an approved indication | |
| FCR | 12.5–50 units, 1 site | Not an approved indication | Not an approved indication | Not an approved indication | |
| FCU | 12.5–50 units, 1 site | Not an approved indication | Not an approved indication | Not an approved indication | |
| FDP | 30–50 units, 1 site | Not an approved indication | Not an approved indication | Not an approved indication | |
| FDS | 30–50 units, 1 site | Not an approved indication | Not an approved indication | Not an approved indication | |
| Total dose | 75–360 units | Not an approved indication | Not an approved indication | Not an approved indication | |

(continued)

**TABLE 11.1 BoNT for UMNS-Related Upper Limb Muscle Hypertonia: Manufacturer Recommended Dosage/Dilution Table (Adults ≥18 Years of Age) (*continued*)**

| BoNT Preparation | OBTA (Botox®) | ABTA (Dysport®) | IBTA (Xeomin®) | RBTB (Myobloc®) | Notes |
|---|---|---|---|---|---|
| Dilution (concentration) | 100 units in 2-mL PFNS or 200 units in 4-mL PFNS (50 units/mL or 5 units/0.1 mL) | Not an approved indication | Not an approved indication | Not an approved indication | |
| **Outside the United States: Approved Muscles and Dosage** | | | | | |
| Biceps brachii | 100–200 units[2,3] | 300–400 units[1,2] (0.6–0.8 mL) | 80 units[1] (for initial treatment) | Not an approved indication | The optimum dose is patient specific. Use a lower dose for small muscles or if a higher dose may cause weakness. |
| | | | 75–200 units[1,3] (for repeat treatment(s)[1]) | — | |
| Injection sites | Up to 4[3] | 2[1] | 1–4[1,3] | | |
| Brachialis | N/A | N/A | 60 units[1,3] (for initial treatment) | Not an approved indication | |
| | | | 25–100 units[1] (for repeat treatment(s)[1]) | — | |
| Injection sites | N/A | N/A | 1–2[1] | | |
| Brachioradialis | N/A | N/A | 50 units[1,3] (for initial treatment) | Not an approved indication | |
| | | | 25–100 units[1] (for repeat treatment(s)[1]) | — | |
| Injection sites | N/A | N/A | 1–3[1] | | |
| Pronator quadratus | | | 25 units[1,3] (for initial treatment) | Not an approved indication | |
| | | | 10–50 units[1,3] (for repeat treatment(s)[1]) | — | |
| Injection sites | N/A | N/A | 1[1] | | |

(*continued*)

**TABLE 11.1 BoNT for UMNS-Related Upper Limb Muscle Hypertonia: Manufacturer Recommended Dosage/Dilution Table (Adults ≥18 Years of Age) (*continued*)**

| BoNT Preparation | OBTA (Botox®) | ABTA (Dysport®) | IBTA (Xeomin®) | RBTB (Myobloc®) | Notes |
|---|---|---|---|---|---|
| **Outside the United States: Approved Muscles and Dosage (*continued*)** | | | | | |
| Pronator teres | N/A | N/A | 40 units[1,3] (for initial treatment)<br>25–75 units[1] (for repeat treatment[s][1]) | Not an approved indication | |
| Injection sites | N/A | N/A | 1–2[1] | — | |
| FCR | 50 units[1–4] | 150 units[1,2](0.3 mL) | 50 units[1,3] (for initial treatment)<br>25–100 units[1] (for repeat treatment[s][1]) | Not an approved indication | |
| Injection sites | 1–2[2–4] | 1[1] | 1–2[1,3] | — | |
| FCU | 50 units[1]<br>10–50 units[2–4] | 150 units[1,2] (0.3 mL) | 40 units[1,3] (for initial treatment)<br>20–100 units[1] (for repeat treatment[s][1]) | Not an approved indication | |
| Injection sites | 1–2[2–4] | 1[1] | 1–2[1,3] | — | |
| FDP | 50 units[1]<br>15–50 units[2–4] | 150 units[1,2] (0.3 mL) | 40 units[1,3] (for initial treatment)<br>40–100 units[1] (for repeat treatment[s][1]) | Not an approved indication | |
| Injection sites | 1–2[2–4] | 1[1] | 2[1,3] | — | |
| FDS | 50 units[1]<br>15–50 units[2–4] | 150–250 units[1,2](0.3–0.5 mL) | 40 units[1] (for initial treatment)<br>40–100 units[1] (for repeat treatment[s][1]) | Not an approved indication | |
| Injection sites | 1–2[2,3] | 1[1] | 2[1,3] | — | |

(*continued*)

**TABLE 11.1 BoNT for UMNS-Related Upper Limb Muscle Hypertonia: Manufacturer Recommended Dosage/Dilution Table (Adults ≥18 Years of Age) (*continued*)**

| BoNT Preparation | OBTA (Botox®) | ABTA (Dysport®) | IBTA (Xeomin®) | RBTB (Myobloc®) | Notes |
|---|---|---|---|---|---|
| **Outside the United States: Approved Muscles and Dosage (*continued*)** | | | | | |
| FPL | 20 units[1–4] | N/A | 20 units[1,3] (for initial treatment)<br>10–50 units[1] (for repeat treatment[s][1]) | Not an approved indication | |
| Injection sites | 1–2[2–4] | N/A | 1[1,3] | — | |
| Adductor pollicis | 20 units[1–4] | N/A | 10 units[1,3] (for initial treatment)<br>5–30 units[1] (for repeat treatment[s][1]) | Not an approved indication | |
| Injection sites | 1–2[2,3] | — | 1[1,3] | — | |
| Opponens pollicis | 20 units[1–4] | N/A | 10 units[1,3] (for initial treatment)<br>5–30 units[1] (for repeat treatment[s][1]) | Not an approved indication | |
| Injection sites | 1[2,3] | — | 1[1,3] | — | |
| Maximum dose | 240 units[1]<br>360 units[2,3]<br>200–240 units[4] | 1,000 units[1,2] | 170–400 units[1–4] | Not an approved indication | |
| Dilution (concentration) | Not specified<br>100 units in 2-mL PFNS (50 units/mL or 5 units/0.1 mL)[6] | 300-unit vial with 0.6-mL PFNS[1]<br>500-unit vial with 1-mL PFNS[1](500 units/mL or 50 units/0.1 mL)<br>300 units in 1.5-mL PFNS or 500 units in 2.5-mL PFNS (200 units/mL or 20 units/0.1 mL)[6] | Not specified<br>100 units in 1- to 2-mL PFNS is common | RBTB is provided in solution (5,000 units/mL), reconstitution not required If desired, product may be diluted with normal saline. | Reconstitute only with PFNS<br>[6]The most commonly reported dilution in the literature. Higher dilutions have been reported. |

(*continued*)

**TABLE 11.1 BoNT for UMNS-Related Upper Limb Muscle Hypertonia: Manufacturer Recommended Dosage/Dilution Table (Adults ≥18 Years of Age) (*continued*)**

| BoNT Preparation | OBTA (Botox®) | ABTA (Dysport®) | IBTA (Xeomin®) | RBTB (Myobloc®) | Notes |
|---|---|---|---|---|---|
| **Outside the United States: Approved Muscles and Dosage (*continued*)** | | | | | |
| Localization | EMG or e-stim suggested as useful | Standard EMG sites, EMG may be useful[1,2] | EMG or e-stim suggested as useful | Not reported, currently not an approved indication | |
| Re-injection | 12–16 weeks[3] | 12–16 weeks | 12–16 weeks | Not reported, currently not an approved indication | |
| Adverse events | Injection site pain, bruising, fever, flu-like illness, dysphagia, hypertonia, and others | Injection site pain, bruising, fever, flu-like illness, dysphagia, and others | Injection site pain, bruising, fever, flu-like illness, dysphagia, and others | Not reported, currently not an approved indication | |

*Abbreviations:* ABTA, abobotulinumtoxinA; CP, cerebral palsy; EMG, electromyography; e-stim, electrical stimulation; FCR, flexor carpi radialis; FCU, flexor carpi ulnaris; FDA, Food and Drug Administration; FDP, flexor digitorum profundus; FDS, flexor digitorum superficialis; FPL, flexor pollicis longus; IBTA, incobotulinumtoxinA; PFNS, preservative-free normal saline (0.9%); OBTA, onabotulinumtoxinA; RBTB, rimabotulinumtoxinB.

*Sources:* Refs. 34–36, 38, 40, 240–244, 246, 247, 491.

**TABLE 11.2 BoNT for UMNS-Related Upper Limb Muscle Hypertonia: Published Studies Dosage/Dilution Table***

| BoNT Preparation | OBTA (Botox®) | ABTA (Dysport®) | IBTA (Xeomin®) | RBTB (Myobloc®) | Notes |
|---|---|---|---|---|---|
| Typical dosage range | 300–500 units | 500–1,000 units | 300–500 units | 2,500–10,000 units<br>Up 20,000 units reported[1] | [1](238) |
| Published maximum | 850–1,200 units[2,3] | 1,500 units | 840 units[3,4] | 17,500–20,000 units | [2]The safety/efficacy of doses >500 units is not established (239)<br>[3](494)[4](493) [5](492) |
| Paraspinal muscles | 100 units | — | — | — | |
| **Upper Limb Muscles** | | | | | |
| **Shoulder/Pectoral Muscles** | | | | | |
| Deltoid<br>Injection sites | 50–75 units<br>1–3 | 100–200 units<br>1–3 | 50 units[1]<br>1–3 | —<br>— | [1](96)<br>[2](495) |
| Infraspinatus<br>Injection sites | 50–60 units<br>1–2 | 100–150 units<br>1–2 | 20–40 units[1]<br>1–2 | —<br>— | |
| Latissimus dorsi<br>Injection sites | 50–150 units<br>1–3 | 150–500 units<br>1–3 | 20–100 units[1]<br>1–3 | 2,500–7,500 units[2]<br>1–3 | |
| Levator scapulae<br>Injection sites | 10–60 units<br>1–2 | 50–200 units<br>1–2 | 10–60 units[1]<br>1–2 | —<br>— | |
| Pectoralis major<br>Injection sites | 50–150 units<br>1–3 | 60–600 units<br>1–3 | 40–80 units<br>1–3 | —<br>— | |
| Pectoralis major and minor<br>Injection sites | 50–100 units[2]<br>2–4 | 100–300 units[2]<br>2–4 | —<br>— | 2,500–7,500 units[2]<br>2–4 | |

*(continued)*

**TABLE 11.2 BoNT for UMNS-Related Upper Limb Muscle Hypertonia: Published Studies Dosage/Dilution Table* (*continued*)**

| BoNT Preparation | OBTA (Botox®) | ABTA (Dysport®) | IBTA (Xeomin®) | RBTB (Myobloc®) | Notes |
|---|---|---|---|---|---|
| **Upper Limb Muscles (*continued*)** | | | | | |
| **Shoulder/Pectoral Muscles (*continued*)** | | | | | |
| Pectoralis minor<br>Injection sites | 40 units<br>1–2 | 150–500 units<br>1–2 | 20–40 units[1]<br>1 | —<br>— | |
| Rhomboids<br>Injection sites | 50–60 units<br>1–2 | 80–150 units<br>1–2 | 20–40 units[1]<br>1–2 | —<br>— | |
| Serratus anterior<br>Injection sites | 60–70 units<br>1–6 | 150–300 units<br>1–6 | 10–60 units[1]<br>1–6 | —<br>— | |
| Subscapularis<br>Injection sites | 50–100 units<br>1–2 | 100–500 units<br>1–2 | —<br>— | —<br>— | |
| Supraspinatus<br>Injection sites | 40 units<br>1–2 | 100–150 units<br>1–2 | 20–40 units<br>1–2 | —<br>— | |
| Teres major<br>Injection sites | 25–100 units<br>1–2 | 100 units<br>1–2 | 40 units[1]<br>1–2 | 1,500–2,500 units[2]<br>1–2 | |
| Teres minor<br>Injection sites | 25–50 units<br>1–2 | 100 units<br>1–2 | 20 units<br>1–2 | —<br>— | |
| Trapezius<br>Injection sites | 60 units<br>1–3 | 100–250 units<br>1–3 | 15–60 units<br>1–3 | —<br>— | |
| **Elbow Flexors/Extensor** | | | | | |
| Biceps<br>Injection sites | 25–200 units<br>2–4 | 60–600 units, up to 980 units[1] (1,500 units in the United Kingdom)[2]<br>2–4 | 55–200 units<br>2–4 | 833–3,750 units<br>2–4 | [1](497) [2](496)<br>[3](496) [4](495) |

(*continued*)

**TABLE 11.2 BoNT for UMNS-Related Upper Limb Muscle Hypertonia: Published Studies Dosage/Dilution Table* (*continued*)**

| BoNT Preparation | OBTA (Botox®) | ABTA (Dysport®) | IBTA (Xeomin®) | RBTB (Myobloc®) | Notes |
|---|---|---|---|---|---|
| **Elbow Flexors/Extensor (*continued*)** | | | | | |
| Brachialis | 20–100 units | 40–400 units (15,00 units in the United Kingdom)[3] | 25–100 units | 833–1,667 units | |
| Injection sites | 1–2 | 1–2 | 1–2 | 1–2 | |
| Biceps/brachialis | 25–100 units[4] | 100–300 units[2,4] | Not reported | 1,500–5,000 units[4] | |
| Injection sites | 2–3 | 2–3 | Not reported | 2–3 | |
| Brachioradialis | 15–100 units | 75–400 units | 25–100 units | 833–2,500 units | |
| Injection sites | 1–3 | 1–3 | 1–3 | 1–2 | |
| Coracobrachialis | 40 units | 120 units | — | — | |
| Injection sites | 1 | 1 | — | — | |
| Triceps | 50–200 units | 100–500 units | 50–120 units | 250–750 units[4] | |
| Injection sites | 1–3 | 1–3 | 1–3 | — | |
| **Forearm Extensor Muscle Groups** | | | | | |
| EDC | 30–40 units | 100–150 units | 5–30 units[1] | — | [1](96) |
| Injection sites | 1 | 1–2 | 1 | — | [2](495) |
| ECRB | 20–30 units | 60–100 units | 5–20 units[1] | — | |
| Injection sites | 1 | 1–2 | 1 | — | |
| ECRL | 30–40 units | 100–200 units | 5–20 units[1] | — | |
| Injection sites | 1 | 1–2 | 1 | — | |
| ECR | Not reported | Not reported | Not reported | 50–100 units[2] | |
| Injection sites | Not reported | Not reported | Not reported | 1–2 | |
| ECU | 30–40 units | 100–150 units | 5–20 units[1] | 50–100 units[2] | |
| Injection sites | 1–2 | 1–2 | 1–2 | 1–2 | |
| EDM | 30–40 units | 50–100 units | 10 units[1] | 50–100 units[2] | |
| Injection sites | 1 | 1 | 1 | 1 | |

(*continued*)

**TABLE 11.2 BoNT for UMNS-Related Upper Limb Muscle Hypertonia: Published Studies Dosage/Dilution Table* (*continued*)**

| BoNT Preparation | OBTA (Botox®) | ABTA (Dysport®) | IBTA (Xeomin®) | RBTB (Myobloc®) | Notes |
|---|---|---|---|---|---|
| **Forearm Extensor Muscle Groups (*continued*)** | | | | | |
| EIP<br>Injection sites | 20–30 units<br>1 | 50–100 units<br>1 | 5–10 units[1]<br>1 | 50–100 units<br>1 | |
| EPB<br>Injection sites | 5–20 units[1]<br>1 | 20–80 units[1]<br>1 | 5–20 units[1]<br>1 | 50–100 units<br>1 | |
| EPL<br>Injection sites | 20–40 units<br>1 | 50–100 units<br>1 | 5–20 units[1]<br>1 | 50–100 units<br>1 | |
| **Forearm Flexor Muscle Groups** | | | | | |
| FCR<br>Injection sites | 25–120 units<br>1–2 | 75–250 units<br>1–2 | 25–100units<br>1–2 | 1,000–2,500 units<br>1–2 | [1](96) |
| FCU<br>Injection sites | 25–120 units<br>1–2 | 75–250 units<br>1–2 | 20–100 units<br>1–2 | 1,000–2,500 units<br>1–2 | |
| FDP<br>Injection sites | 30–120 units<br>1–4 | 20–300 units<br>1–4 | 40–100 units<br>1–4 | 625 units<br>1–4 | |
| FDS<br>Injection sites | 25–120 units<br>1–4 | 75–500 units<br>1–4 | 40–120 units<br>1–4 | 625–2,500 units<br>1–4 | |
| FPL<br>Injection sites | 15–40 units<br>1 | 40–250 units<br>1–2 | 10–50 units<br>1 | 250–1,000 units<br>1–2 | |
| Palmaris longus<br>Injection sites | 20–25 units<br>1 | 80–100 units<br>1 | 10 units[1]<br>1 | —<br>— | |
| "Forearm finger flexors"<br>Injection sites | 80 units<br>1–4 | Not reported<br>Not reported | Not reported<br>Not reported | Not reported<br>Not reported | |

(*continued*)

**TABLE 11.2 BoNT for UMNS-Related Upper Limb Muscle Hypertonia: Published Studies Dosage/Dilution Table* (*continued*)**

| BoNT Preparation | OBTA (Botox®) | ABTA (Dysport®) | IBTA (Xeomin®) | RBTB (Myobloc®) | Notes |
|---|---|---|---|---|---|
| **Forearm Flexor Muscle Groups (*continued*)** | | | | | |
| "Wrist flexors" dose divided<br>Injection sites | 50–120 units<br>1–2 | Not reported<br>Not reported | Not reported<br>Not reported | Not reported<br>Not reported | |
| **Pronators/Supinators** | | | | | |
| Pronator quadratus<br>Injection sites | 10–50 units<br>1 | 100–150 units<br>1–2 | 10–55 units<br>1 | —<br>— | [1](96) |
| Pronator teres<br>Injection sites | 25–120 units<br>1–3 | 50–350 units<br>1–2 | 10–120 units<br>1–2 | —<br>— | |
| Supinator<br>Injection sites | 5–40 units<br>1–2 | 100–200 units<br>1–2 | 5–30 units[1]<br>1–2 | —<br>— | |
| **Hand: Finger/Thumb Muscles** | | | | | |
| AbPB<br>Injection sites | 2.5–10 units[1]<br>1 | 20–40 units[1]<br>1 | 2.5–30 units<br>1 | 250–500 units[2]<br>1 | [1](96)<br>[2](495) |
| AbPL<br>Injection sites | 10 units<br>1 | 30–80 units<br>1 | 5–30 units<br>1 | 250–500 units[2]<br>1 | |
| AbDM<br>Injection sites | 2.5–5 units[1]<br>1 | 10–20 units[1]<br>1 | 2.5–5 units[1]<br>1 | 250–500 units[2]<br>1 | |
| AdP<br>Injection sites | 10–40 units<br>1 | 40–100 units<br>1 | 5–30 units<br>1 | 250–500 units[2]<br>— | |
| EDM<br>Injection sites | 30–40 units<br>1 | 50–100 units<br>1 | 15–30 units<br>1 | —<br>— | |
| FDM<br>Injection sites | 2.5–10 units[1]<br>1 | 10–20 units[1]<br>1 | 2.5–5 units[1]<br>1 | —<br>— | |

(*continued*)

**TABLE 11.2 BoNT for UMNS-Related Upper Limb Muscle Hypertonia: Published Studies Dosage/Dilution Table* (*continued*)**

| BoNT Preparation | OBTA (Botox®) | ABTA (Dysport®) | IBTA (Xeomin®) | RBTB (Myobloc®) | Notes |
|---|---|---|---|---|---|
| **Hand: Finger/Thumb Muscles (*continued*)** | | | | | |
| EPB<br>Injection sites | 5–20 units<br>1 | 50–75 units<br>1 | 5–20 units<br>1 | —<br>— | |
| FPB<br>Injection sites | 5–25 units<br>1 | 50 units<br>1 | 5–30 units<br>1 | 250–500 units[2]<br>1 | |
| Interossei dorsal/volar<br>Injection sites | 2.5–5 units per muscle belly<br>1 per muscle belly | 10–20 units per muscle belly<br>1 per muscle belly | 2.5–5 units per muscle belly<br>1 per muscle belly | 75–100 units per muscle belly[3]<br>1 per muscle belly | [3]First author's dosage range |
| Interossei, palmar<br>Injection sites | 2.5–5 units per muscle belly<br>1 per muscle belly | 10–20 units per muscle belly<br>1 per muscle belly | 2.5–5 units per muscle belly<br>1 per muscle belly | 75–100 units per muscle belly[3]<br>1 per muscle belly | |
| Lumbricals<br>Injection sites | 2.5–10 units per lumbrical<br>1 per lumbrical | 10–20 units per lumbrical<br>1 per lumbrical | 2.5–10 units per lumbrical<br>1 per lumbrical | 75 units per lumbrical[3]<br>1 per lumbrical | |
| OP<br>Injection sites | 5–25 units<br>1 | 10–40 units<br>1 | 5–30 units<br>1 | 75–100 units[3]<br>1 | |
| ODM<br>Injection sites | 2.5–5 units<br>1 | 10–20 units<br>1 | 2.5–5 units<br>1 | 75 units[3]<br>1 | |
| Mean total dose | Not reported | 600–832 units[4] | Not reported | Not reported | [4](496) |
| Maximum published dose | Up to 850 units[5] | 1500 units | Up to 840–850 units[5] | Up to 19,800 units | [5](494) |
| Dilution (concentration) | 50 units in 1-mL PFNS, 100 units in 2-mL PFNS, or 200 units in 4-mL PFNS (50 units/mL, 5 units/0.1 mL) | 300 units in 1.5-mL PFNS 500 units in 2.5-mL PFNS (200 units/mL, 20 units/0.1 mL) | 100 units in 2-mL PFNS or 200 units in 4-mL PFNS (25 units/mL, 1.5 units/0.1 mL) | Provided in solution (5,000 units/mL). If desired, dilute with PFNS | Optimal dilution has not been established |
| Localization | EMG, e-stim, US | EMG, e-stim, US | EMG, e-stim, US | EMG, e-stim, US | |
| Re-injection | 12–16 weeks | 12–16 weeks | 12–16 weeks | 12–16 weeks | |

(*continued*)

**TABLE 11.2 BoNT for UMNS-Related Upper Limb Muscle Hypertonia: Published Studies Dosage/Dilution Table* (*continued*)**

| BoNT Preparation | OBTA (Botox®) | ABTA (Dysport®) | IBTA (Xeomin®) | RBTB (Myobloc®) | Notes |
|---|---|---|---|---|---|
| **Hand: Finger/Thumb Muscles (*continued*)** | | | | | |
| Adverse events | Injection site pain, bruising, fever, flu-like illness, dysphagia, dry mouth (see full PI) | Injection site pain, bruising, fever, flu-like illness, dysphagia, dry mouth (see full PI) | Injection site pain, bruising, fever, flu-like illness, dysphagia, dry mouth (see full PI) | Injection site pain, bruising, fever, flu-like illness, dysphagia, dry mouth (see full PI) | |
| **Other Muscles** | | | | | |
| Masseter (trismus, poststroke) | Not reported for this indication | Not reported for this indication | Not reported for this indication | 2,500 units/side[1] | [1](273) |
| Oromandibular dosage range | 5–20 units[1] | 20–60 units[1] | 5–20 units[1] | 150–600 units[1] | |

**Note:** The published total dose and dose per muscle group in this table are taken from published clinical studies and texts. The optimal starting dose and retreatment dose are not well established, other than for a limited number of muscles. When calculating the dose per muscle and total dose per treatment session, clinicians should consider the following factors as potential dose modifiers: the BoNT product to be used, the etiology and severity of muscle hypertonia, clinical findings/level of function, treatment goals, medical comorbidities, whether the patient is toxin-naïve, response to prior treatment, number and size of muscles to be injected, and number of injection sites per muscle.

Clinicians should be aware that although doses >400 units of OBTA or IBTA, >1,000 units of ABTA, or >10,000 units of RBTB are reported, these high dosage ranges *may* be associated with an increased incidence of adverse events. The dose on any BoNT product should be increased incrementally based on the patient's clinical condition and response to prior injection(s).

*Unless otherwise noted, the dosage range per muscle reported here is compiled from published studies.

*Abbreviations:* ABTA, abobotulinumtoxinA; AdP, adductor pollicis; AdPB, adductor pollicis brevis; AbDM, abductor digiti minimi; AbPB, abductor pollicis brevis; AbPL, abductor pollicis longus; BoNT, botulinum toxin; ECR, extensor carpi radialis; ECRB, extensor carpi radialis brevis; ECRL, extensor carpi radialis longus; ECU, extensor carpi ulnaris; EDC, extensor digitorum communis; EDM, extensor digiti minimi; EIP, extensor indices proprius; EMG, electromyography; EPB, extensor pollicis brevis; EPL, extensor pollicis longus; e-stim, electrical stimulation; FCR, flexor carpi radialis; FCU, flexor carpi ulnaris; FDM, flexor digiti minimi; FDP, flexor digitorum profundus; FDS, flexor digitorum superficialis; FPB, flexor pollicis brevis; FPL, flexor pollicis longus; IBTA, incobotulinumtoxinA; OBTA, onabotulinumtoxinA; ODM, opponens digiti minimi; OP, opponens pollicis; RBTB, rimabotulinumtoxinB; PFNS, preservative-free normal saline; PI, prescribing information; UMNS, upper motor neuron syndrome; US, ultrasound.

*Sources:* 96, 125, 212, 214–216, 226, 231, 234, 235, 238, 239, 454, 456, 492–527.

**TABLE 11.3 BoNT for UMNS-Related Lower Limb Muscle Hypertonia: Manufacturer Recommended Dosage/Dilution Table (Adults ≥18 Years of Age)**

| BoNT Preparation | OBTA (Botox®) | ABTA (Dysport®) | IBTA (Xeomin®) | RBTB (Myobloc®) | Notes |
|---|---|---|---|---|---|
| U.S. FDA approval | Currently not FDA approved | Currently not FDA approved | Currently not FDA approved | Currently not FDA approved | [1]Approval for lower limb spasticity in adults |
| Approvals in countries outside the United States[1] | New Zealand[2] | Currently not an approved indication | Currently not an approved indication | Currently not an approved indication | |
| **Approved Muscles and Dosage in Countries Outside the United States** | | | | | |
| Gastrocnemius<br>Injection sites | 50–200 units[2]<br>up to 4[2] | N/A<br>N/A | N/A<br>N/A | N/A<br>N/A | [2]Total dose determined by severity of spasticity, weakness, and response to prior injection(s) |
| Soleus<br>Injection sites | 80–125 units[2]<br>1–2[2] | N/A<br>N/A | N/A<br>N/A | N/A<br>N/A | |
| Tibialis posterior<br>Injection sites | 70–100 units[2]<br>1–2[2] | N/A<br>N/A | N/A<br>N/A | N/A<br>N/A | |
| FD<br>Maximum dose<br>Injection sites | 50–100 units[2]<br><br>2–4[2] | N/A<br>N/A<br>N/A | N/A<br>N/A<br>N/A | N/A<br>N/A<br>N/A | |

*(continued)*

**TABLE 11.3 BoNT for UMNS-Related Lower Limb Muscle Hypertonia: Manufacturer Recommended Dosage/Dilution Table (Adults ≥18 Years of Age) (*continued*)**

| BoNT Preparation | OBTA (Botox®) | ABTA (Dysport®) | IBTA (Xeomin®) | RBTB (Myobloc®) | Notes |
|---|---|---|---|---|---|
| **Approved Muscles and Dosage in Countries Outside the United States (*continued*)** | | | | | |
| Dilution | Not specified.<br>50 units in 1-mL PFNS (100 units in 2-mL PFNS or 200 units in 4-mL PFNS) is typical | N/A | N/A | N/A | |
| Localization | EMG, e-stim, or US[2] | N/A | N/A | N/A | |
| Re-injection Interval | Minimum 12 weeks | N/A | N/A | N/A | |
| Adverse events | See full PI and Medsafe.NZ.gov | N/A | N/A | N/A | |

*Abbreviations:* ABTA, abobotulinumtoxinA; BoNT, botulinum toxin; FD, flexor digitorum; FDA, Food and Drug Administration; EMG, electromyography; e-stim, electrical stimulation; IBTA, incobotulinumtoxinA; OBTA, onabotulinumtoxinA; PFNS, preservative-free normal saline; RBTB, rimabotulinumtoxinB; PI, prescribing information; UMNS, upper motor neuron syndrome; US, ultrasound.

*Source:* Ref. 240. Botox NZ Data Sheet Version 11. Medsafe: New Zealand Medicines and Medical Devices Safety Authority. Available at http://www.medsafe.govt.nz/profs/datasheet/b/Botoxinj.pdf. Updated December 2013.

**TABLE 11.4 BoNT for UMNS-Related Lower Limb Muscle Hypertonia: Published Studies Dosage/Dilution Table (Adults ≥18 Years of Age)***

| BoNT Preparation | OBTA (Botox®) | ABTA (Dysport®) | IBTA (Xeomin®) | RBTB (Myobloc®) | Notes |
|---|---|---|---|---|---|
| Typical dose | 300–600 units | 500–1,000 units | 300–500 units | 1,000–10,000 units | |
| Maximum reported dose | 850–1,200 units[1,2] | 1,500 units | 750–840 units reported for combined upper and lower limb injections[2–4] | 17,500[1]–20,000[5] units reported | [1]The safety and efficacy of doses >500 units is not established (239)<br>[2](494)<br>[3](493)<br>[4](492)<br>[5](238) |
| **Hip Girdle and Adductor Muscles** | | | | | |
| Hip adductors | 200–400 units | 850 units | 60–80 units per muscle<br>Total dose: 60–120 units[1] | 5,000–7,500 divided (brevis, longus, and magnus) or 8–22,000 units, divided bilaterally | [1](492) |
| Adductor brevis | 50–100 units | 100–250 units | 20–80 units | 1,500–2,000 units[2] | [2]First author's dosage range |
| Injection sites | 1–2 | 1–2 | 1–2 | 1–2 | |
| Adductor longus | 50–100 units | 100–300 units | 20–100 units | 1,500–2,000 units[2] | |
| Injection sites | 1–3 | 1–3 | 1–3 | 1–3 | |
| Adductor magnus | 30–200 units | 100–500 units | 30–150 units | 1,500–2,000 units[2] | |
| Injection sites | 2–4 | 2–4 | 2–4 | 1–3 | |
| Gluteus maximus | 50–100 units | 100–650 units | 40–100 units | — | Rarely injected |
| Injection sites | 2–4 | 2–4 | 2–4 | — | |

**TABLE 11.4 BoNT for UMNS-Related Lower Limb Muscle Hypertonia: Published Studies Dosage/Dilution Table (Adults ≥18 Years of Age)* (*continued*)**

| BoNT Preparation | OBTA (Botox®) | ABTA (Dysport®) | IBTA (Xeomin®) | RBTB (Myobloc®) | Notes |
|---|---|---|---|---|---|
| **Hip Girdle and Adductor Muscles (*continued*)** | | | | | |
| Gluteus medius | 40–100 units | 70–300 units | 40–60 units | — | |
| Injection sites | 2–3 | 2–3 | 2–3 | — | |
| Gluteus minimus | 20–60 units | 70–100 units | 20–60 units | — | Rarely injected |
| Injection sites | 1–2 | 1–2 | 1–2 | — | |
| Gracilis | 80–120 units | 100–300 units | 60–100 units | 500–1,000 units | |
| Injection sites | 1–3 | 1–3 | 1–3 | — | |
| Hip flexors | 50–200 units | 400–850 units | — | — | |
| Injection sites | 1–2 | 1–2 | — | — | |
| Iliopsoas | 40–200 units | 300–300 units | 25–200 units | 5,000–7,500 units[3] | [3](495) |
| Injection sites | 1–4 | 2–4 | 1–4 | 1–4 | |
| Pectineus | 50–100 units | 150–400 units | 50–80 units | 750–1,000 units[2] | |
| Injection sites | 1 | 1 | 1 | 1 | |
| Piriformis | 50–100 units | 200–500 units | 50–100 units[2] | 750–1,000 units[2] | |
| Injection sites | 1–2 | 1–2 | 1–2 | 1–2 | |
| Psoas major | 50–200 units | 300–400 units | 50–150 units[2] | 750–1,500 units[2] | |
| Injection sites | 1–2 | 1–2 | 1–2 | 1–2 | |
| Rectus femoris | 30–200 units | 100–500 units | 50–100 units | 750–2,000 units[2] | |
| Injection sites | 1–3 | 1–3 | 1–2 | 1–3 | |
| Quadratus lumborum | 100 units | 300 units | 50–100 units | 750–1,000 units[2] | |
| Injection sites | 1–2 | 1–2 | 1–2 | 1–2 | |
| Sartorius | 20–40 units | 70–140 units | 20–40 units | 500–750 units[2] | |
| Injection sites | 1–2 | 1–2 | 1–2 | 1–2 | |

(*continued*)

**TABLE 11.4 BoNT for UMNS-Related Lower Limb Muscle Hypertonia: Published Studies Dosage/Dilution Table (Adults ≥18 Years of Age)* (*continued*)**

| BoNT Preparation | OBTA (Botox®) | ABTA (Dysport®) | IBTA (Xeomin®) | RBTB (Myobloc®) | Notes |
|---|---|---|---|---|---|
| **Hip Girdle and Adductor Muscles (*continued*)** | | | | | |
| Tensor fascia lata | 20–60 units | 70–300 units | 20–60 units | 500–750 units[2] | |
| Injection sites | 1–2 | 1–2 | 1–2 | 1–2 | |
| **Knee Flexors** | | | | | |
| Hamstrings | 50–200 units | Not reported | Not reported | 8–16,000 units, divided | |
| Injection sites | 1–4 | Not reported | Not reported | Not reported | |
| Biceps femoris | 30–200 units | 100–500 units | 50–140 units | 500–1,000 units[1] | [1]First author's dosage range |
| Injection sites | 1–4 | 1–4 | 1–4 | — | |
| Popliteus | 30 units | 100 units | 25–30 units[1] | 250–500 units[1] | |
| Injection sites | 1 | 1–2 | 1–2 | 1–2 | |
| Semimembranosus | 40–200 units | 200–400 units | 40–100 units | 750–1,500 units[1] | |
| Injection sites | 1–4 | 1–4 | 1–4 | 1–4 | |
| Semitendinosus | 30–200 units | 200–400 units | 20–80 units[2] | 750–1,500 units[1] | [2](96) |
| Injection sites | 1–4 | 1–4 | 1–3 | 1–3 | |
| **Knee Extensors** | | | | | |
| Quadriceps | 50–200 units | 350–500 units | 50–70 units | 5,000–7,500 units[1] | [1](495) |
| Injection sites | 1–4 | 1–4 | 1–4 | 1–4 | |
| Rectus femoris | 30–200 units | 300–500 units | 50–100 units | 750–1,000 units[2] | [2]First author's dosage range |
| Injection sites | 1–3 | 1–3 | 1–3 | 1–3 | |
| Vastus intermedius | 20–80 units[3] | 50–300 units[3] | 20–80 units[3] | 500–750 units[2] | [3](96) |
| Injection sites | 1–2 | 1–2 | 1–2 | 1–2 | |

(continued)

**TABLE 11.4 BoNT for UMNS-Related Lower Limb Muscle Hypertonia: Published Studies Dosage/Dilution Table (Adults ≥18 Years of Age)* (*continued*)**

| BoNT Preparation | OBTA (Botox®) | ABTA (Dysport®) | IBTA (Xeomin®) | RBTB (Myobloc®) | Notes |
|---|---|---|---|---|---|
| **Knee Extensors (*continued*)** | | | | | |
| Vastus lateralis<br>Injection sites | 25–60 units<br>1–4 | 50–300 units<br>1–4 | 20–80 units<br>1–4 | 500–750 units[2]<br>1–4 | |
| Vastus medialis<br>Injection sites | 30–80 units<br>1–4 | 50–300 units<br>1–4 | 30–80 units<br>1–4 | 500–750 units[2]<br>1–4 | |
| **Calf Muscles** | | | | | |
| EDL<br>Injection sites | 50–80 units<br>1–2 | 150–250 units<br>1–2 | 40–80 units<br>1–2 | 250–1,000 units[1]<br>1–2 | [1]First author's dosage range |
| EHL<br>Injection sites | 25–160 units<br>1–2 | 100–170 units<br>1–2 | 30–40 units<br>1–2 | 1,000–3,000 units<br>1–2 | |
| FDL<br>Injection sites | 25–125 units<br>1–2 | 150–300 units<br>1–2 | 30–100 units<br>1–2 | 250–1,000 units[1]<br>1–2 | |
| FHL<br>Injection sites | 15–95 units<br>1–2 | 100–200 units<br>1–2 | 15–60 units<br>1–2 | 500–750 units[1]<br>1–2 | |
| Fibularis brevis<br>Injection sites | 30–40 units<br>1 | 80–120 units<br>1–2 | 30–50 units[1]<br>1–2 | 250–500 units[1]<br>1–2 | |
| Fibularis longus<br>Injection sites | 50–80 units<br>1–2 | 100–250 units<br>1–2 | 40 units<br>1–2 | 250–750 units[1]<br>1–2 | |
| Fibularis tertius<br>Injection sites | 30–40 units<br>1 | 80–120 units<br>1 | 30–40 units[1]<br>— | 250–500 units[1]<br>1–2 | |
| Gastrocnemius (medial/lateral) | 50–250 units,[1] divided | 500–1,000 units,[1] divided | 60–200 units | Up to 10,000 units, divided | |
| Gastrocnemius, lateral<br>Injection sites | 50–100 units<br>2–4 | 150–400 units<br>2–4 | 30–100 units<br>2–4 | 1,000–3,000 units[1]<br>2–4 | |

(*continued*)

**TABLE 11.4 BoNT for UMNS-Related Lower Limb Muscle Hypertonia: Published Studies Dosage/Dilution Table (Adults ≥18 Years of Age)* (*continued*)**

| BoNT Preparation | OBTA (Botox®) | ABTA (Dysport®) | IBTA (Xeomin®) | RBTB (Myobloc®) | Notes |
|---|---|---|---|---|---|
| **Calf Muscles (*continued*)** | | | | | |
| Gastrocnemius, medial<br>Injection sites | 50–150 units<br>2–4 | 150–400 units<br>2–4 | 30–150 units<br>2–4 | 1,000–5,000 units[1]<br>2–4 | |
| Soleus<br>Injection sites | 50–200 units<br>1–3 | 250–500 units<br>1–2 | 40–100 units<br>1–2 | 1,000–3,000 units[1]<br>1–2 | |
| Tibialis anterior<br>Injection sites | 30–150 units<br>1–3 | 200–400 units<br>1–3 | 30–80 units<br>1–3 | 1,000–2,500 units[2]<br>1–3 | [2](495) |
| Tibialis posterior<br>Injection sites | 50–100 units<br>1–3 | 100–350 units<br>1–2 | 30–200 units<br>1–2 | 6–8,000 units<br>1–2 | |
| Triceps surae (gastrocnemius and soleus)<br>Injection sites | Not reported<br>Not reported | 500–1,000 units, divided<br>4–6 | Not reported<br>Not reported | 5,000–7,500 units,[2] divided<br>4–6 | |
| **Foot Muscles** | | | | | |
| AbdH<br>Injection sites | 10–20 units[1]<br>1 | 30–80 units[1]<br>1 | 5–20 units[1]<br>1 | 50–100 units<br>1 | [1](96) |
| AdH<br>Injection sites | 5–20 units<br>1 | 30–50 units<br>1 | 5–20 units<br>1 | 50–100 units[2]<br>1 | [2]First author's dosage range |
| AbDM<br>Injection sites | 5–20 units<br>1 | 30–50 units<br>1 | 5–20 units<br>1 | 50–100 units<br>1–2 | |
| EDB<br>Injection sites | 4–70 units<br>1–2 | 50–100 units<br>1–2 | 5–30 units<br>1–2 | 50–100 units<br>1–2 | |
| FDB<br>Injection sites | 20–80 units<br>1–2 | 40–200 units<br>1–2 | 20–80 units<br>1–2 | 50–100 units<br>1–2 | |

(*continued*)

**TABLE 11.4 BoNT for UMNS-Related Lower Limb Muscle Hypertonia: Published Studies Dosage/Dilution Table (Adults ≥18 Years of Age)* (*continued*)**

| BoNT Preparation | OBTA (Botox®) | ABTA (Dysport®) | IBTA (Xeomin®) | RBTB (Myobloc®) | Notes |
|---|---|---|---|---|---|
| **Foot Muscles (*continued*)** | | | | | |
| FHB<br>Injection sites | 10–50 units<br>1–2 | 30–80 units<br>1–2 | 20–50<br>1–2 | 50–250 units<br>1–2 | |
| Interossei, dorsal<br>1–4<br>Injection sites | 5–10 units per muscle[1]<br>1 per muscle belly | 20–40 units per muscle[1]<br>1 per muscle belly | 5–10 units per muscle[1]<br>1 per muscle belly | 50–100 units per muscle belly[2]<br>1 per muscle belly | |
| Interossei, plantar<br>1–3<br>Injection sites | 5–20 units per muscle belly[1]<br>1 per muscle belly | 20–80 units per muscle belly<br>1 per muscle belly | 5–20 units per muscle[1]<br>1 per muscle belly | 50–100 units per muscle belly[2]<br>1 per muscle belly | |
| Lumbricals pedis<br>1–4<br>Injection sites | 5–10 units per muscle belly[1]<br>1 per muscle belly | 20–40 units per muscle[1]<br>1 per muscle belly | 5–10 units per muscle[1]<br>1 per muscle belly | 50–100 units per muscle belly[2]<br>1 per muscle belly | |
| Mean total dose | Not reported | 508–773 units[3] | Not reported | | [3](496) |
| Maximum published dose | 840–850 units | 1,000–1,500 units | 400–500 units is common[4]<br>750–840 units has been reported when both upper and lower limbs were injected[5] | 19,800 units | [4](494)<br>[5](493) |
| Dilution (concentration) | 50 units with 1-mL PFNS, 100 units with 2-mL PFNS, or 200 units with 4-mL PFNS is typical | 500 units in 2.5-mL PFNS (200 units/mL, 20 units/0.1 mL) | 100 units in 2-mL PFNS or 200 units with 4-mL PFNS is typical<br>100 units in 8-mL PFNS has been reported (12.5 units/mL, 1.25 units/0.1 mL) | Provided in solution (5,000 units/mL).<br>If desired, may be further diluted with PFNS | |

(*continued*)

**TABLE 11.4 BoNT for UMNS-Related Lower Limb Muscle Hypertonia: Published Studies Dosage/Dilution Table (Adults ≥18 Years of Age)* (*continued*)**

| BoNT Preparation | OBTA (Botox®) | ABTA (Dysport®) | IBTA (Xeomin®) | RBTB (Myobloc®) | Notes |
|---|---|---|---|---|---|
| **Foot Muscles (*continued*)** | | | | | |
| Localization | Palpation, reference guides, EMG, e-stim, or US | Palpation, reference guides, EMG, e-stim, or US | Palpation, reference guides, EMG, e-stim, or US | Palpation, reference guides, EMG, e-stim, or US | |
| Re-injection interval | 12–16 weeks | 12–16 weeks | 12–16 weeks | 12–16 weeks | |
| Adverse events | Injection site pain, bruising, fever, flu-like illness, dysphagia, dry mouth (see full PI) | Injection site pain, bruising, fever, flu-like illness, dysphagia, dry mouth (see full PI) | Injection site pain, bruising, fever, flu-like illness, dysphagia, dry mouth (see full PI) | Injection site pain, bruising, fever, flu-like illness, dysphagia, dry mouth (see full PI) | |

**Note:** The published total dose and dose per muscle group in this table are taken from published clinical studies and texts. The optimal starting dose and retreatment dose are not well established, other than for a limited number of muscles. When calculating the dose per kilogram and total dose per treatment session, considerations should include: BoNT product to be used, etiology of UMNS, number and size of muscles to be injected, number of injection sites per muscle, clinical findings on examination, severity of hypertonia, treatment goals, medical comorbidities, response to prior treatment, toxin-naïve patients, and other dose modifiers.

Clinicians should be aware that although doses >400 units of OBTA or of IBTA, >1000 units of ABTA, or >10,000 units of RBTB are reported, these high-dose ranges *may* be associated with an increased incidence of adverse events. The dose of any BoNT product should be increased incrementally based on the patient's clinical condition and response to prior injection.

*Unless otherwise noted, the dosage range per muscle reported here is compiled from published studies.

*Abbreviations:* AbDM, abductor digiti minimi; ABTA, abobotulinumtoxinA; AbdH, abductor halluces; AdH, adductor halluces; BoNT, botulinum toxin; EDB, extensor digitorum brevis; EDL, extensor digitorum longus; EHL, extensor hallucis longus; EMG, electromyography; e-stim, electrical stimulation; FDB, flexor digitorum brevis; FDL, flexor digitorum longus; FHB, flexor hallucis brevis; FHL, flexor hallucis longus; IBTA, incobotulinumtoxinA; OBTA, onabotulinumtoxinA; PFNS, preservative-free normal saline; RBTB, rimabotulinumtoxinB; UMNS, upper motor neuron syndrome; US, ultrasound.

*Sources:* Refs. 96, 126, 214, 215, 226, 234, 235, 238, 239, 454, 492, 493–496, 510, 511, 516–518, 520, 521, 527–534, 536–539.

**TABLE 11.5 BoNT for Cerebral Palsy–Associated Muscle Hypertonia: Evolution in Dosage Recommendations: 1997–2014 (Pediatrics <18 Years of Age)**

| BoNT Preparation | OBTA (Botox®) | ABTA (Dysport®) | IBTA (Xeomin®) | RBTB (Myobloc®) | Notes |
|---|---|---|---|---|---|
| **Upper Limb Only: Starting Dose** | | | | | |
| Median starting dose[1] | 4.1 units/kg[1] | 7.3 units/kg[1] | Not reported | Not reported | [1](540) |
| Median starting dosage range[1] | 2.7–6.25 units/kg[1] | 4.7–11.4 units/kg[1] | Not reported | Not reported | |
| Maximum starting dose[1] | 19.3 units/kg[1] | 34.7 units/kg[1] | Not reported | Not reported | |
| **Maximum Recommended Dose: Upper Limb** | | | | | |
| 2012 (upper limb) | 19.3 units/kg[1] | 34.7 units/kg[1] | Not reported | Not reported | [1](540) |
| **Lower Limbs Only** | | | | | |
| Distal lower limbs, mean dosage | 18.6 units/kg (±6.5 units)[1] | | | | [1](541) |
| **Maximum Dose: Combined Upper and Lower Limbs** | | | | | |
| 2014[2] (based on 2009 consensus recommendation) | 20 units/kg[2] 400 units (±600 units) | 30 units/kg[2–4] 1,000 units | Adult studies *suggested* dose is equivalent to OBTA. However, data to support this are limited, particularly in children[2] | | [2](250) [3](499) [4](515) |

*(continued)*

**TABLE 11.5 BoNT for Cerebral Palsy–Associated Muscle Hypertonia: Evolution in Dosage Recommendations: 1997–2014 (Pediatrics <18 Years of Age) (*continued*)**

| BoNT Preparation | OBTA (Botox®) | ABTA (Dysport®) | IBTA (Xeomin®) | RBTB (Myobloc®) | Notes |
|---|---|---|---|---|---|
| **Maximum Dose: Combined Upper and Lower Limbs (*continued*)** | | | | | |
| 2013[5] | 20–30 units/kg<br>500 units maximum dose per treatment session[5] | 30 units/kg<br>1,500 units maximum dose per treatment session[5] | | Mean: 343.4 units/kg<br>Range: 73.7–657.9 units/kg[6] Mean: 8,959 units[7]<br>Range: 300–22,000[6] | [5](254) [6](543)<br>[7](542) |
| 2009[2]<br>Dosage range | 1–20 units/kg (±25) | 1–20 (±25) units/kg | Adult studies *suggested* dose is equivalent to OBTA.[2] However, data to support this are limited, particularly in children | Not established. Up to 400 units/kg used in small pilot[8] | |
| Max dose | 400 units (up to 600 units is reported; use doses >400 units with caution in vulnerable patients) | 500–1,000 units | | Not established | |
| Max dose per injection site | 10–50 units | 50–250 units | | Not established | |
| 2007 | | | | 50–200 units/kg, upper limbs only[6] | |

(*continued*)

**TABLE 11.5 BoNT for Cerebral Palsy–Associated Muscle Hypertonia: Evolution in Dosage Recommendations: 1997–2014 (Pediatrics <18 Years of Age) (*continued*)**

| BoNT Preparation | OBTA (Botox®) | ABTA (Dysport®) | IBTA (Xeomin®) | RBTB (Myobloc®) | Notes |
|---|---|---|---|---|---|
| **Maximum Dose: Combined Upper and Lower Limbs (*continued*)** | | | | | |
| 2006[9] | 6–25 units/kg[9]<br>400–600 units[9] | 11–25 units/kg[9] 900 units[9] | | 150–400 units/kg[9]<br>10,000 units[9] | [8](546) [9](253)<br>[10](544)<br>[11](545) |
| 2006[10] | 30 units/kg | | | | |
| 2004[11]<br>Upper and lower limbs | 13–17 units/kg[11] | | | Maximum<br>400 units/kg[8] Maximum dose 10,000 units | |
| 1999–2005[8] | 12–20 units/kg<br>400 units maximum dose per treatment session[12] | 30–50 units/kg<br>2,000 units maximum per treatment session[12] | | | [12](254) |
| 1997[12]<br>Upper and lower limbs | 4–7 units/kg[13]<br>(90–250 units)[13] | 8–9 units/kg[13]<br>160–400 units[13] | | | [13](509) |

*Abbreviations:* ABTA, abobotulinumtoxinA; BoNT, botulinum toxin; IBTA, incobotulinumtoxinA; OBTA, onabotulinumtoxinA; RBTB, rimabotulinumtoxinB.

*Sources:* Refs. 250, 253, 254, 499, 509, 540–547.

**TABLE 11.6 BoNT for Cerebral Palsy–Associated Upper Limb Muscle Hypertonia: Manufacturer Recommended Dosage/Dilution Table (Pediatrics < 18 Years of Age)**

| BoNT Preparation | OBTA (Botox®) | ABTA (Dysport®) | IBTA (Xeomin®) | RBTB (Myobloc®) | Notes |
|---|---|---|---|---|---|
| U.S. FDA approval | Currently not FDA approved | Currently not FDA approved | Currently not FDA approved | Currently not FDA approved | |
| Approvals in countries outside the United States[1] | New Zealand[2] | Currently not an approved indication | Currently not an approved indication | Currently not an approved indication | [1]Approved for pediatric upper limb spasticity |
| **Countries Outside the United States** | | | | | |
| Biceps | 0.5–2 units/kg[2] | Not an approved indication | Not an approved indication | Not an approved indication | [2]The number of injection sites and location in each muscle is determined by the size of the muscle and the specific muscle group. |
| Brachialis | 0.5–2 units/kg[2] | Not an approved indication | Not an approved indication | Not an approved indication | |
| Brachioradialis | 0.5–2 units/kg[2] | Not an approved indication | Not an approved indication | Not an approved indication | |
| Pronator quadratus | 0.5–2 units/kg[2] | Not an approved indication | Not an approved indication | Not an approved indication | |
| Pronator teres | 0.5–2 units/kg[2] | Not an approved indication | Not an approved indication | Not an approved indication | |
| FCR | 0.5–2 units/kg[2] | Not an approved indication | Not an approved indication | Not an approved indication | |
| FCU | 0.5–2 units/kg[2] | Not an approved indication | Not an approved indication | Not an approved indication | |
| FDP | 0.5–2 units/kg[2] | Not an approved indication | Not an approved indication | Not an approved indication | |
| FDS | 0.5–2 units/kg[2] | Not an approved indication | Not an approved indication | Not an approved indication | |

*(continued)*

**TABLE 11.6 BoNT for Cerebral Palsy–Associated Upper Limb Muscle Hypertonia: Manufacturer Recommended Dosage/Dilution Table (Pediatrics < 18 Years of Age) (*continued*)**

| BoNT Preparation | OBTA (Botox®) | ABTA (Dysport®) | IBTA (Xeomin®) | RBTB (Myobloc®) | Notes |
|---|---|---|---|---|---|
| **Countries Outside the United States (*continued*)** | | | | | |
| FPB | 0.5–2 units/kg[2] | Not an approved indication | Not an approved indication | Not an approved indication | |
| FPL | 0.5–2 units/kg[2] | Not an approved indication | Not an approved indication | Not an approved indication | |
| Opponens pollicis | 0.5–2 units/kg[2] | Not an approved indication | Not an approved indication | Not an approved indication | |
| Adductor pollicis | 0.5–2 units/kg[2] | Not an approved indication | Not an approved indication | Not an approved indication | |
| Total dose | 3–8 units/kg or 300 units[2] | Not an approved indication | Not an approved indication | Not an approved indication | |
| Dilution (concentration) | 100 units in 2-mL PFNS or 200 units in 4-mL PFNS (50 units/mL, 5 units/0.1 mL) | N/A | N/A | N/A | |
| Re-injection interval | ≥12 weeks | N/A | N/A | N/A | |
| Localization | EMG, e-stim, US | N/A | N/A | N/A | |
| Adverse events | | N/A | N/A | N/A | |

*Abbreviations:* ABTA, abobotulinumtoxinA; BoNT, botulinum toxin; EMG, electromyography; e-stim, electrical stimulation; FCR, flexor carpi radialis; FCU, flexor carpi ulnaris; FDA, Food and Drug Administration; FDP, flexor digitorum profundus; FDS, flexor digitorum superficialis; FPB, flexor pollicis brevis; FPL, flexor pollicis longus; IBTA, incobotulinumtoxinA; OBTA, onabotulinumtoxinA; PFNS, preservative-free normal saline; RBTB, rimabotulinumtoxinB; US, ultrasound.

*Source:* Ref. 240. Botox NZ Data Sheet Version 11. Medsafe: New Zealand Medicines and Medical Devices Safety Authority. Available at http://www.medsafe.govt.nz/profs/datasheet/b/Botoxinj.pdf. Updated December 2013.

**TABLE 11.7 BoNT for Cerebral Palsy/Acquired Brain Injury–Associated Upper Limb Muscle Hypertonia: Published Studies Dosage/Dilution Table (Pediatrics < 18 Years of Age)**

| BoNT Preparation | OBTA (Botox®) | ABTA (Dysport®) | IBTA (Xeomin®) | RBTB (Myobloc®) | Notes |
|---|---|---|---|---|---|
| **Upper limb: Starting Dose** | | | | | |
| Median starting dose[1] | 4.1 units/kg[1] | 7.3 units/kg[1] | Not reported | Not reported | [1](540) |
| Median starting dose range[1] | 2.7–6.25 units/kg[1] | 4.7–11.4 units/kg[1] | Not reported | Not reported | |
| Maximum starting dose[1] | 19.3 units/kg[1] | 34.7 units/kg[1] | Not reported | Not reported | |
| **Average Dose In Patients <3 Years of Age** | | | | | |
| Age <12 months Dose divided (≥6 upper limb muscles and/or ≥4 lower limb muscles) | 10.98 units/kg[1] | Not reported | Not reported | Not reported | [1](548) |
| Age 12–24 months Dose divided (≥6 upper limb muscles and/or ≥4 lower limb muscles) | 11.89 units/kg[1] | Not reported | Not reported | Not reported | |
| Age 25–36 months Dose divided (≥6 upper limb muscles and/or ≥4 lower limb muscles) | 14.07 units/kg[1] | Not reported | Not reported | Not reported | |

*(continued)*

**TABLE 11.7 BoNT for Cerebral Palsy/Acquired Brain Injury–Associated Upper Limb Muscle Hypertonia: Published Studies Dosage/Dilution Table (Pediatrics < 18 Years of Age) (*continued*)**

| BoNT Preparation | OBTA (Botox®) | ABTA (Dysport®) | IBTA (Xeomin®) | RBTB (Myobloc®) | Notes |
|---|---|---|---|---|---|
| **Average Dose In Patients <3 Years of Age (*continued*)** | | | | | |
| Suggested maximum dose for combined upper and lower limbs | 10–20 units/kg up to 400 units (up to 600 units is reported; use doses >400 units with caution in vulnerable patients) | 10–30 units/kg up to 1,000 units (up to 1,500 units is reported; use doses >1,000 units with caution in vulnerable patients) | Dosage range not well established | Mean: 343.4 units/kg<br>Range: 73.7–657.9 units/kg<br>Mean: 8,959 units<br>Range: 300–22,000 units<br>1–10 muscles[2] | [2](542) |
| Note: The optimal starting, retreatment, and maximum doses of BoNTs for pediatric patients are not well established, other than for a limited number of muscles. When calculating the dose per kg and total dose per treatment session, considerations should include: BoNT product to be used, diagnosis, comorbidities, patient age/weight, findings on clinical examination, severity of hypertonia, number/size of the muscles to be injected, treatment goals, if the patient is toxin-naïve, response to prior treatment, and other dose modifiers.<br>Clinicians should be aware that although dosages of >400 units of OBTA or of IBTA, >1000 units of ABTA, or >10,000 units of RBTB have been reported in the literature, the use of these high dosages *may* be associated with an increased incidence of adverse events. | | | | | |
| Latissimus dorsi | 1.13–3 units/kg[1]<br>1–3 units/kg[2] | 3–5 units/kg[2] | 1–3 units/kg[2] | 10–25 units/kg[2] | [1]New Zealand Medsafe reported dose<br>[2]First author's initial dosage range<br>[3](543) |
| Pectoralis major | 0.6–3 units/kg | 3–5 units/kg[2] | 1–3 units/kg[2] | 12–25 units/kg[2] | |
| Teres major | 0.5–3 units/kg | 3–5 units/kg[2] | 1–3 units/kg[2] | 17.8 units/kg<br>10–15 units/kg[2] | |
| Biceps brachii | 0.5–3 units/kg[3]<br>1–3 units/kg[2] | 3–5 units/kg[2] | 1–3 units/kg[2] | 12.5–50 units/kg[3]<br>10–25 units/kg[2] | |
| Biceps/brachialis | 1.2–2.2 units/kg[1]<br>1–3 units/kg | 3–5 units/kg[2] | 1–3 units/kg[2] | 12.5–50 units/kg[3] | |

(*continued*)

**TABLE 11.7 BoNT for Cerebral Palsy/Acquired Brain Injury–Associated Upper Limb Muscle Hypertonia: Published Studies Dosage/Dilution Table (Pediatrics < 18 Years of Age) (*continued*)**

| BoNT Preparation | OBTA (Botox®) | ABTA (Dysport®) | IBTA (Xeomin®) | RBTB (Myobloc®) | Notes |
|---|---|---|---|---|---|
| **Average Dose in Patients <3 Years of Age (*continued*)** | | | | | |
| Brachialis | 0.5–2.4 units/kg[1] | | | | |
| Elbow flexors (biceps, brachialis, brachioradialis) | 4.6 ± 0.36 units/kg[4] | Not reported | Not reported | Not reported | [4](545) |
| Brachioradialis | 0.5–2 units/kg[1]<br>0.5–2 units/kg[2] | 2.5–15 units/kg[2] | 0.5–2 units/kg[2] | 12.5–50 units/kg[3]<br>7.5–20 units/kg[2] | |
| Pronator quadratus | 0.5–2 units/kg[1]<br>0.5–1.5 units/kg[2] | 2.5–10 units/kg[2] | 0.5–1 units/kg[2] | 7.5–15 units/kg[2] | |
| Pronator teres | 0.5–3.3 units/kg[1]<br>0.5–2 units/kg[2] | 2.5–15 units/kg[2] | 0.5–2 units/kg[2] | 10–25 units/kg[2] | |
| Pronators (pronator teres, pronator quadratus) | 2.03 ± 0.32 units/kg[4] | Not reported | Not reported | Not reported | |
| FCR | 0.5–2.5 units/kg | 2.8–5 units/kg | 0.5–2.5 units/kg[2] | 12–25 units/kg[2] | |
| FCU | 0.5–2.3 units/kg | 2.6–5 units/kg | 0.5–2.5 units/kg[2] | 12–25 units/kg[2] | |
| Wrist flexors (FCR, FCU) | 2.31 ± 0.73 units/kg[4] | Not reported | Not reported | Not reported | |
| FDP | 0.5–2 units/kg<br>0.5–2.5 units/kg[2] | 1.5–5 units/kg | 0.5–2.5 units/kg[2] | 12–25 units/kg[2] | |
| FDS | 0.5–2 units/kg | 2.9–4 units/kg | 0.5–2.5 units/kg[2] | 12–25 units/kg[2] | |
| Finger flexors (FDP, FDS) | 3.13 ± 1.2 units/kg[4] | Not reported | Not reported | Not reported | |

(*continued*)

**TABLE 11.7 BoNT for Cerebral Palsy/Acquired Brain Injury–Associated Upper Limb Muscle Hypertonia: Published Studies Dosage/Dilution Table (Pediatrics < 18 Years of Age) (*continued*)**

| BoNT Preparation | OBTA (Botox®) | ABTA (Dysport®) | IBTA (Xeomin®) | RBTB (Myobloc®) | Notes |
|---|---|---|---|---|---|
| **Average Dose in Patients <3 Years of Age (*continued*)** | | | | | |
| FDI | 0.2–0.8 units/kg or<br>5–10 units[1]<br>2.5–5 units[2] | 5–10 units[2] | 2.5–5 units[2] | 10–25 units[2] | [5](509) |
| FPL | 0.5–2 units/kg[1]<br>0.5–2 units/kg[2]<br>Maximum<br>50–60 units | 2.5–5 units/kg[2]<br>Maximum 75–100 units[2] | 0.5–2 units/kg[2]<br>Maximum 50–60 units[2] | 75–250 units[2] | |
| FPB | 0.5–2 units/kg or<br>5–10 units[1] | 5–10 units[2] | 2.5–5 units[2] | 10–25 units[2] | |
| Opponens pollicis | 0.5–2 units/kg or<br>5–10 units[1] | 2.5–5 units/kg<br>Maximum 75–100 units | 0.5–2 units/kg[2]<br>Maximum 50–60 units | 75–250 units | |
| Adductor pollicis | 0.5–2 units/kg or<br>5–10 units[1] | 2.5–5 units/kg<br>Maximum 75–100 units | 0.5–2 units/kg[2]<br>Maximum 50–60 units | 75–250 units | |
| Thumb (FPL, AdP, OP) | 2.5 units/kg[4] | Not reported | Not reported | Not reported | |
| Upper limb (biceps, brachialis, FCR, FCU, PT, FPL, FPB, AdP) | 4–7 units/kg[5]<br>90–250 units[5] | 8–9 units/kg[5]<br>160–400 units[5] | Not reported | 50–200 units/kg[3] | |
| Total dose (upper limb only) | 3–19 units/kg is common<br>≤300 units[1] | 7.3–34 units/kg | Not reported | 50–200 units/kg[3] | |

(*continued*)

**TABLE 11.7 BoNT for Cerebral Palsy/Acquired Brain Injury–Associated Upper Limb Muscle Hypertonia: Published Studies Dosage/Dilution Table (Pediatrics < 18 Years of Age) (*continued*)**

| BoNT Preparation | OBTA (Botox®) | ABTA (Dysport®) | IBTA (Xeomin®) | RBTB (Myobloc®) | Notes |
|---|---|---|---|---|---|
| **Average Dose in Patients <3 Years of Age (*continued*)** | | | | | |
| Total dose (combined upper and lower limbs) | 12–16 units is common<br>28–32 units/kg has been reported[5] | 10–20 units/kg (≤1,000 units) is common<br>≤30 units/kg (≤30,000 units) has been reported | Limited data on dosage in pediatric patients | Mean: 343.4 units/kg<br>Range: 73.7–657.9 units/kg<br>Mean: 8,959 units<br>Range: 300–22,000 units<br>1–10 muscles[6] | [6](542) |
| Dilution (concentration) | 100 units in 2-mL PFNS or 200 units in 4-mL PFNS (50 units/mL, 5 units/0.1 mL) | 500 units in 1-mL PFNS is most commonly reported dilution (500 units/mL or 50 units/0.1 mL<br>500 units in 2.5-mL PFNS is also reported (200 units/mL, 20 units/0.1 mL) | 100 units in 2-mL PFNS or 200 units in 4-mL PFNS (50 units/mL, 5 units/0.1 mL) | RBTB does not require reconstitution. If desired, saline can be added to increase the dilution | |

(*continued*)

**TABLE 11.7 BoNT for Cerebral Palsy/Acquired Brain Injury–Associated Upper Limb Muscle Hypertonia: Published Studies Dosage/Dilution Table (Pediatrics < 18 Years of Age) (*continued*)**

| BoNT Preparation | OBTA (Botox®) | ABTA (Dysport®) | IBTA (Xeomin®) | RBTB (Myobloc®) | Notes |
|---|---|---|---|---|---|
| **Average Dose in Patients <3 Years of Age (*continued*)** | | | | | |
| Retreatment Interval | ≥12 weeks | ≥12 weeks | ≥12 weeks | ≥12 weeks | |
| Localization | Palpation, reference guides, EMG, e-stim, US | Palpation, reference guides, EMG, e-stim, US | Palpation, reference guides, EMG, e-stim, US | Palpation, reference guides, EMG, e-stim, US | |

Adverse events (see the boxed warning from each manufacturer for a complete list of adverse events): Common: injection site pain, bruising, muscle weakness, flu-like symptoms. Less common: dysphagia, diplopia, generalized weakness.

*Abbreviations:* ABTA, abobotulinumtoxinA; AdP, adductor pollicis; BoNT, botulinum toxin; EMG, electromyography; e-stim, electrical stimulation; FCR, flexor carpi radialis; FCU, flexor carpi ulnaris; FDI, first dorsal interosseous; FDP, flexor digitorum profundus; FDS, flexor digitorum superficialis; FPB, flexor pollicis brevis; FPL, flexor pollicis longus; IBTA, incobotulinumtoxinA; OBTA, onabotulinumtoxinA; OP, opponens pollicis; PFNS, preservative-free normal saline; PT, pronator teres; RBTB, rimabotulinumtoxinB; US, ultrasound.

*Sources:* Refs. 232, 250, 252–254, 510, 540, 542–546, 548–553.

**TABLE 11.8 BoNT for Cerebral Palsy–Associated Lower Limb Muscle Hypertonia: Manufacturer Recommended Dosage/Dilution Table (Pediatrics < 18 Years of Age)**

| BoNT Preparation | OBTA (Botox®) | ABTA (Dysport®) | IBTA (Xeomin®) | RBTB (Myobloc®) | Notes |
|---|---|---|---|---|---|
| U.S. FDA approval | Currently not FDA approved | Currently not FDA approved | Currently not FDA approved | Currently not FDA approved | |
| UK MHRA[1,5]<br>New Zealand[2]<br>Canada[3]<br>EU[4] | Pediatric CP[1–4] | Dynamic equinus, pediatric CP[1,2] | Not currently approved for pediatric spasticity | Currently not FDA approved | [1–4]CP ≥ 2 years of age, ambulatory patients<br>[5]Only hospital specialists with training |
| Gastrocnemius (medial and lateral heads) | 4 units/kg, total dose[1] | 10–30 units/kg (per PI), focus is gastrocnemius.<br>If the soleus and/or tibialis posterior are involved, dose is divided. | Not an approved indication | Not an approved indication | [1]2 units/kg per muscle, if bilateral |
| | 2–4 units/kg per muscle[2] | | | | |
| | 4 units/kg unilateral, up to 6 units/kg if bilateral[3,4] | | | | |

(continued)

**TABLE 11.8 BoNT for Cerebral Palsy–Associated Lower Limb Muscle Hypertonia: Manufacturer Recommended Dosage/Dilution Table (Pediatrics <18 Years of Age) (*continued*)**

| BoNT Preparation | OBTA (Botox®) | ABTA (Dysport®) | IBTA (Xeomin®) | RBTB (Myobloc®) | Notes |
|---|---|---|---|---|---|
| Soleus | Not reported | Focus is gastrocnemius. If the soleus and/or tibialis posterior are involved, dose is divided.[1] | Not an approved indication | Not an approved indication | |
| Tibialis anterior | Not reported | — | Not an approved indication | — | |
| Tibialis posterior | Not reported | Focus is gastrocnemius. If the soleus and/or tibialis posterior are involved, dose is divided.[1] | Not an approved indication | Not an approved indication | |
| Adductor group | 4 units/kg per muscle[2] | — | Not an approved indication | Not an approved indication | |
| Hamstrings | 2–4 units/kg per muscle[2] | — | Not an approved indication | Not an approved indication | |
| Maximum cumulative dose[2] | 4–8 units/kg, Not to exceed 300–400 units[2] | 10–30 units/kg 1,000–1,500 units | Not an approved indication | Not an approved indication | [1,2]Use lower doses for smaller muscles or if there are concerns about weakness |
| Combined upper/lower limb<br>Injection sites | Varies per country 4–8 units/kg[1–3]<br>Not specified | 10–30 units/kg 1,000–1,500 units<br>Not specified | Not an approved indication<br>N/A | Not an approved indication<br>N/A | [3]Higher doses associated with an increased risk of adverse events |

(*continued*)

**TABLE 11.8 BoNT for Cerebral Palsy–Associated Lower Limb Muscle Hypertonia: Manufacturer Recommended Dosage/Dilution Table (Pediatrics < 18 Years of Age) (*continued*)**

| BoNT Preparation | OBTA (Botox®) | ABTA (Dysport®) | IBTA (Xeomin®) | RBTB (Myobloc®) | Notes |
|---|---|---|---|---|---|
| Dilution | Not specified | 500 units with 1-mL PFNS[1,2] | N/A | N/A | |
| Re-injection interval | 12–16 weeks[1–4] | 12–16 weeks | N/A | N/A | |
| Localization | Not specified[1,3,4] EMG, e-stim, or US recommended[2] | EMG suggested to help identify muscles[1,2] | N/A | N/A | [4](242) |
| Adverse events | Muscle weakness, injection site pain, and/or bruising, flu-like symptoms, aspiration-related death | Muscle weakness, injection site pain, and/or bruising, flu-like symptoms, aspiration-related death | N/A | N/A | |

*Abbreviations:* ABTA, abobotulinumtoxinA; BoNT, botulinum toxin; EMG, electromyography; e-stim, electrical stimulation; FDA, Food and Drug Administration; IBTA, incobotulinumtoxinA; OBTA, onabotulinumtoxinA; PFNS, preservative-free normal saline; RBTB, rimabotulinumtoxinB; US, ultrasound.

*Sources:* Refs. 34–36, 38, 40, 240–244, 246, 247.

**TABLE 11.9 BoNT for Cerebral Palsy/Acquired Brain Injury–Associated Lower Limb Muscle Hypertonia: Published Studies Dosage/Dilution Table (Pediatrics < 18 Years of Age)**

| BoNT Preparation | OBTA (Botox®) | ABTA (Dysport®) | IBTA (Xeomin®) | RBTB (Myobloc®) | Notes |
|---|---|---|---|---|---|
| Commonly reported lower dosage ranges | 6–12 units/kg<br>400 units[1] | 10–20 units/kg<br>500–1,000 units[1] | Not established. Adult studies *suggest* dose equivalence to OBTA. This equivalence is *not established* in adults or in children[1] | Not established due to limited data from published studies. In clinical practice, 200–400 units/kg or total dose of 2,500–10,000 are reported. | [1](250) |
| Commonly reported higher dose ranges | 16–19 units/kg (≤30 units/kg reported)[1–4]<br>Maximum dose 400 units (≤600 units reported)[1–4] | 20–30 units/kg[1,5–8]<br>375–700 units[9]<br>1000 units[1,5–7]<br>1200 units[12] (≤1500 units reported)[9] | Not established[1]<br>16–19 units/kg reported.<br>Maximum dose: Not established. Adult studies *suggest* dose equivalence to OBTA. This equivalence is *not established* in adults or in children[1] | 343–400 units/kg[10,11]<br>Maximum dose:<br>8–10,000 units[10]<br>9–22,000 units[11] | [2](252)<br>[3](253)<br>[4](541)<br>[5](499)<br>[6](547)<br>[7](554)<br>[8](556)<br>[9](496)<br>[10](546)<br>[11](542)<br>[12](555) |

(continued)

**TABLE 11.9 BoNT for Cerebral Palsy/Acquired Brain Injury–Associated Lower Limb Muscle Hypertonia: Published Studies Dosage/Dilution Table (Pediatrics < 18 Years of Age) (*continued*)**

| BoNT Preparation | OBTA (Botox®) | ABTA (Dysport®) | IBTA (Xeomin®) | RBTB (Myobloc®) | Notes |
|---|---|---|---|---|---|
| **Patients <2 Years of Age: Reported Dosage Range, Lower Limbs** | | | | | |
| Average dose<br>Age 0–1 year | 7.2 units/kg[1] | 19.5 units/kg[1] | Not reported | Not reported | [1](256) |
| Age 1–2 years | 8.8 units/kg[1] | 23.6 units/kg[1] | Not reported | Not reported | |
| Maximum dose<br>Age 0–2 years | 14.29 units/kg[1] | 37.5 units/kg[1] | Not reported | Not reported | |
| Average dosage (combined for upper and lower limbs)<br>Age 0–1 year | 10.98 units/kg[2] | | Not reported | Not reported | [2](548) |
| Age 1–2 years | 11.89 units/kg[2] | | Not reported | Not reported | |
| Note: The optimal starting, retreatment, and maximum doses of BoNTs for pediatric patients are not well established, other than for a limited number of muscles. When calculating the dose per kilogram and total dose per treatment session, considerations should include BoNT product to be used, diagnosis, comorbidities, patient age/weight, findings on clinical examination, severity of hypertonia, number/size of the muscles to be injected, treatment goals, if the patient is toxin-naïve, response to prior treatment, and other dose modifiers. Clinicians should be aware that although dosages of >400 units of OBTA or of IBTA, >1000 units of ABTA, or >10,000 units of RBTB have been reported in the literature, the use of these high dosages *may* be associated with an increased incidence of adverse events. | | | | | |
| **Published Dosage Ranges, Lower Limb Muscles (Pediatric Patient, <18 Years of Age)** | | | | | |
| Large muscle groups | 3–6 units/kg[1] | Not reported | Not reported | 1,000–5,000 units[2] | [1](550) |
| Small muscle groups | 0.5–2 units/kg[1] | Not reported | Not reported | 500–1,000 units[2] | [2](546) |

(*continued*)

**TABLE 11.9 BoNT for Cerebral Palsy/Acquired Brain Injury–Associated Lower Limb Muscle Hypertonia: Published Studies Dosage/Dilution Table (Pediatrics <18 Years of Age) (*continued*)**

| BoNT Preparation | OBTA (Botox®) | ABTA (Dysport®) | IBTA (Xeomin®) | RBTB (Myobloc®) | Notes |
|---|---|---|---|---|---|
| **Hip Girdle** | | | | | |
| Adductor group | 3–6 units/kg, divided | 7.5–15 units/kg per limb (up to 20 units/kg per limb, if unilateral) | Not reported | 1,000–5,000 units[1] | [1](546)<br>[2]First author's initial dosage range |
| Adductor brevis | 1.5–2 units/kg | 5 units/kg | 1.5–2 units/kg[2] | 1,000–5,000 units[1] | |
| Adductor longus | 1.6–2.4 units/kg | 5 units/kg | 1.5–2.5 units/kg[2] | 1,000–5,000 units[1] | |
| Adductor magnus | 2–3 units/kg | 5 units/kg | 2–3 units/kg[2] | 1,000–5,000 units[1] | |
| Gracilis | 1.5–2.2 units/kg | 5 units/kg | 1.5–2.5 units/kg[2] | 1,000–5,000 units[1] | |
| Iliopsoas | 2–6 units/kg | 12 units/kg | 2–5 units/kg[2] | 1,000–5,000 units[1] | |
| Pectineus | 2–3 units/kg | 5 units/kg | 2–3 units/kg[2] | 1,000–5,000 units[1] | |
| Psoas | 2–6 units/kg | 3–7.5 units/kg[2] | 2–5 units/kg[2] | 1,000–5,000 units[1] | |
| **Knee Flexors/Extensors** | | | | | |
| Hamstrings | 2–6 units/kg/muscle | 7.5–13 units/kg | 2–5 units/kg/muscle[1] | 1,000–5,000 units[2] | [1]First author's initial dosage range<br>[2](546) |
| Semimembranosis | 2–6 units/kg/muscle | 5–6.5 units/kg | 2–5 units/kg/muscle[1] | 1,000–5,000 units[2] | |

(*continued*)

**TABLE 11.9 BoNT for Cerebral Palsy/Acquired Brain Injury–Associated Lower Limb Muscle Hypertonia: Published Studies Dosage/Dilution Table (Pediatrics <18 Years of Age) (*continued*)**

| BoNT Preparation | OBTA (Botox®) | ABTA (Dysport®) | IBTA (Xeomin®) | RBTB (Myobloc®) | Notes |
|---|---|---|---|---|---|
| **Knee Flexors/Extensors (*continued*)** | | | | | |
| Semitendinosis | 2–6 units/kg/muscle | 5–6.5 units/kg | 2–5 units/kg/muscle[1] | 1,000–5,000 units[2] | |
| Biceps femoris | 2–6 units/kg/muscle | 5–7.5 units/kg[1] | 2–5 units/kg/muscle[1] | 1,000–5,000 units[2] | |
| Quadriceps | 2–6 units/kg/limb, divided | 5–10.5 units/kg | 2–5 units/kg/limb, divided[1] | 1,000–5,000 units[2] | |
| Rectus femoris | 3–6 units/kg/muscle | 6–8 units kg | 2.5 units/kg/muscle[1] | 1,000–5,000 units[2] | |
| Vastus lateralis | 1.5–2 units/kg[1] | 5 units/kg | 1.5–2 units/kg[1] | 1,000–5,000 units[2] | |
| Vastus medialis | 1.5–2 units/kg[1] | 3–5 units/kg[1] | 1.5–2 units/kg[1] | 1,000–5,000 units[2] | |
| **Calf Muscles** | | | | | |
| Flexor digitorum longus | 2–3 units/kg | 3–5 units/kg[1] | 1.5–3 units/kg[1] | 500–1000 units[2] | [1]First author's initial dosage range<br>[2](546) |
| Flexor hallucis longus | 2–3 units/kg | 3–5 units/kg | 2–3 units/kg[1] | 500–1000 units[2] | |
| Gastrocnemius (medial and lateral) | 2–6 units per limb, divided | 10–30 units/kg, divided[3] | 2–6 units per limb, divided[1] | 1,000–5,000 units[2] | [3](499) |
| Gastrocnemius, lateral head | 0.5–3 units/kg | 5–7.5 units/kg | 0.5–3 units/kg[1] | 1,000–5,000 units[2] | |

(*continued*)

**TABLE 11.9 BoNT for Cerebral Palsy/Acquired Brain Injury–Associated Lower Limb Muscle Hypertonia: Published Studies Dosage/Dilution Table (Pediatrics < 18 Years of Age) (*continued*)**

| BoNT Preparation | OBTA (Botox®) | ABTA (Dysport®) | IBTA (Xeomin®) | RBTB (Myobloc®) | Notes |
|---|---|---|---|---|---|
| **Calf Muscles (*continued*)** | | | | | |
| Gastrocnemius, medial head | 1.5–3.9 units/kg | 5–7.5 units/kg | 1.5–4 units/kg[1] | 1,000–5,000 units[2] | |
| Soleus | 1.5–6 units/kg | 3–7.5 units/kg | 1.5–6 units/kg[1] | 1,000–5,000 units[2] | |
| Triceps surae (gastrocnemius and soleus) | 12 units/kg, divided (6 units/kg per side)[4,5] | — | 12 units/kg, divided (6 units/kg per side)[1] | 1,000–5,000 units[2] | [4](557)<br>[5](558) |
| Tibialis anterior | 0.5–2 units/kg per muscle | 1.5–5 units/kg[1] | 0.5–2 units/kg[1] | 1,000–5,000 units[2] | |
| Tibialis posterior | 0.5–6 units/kg per muscle | 7.2–12.5 units/kg | 0.5–3 units/kg per muscle[1] | 1,000–5,000 units[2] | |
| Adducutor hallucis | 0.5–1 units/kg | 2–9 units/kg | 0.5–1 units/kg[1] | 500–1000 units[2] | |
| Flexor hallucis brevis/ flexor digitorum brevis/interossei | 5–10 units per muscle | | 5–10 units per muscle[1] | 500–1000 units[2] | |
| | | | | | |
| Total dose | 4 units/kg<br>3–8 units/kg, not to exceed 300 units[7]<br>4–6 units/kg,[8,9] not to exceed 200 units[6,8,9] | Initial: 10 units/kg, if unilateral<br>20 units/kg, if bilateral<br>Repeat: titrate to 30 units/kg[6,7]<br>Maximum 1,000 units[6,7] 8 or 24 units/kg, maximum dose 1,200 units[11] | Not well established | 3–20,0000 units<br>Dose/muscle: 1,000–5,000 units[10] for large muscles<br>500–1,000 units for small muscles | [6,7]Consider a lower dose for smaller muscles or for concerns about weakness<br>[6](243); [7](240)<br>[8](241)<br>[9](242)<br>[10](546)<br>[11](555) |

(*continued*)

**TABLE 11.9 BoNT for Cerebral Palsy/Acquired Brain Injury–Associated Lower Limb Muscle Hypertonia: Published Studies Dosage/Dilution Table (Pediatrics <18 Years of Age) (*continued*)**

| BoNT Preparation | OBTA (Botox®) | ABTA (Dysport®) | IBTA (Xeomin®) | RBTB (Myobloc®) | Notes |
|---|---|---|---|---|---|
| **Calf Muscles (*continued*)** | | | | | |
| Published total dose (units/kg) | 19–20 units/kg or 400 units (use caution with >400 units)[12] | 30 units/kg or 1,000–1,500 units | Up to 19–20 units/kg is reported (up to 400 units total) | Mean 343.4 units/kg[13]<br>Range: 73.7 units/kg (1 muscle injected) 657.9 units/kg (10 muscles injected)<br>110–970 units/kg, mean 350 units/kg, maximum dose 10,000 units[14] | [12](250)<br>[13](542)<br>[14](496) |
| Maximum dose (units per injection site) | 50 units | 100–125 units | Maximum dosage is not established. Dose equivalence to OBTA is reported in adult studies. Equivalence has not been established in head-to-head clinical trials in either pediatric or adult patients. | — | |
| Injection sites | Large/long muscles: 2–4<br>Medium muscles: 2–3<br>Small muscles: 1 | Large/long muscles: 2–4<br>Medium muscles: 2–3<br>Small muscles: 1 | Large/long muscles: 2–4<br>Medium muscles: 2–3<br>Small muscles: 1 | Large/long muscles: 2–4<br>Medium muscles: 2–3<br>Small muscles: 1 | |

(*continued*)

**TABLE 11.9 BoNT for Cerebral Palsy/Acquired Brain Injury–Associated Lower Limb Muscle Hypertonia: Published Studies Dosage/Dilution Table (Pediatrics <18 Years of Age) (*continued*)**

| BoNT Preparation | OBTA (Botox®) | ABTA (Dysport®) | IBTA (Xeomin®) | RBTB (Myobloc®) | Notes |
|---|---|---|---|---|---|
| **Calf Muscles (*continued*)** | | | | | |
| Dilution | Weight <20–25 kg: 100 units in 1-mL PFNS<br>Weight >20–25 kg: 100 units in 2-mL PFNS is commonly reported | 500 units/1-mL PFNS is common<br>200 units in 2.5-mL PFNS for larger patients (weight >20–25 kg) | 100 units in 1-mL PFNS | Does not require reconstitution/dilution | |
| Retreatment Interval | 12–16 weeks | 12–16 weeks | 12–16 weeks | 12–16 weeks | |
| Localization[15,16,17,18] | EMG, e-stim, US, and/or motor point localization | EMG, e-stim, US, and/or motor point localization | EMG, e-stim, US, and/or motor point localization | EMG, e-stim, US, and/or motor point localization | [15](541)<br>[16](233)<br>[17](90)<br>[18](107) |
| Adverse events | Muscle weakness, injection site pain/bruising, flu-like symptoms, aspiration-related deaths | Muscle weakness, injection site pain/bruising, flu-like symptoms, aspiration-related deaths | Muscle weakness, injection site pain/bruising, flu-like symptoms, aspiration-related deaths | Muscle weakness, injection site pain/bruising, flu-like symptoms, aspiration-related deaths | |

Note: The published dosage range and dose per muscle groups are *suggestions, not absolute recommendations*. Other than for a few select muscles, the optimal starting dose, retreatment dose, and maximum doses for pediatric patients are not established. When calculating the dose per kilogram of BoNT product, if the calculated dose per kilogram exceeds the recommended or typically prescribed adult dose, the lower dose should be used.

When calculating the dose per kilogram and total dose per treatment session, considerations should include BoNT product to be used, number of muscles to be injected, number of injection sites per muscle, physical examination findings, severity of hypertonia, size of muscle to be injected, treatment goals, medical comorbidities, if the patient is toxin-naïve, the response to prior treatment, and other dose modifiers.

*Abbreviations:* ABTA, abobotulinumtoxinA; BoNT, botulinum toxin; EMG, electromyography; e-stim, electrical stimulation; FDA, Food and Drug Administration; IBTA, incobotulinumtoxinA; OBTA, onabotulinumtoxinA; PFNS, preservative-free normal saline; RBTB, rimabotulinumtoxinB; US, ultrasound.

*Sources:* Refs. 7, 86, 232, 250, 252–254, 256, 496, 499, 504, 510, 541, 542, 544–564.

# 12

# *Botulinum Neurotoxin for the Treatment of Trunk Dystonia/Camptocormia*

*Katharine E. Alter, MD*
*Codrin Lungu, MD*

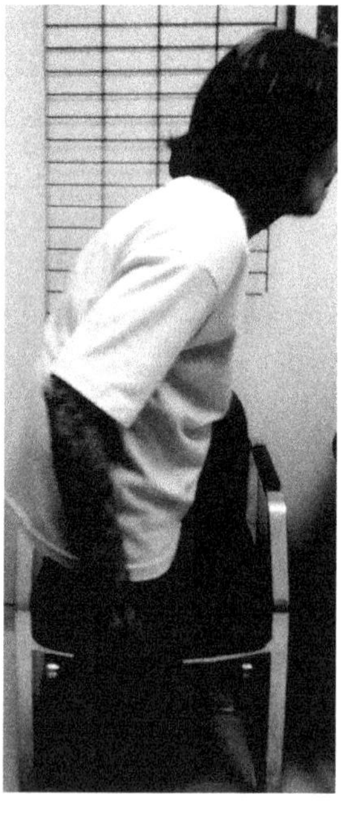

## Condition

Dystonia is a movement disorder characterized by involuntary muscle contraction leading to sustained or intermittent postures. Dystonia involving trunk muscles (chest, back, abdominals) is seen in patients presenting with idiopathic generalized primary dystonia, primary segmental dystonia, and secondary dystonia. These include motor neuron syndromes (amyotrophic lateral sclerosis [ALS], etc.), neurodegenerative conditions (Parkinson disease [PD], multisystem atrophy [MS]), and dementia, and may be seen in patients with dystonia associated with upper motor neuron syndromes (UMNS). Other potential causes of trunk dystonia include side effects from medications, including neuroleptic medications and anticholinesterase inhibitors (188, 259).

Patients rarely present with isolated trunk dystonia and the majority of patients with trunk dystonia also have dystonia involving other body segments. Bent spine syndrome, or camptocormia with trunk flexion greater than 45 degrees, and Pisa syndrome (axial deviation) are two types of trunk dystonia (188, 260, 261). Trunk dystonia is reported to be present in 39% to 50% of patients with cervical dystonia and in 3% to 12% of patients with PD (260, 262). Idiopathic scoliosis is also believed to be a form of dystonia, although this association is not fully established (263).

Nondystonic causes of excessive trunk flexion include primary or secondary myopathies, myositis, mitochondrial disorders, polyneuropathy, spinal muscular atrophy, and ALS. In these patients, trunk flexion is due to weakness in the trunk extensors, rather than due to dystonic contraction of the trunk flexors (264–267). Musculoskeletal causes of trunk flexion also include spondyloarthropathies (e.g., ankylosing spondylitis and Scheuermann's disease). Rarely, camptocormia may be seen due to psychiatric conditions or may be psychogenic (264).

### *Clinical/Functional Impact*

In patients with trunk dystonia, excessive muscle contraction leads to abnormal postures, including trunk flexion, rotation, extension, and/or combinations of these positions. Dystonia may cause pain, interfere with breathing/swallowing, lead to spinal deformity, and affect appearance. Abnormal postures may affect sitting, standing, walking, and various activities of daily living (ADLs). An inability to stand erect may also affect vision, further limiting ADLs, reading, watching TV, or walking. Abnormal postures may occur at rest, may be positional or task specific, and/or may be present in multiple positions/activities (260, 264, 268).

### *Pattern of Involvement*

A patient's posture/trunk position is determined by the specific muscles involved in maintaining that posture. Patients present with various abnormal postures, including flexion, rotation, extension, and combinations of these postures/movements. Pure flexion occurs with symmetrical involvement of abdominal muscles, primarily the rectus abdominis, but also with symmetric contraction of the internal/external oblique muscles. Asymmetric involvement of the rectus abdominis and/or the internal/external oblique muscles will lead to flexion and rotation in the direction of the more active muscles. Pure rotation can also occur, typically with unilateral external or internal oblique involvement. Extension and/or extension and rotation may occur with involvement of the erector spinae group and the deep and superficial rotators of the spine. Excessive flexion may also be due to flexion at the hip joint with dystonic contraction in the hip flexor muscles (e.g., iliacus, psoas and pectineus). Evaluation of the patient at rest, sitting, and walking will assist in determining the pattern of involvement.

### *Evaluation*

Evaluation starts with a detailed medical history and physical examination. In many patients, the history and physical examination will point to the diagnosis. If the history or physical examination is suggestive of a peripheral nervous system disorder (i.e., polyneuropathy or myopathy), the patient should be referred for electrodiagnostic testing and/or needle electromyography (EMG) and blood work/genetic testing (264, 268). In patients with trunk dystonia, brain imaging may reveal atrophy or calcification of the basal ganglia or other abnormalities. Spine MRI is useful to rule out musculoskeletal causes of trunk flexion or atrophy of the extensor muscles. In patients with myositis or myopathy, needle EMG may reveal myopathic motor units, positive sharp waves, fibrillations, and complex repetitive discharges (269, 270). A muscle biopsy may be required to establish a diagnosis of myopathy, although the role of muscle MRI imaging for establishing a diagnosis of myopathy is expanding. Gait analysis may be helpful in evaluating kinematic and EMG abnormalities in patients with trunk dystonia. The findings on EMG may be helpful in muscle selection for botulinum neurotoxin (BoNT) treatment.

### *Treatment*

Selection of the most appropriate treatment option requires establishing the correct etiology of a patient's posture. Patients with trunk flexion due to extensor weakness or myopathy will not benefit from treatment options that reduce involuntary or excessive muscle contraction. For an established diagnosis of trunk dystonia, treatment options include rehabilitation therapy (strengthening, range of motion, gait training, splinting/braces, and others). Oral medications, including anticholinergics and L-dopa, are rarely effective for the treatment of trunk muscle dystonia, but may be useful for some patients (264, 268). Most patients discontinue oral medications due to intolerable side effects or limited benefits. Intrathecal baclofen therapy or deep brain stimulation should be considered for patients who fail or have a less-than-optimal response to less invasive treatment options (188, 264).

BoNT injections have been used for many years for the treatment of primary and secondary dystonia, including trunk dystonia. BoNT injections may provide symptomatic relief from the dystonic movements, reduce involuntary movements/postures, and improve pain, quality of life, and function (23, 264, 268, 271, 272). Target muscles include abdominal flexors (rectus abdominis), flexors/rotators (internal/external obliques), hip flexors (iliopsoas, psoas, iliacus, pectineus), spinal rotators (multifidus), and trunk extensors (the erector spinae group).

### *BoNTs Approved for the Treatment of Trunk Dystonia*

None of the four BoNT products that are currently approved by the FDA in the United States (abobotulinumtoxinA [ABTA], incobotulinumtoxinA [IBTA], onabotulinumtoxinA [OBTA], and rimabotulinumtoxinB [RBTB]) carry approval specifically for the treatment of trunk muscle dystonia. Therefore, the use of BoNTs for the treatment of the various forms of trunk dystonia is off-label (34, 36, 38, 44).

### Approvals Outside the United States

None of the four FDA-approved BoNT products are approved outside the United States for the treatment of trunk muscle dystonia. In addition, none of the other BoNT products available outside the United States are currently approved for the treatment of trunk muscle dystonia. Therefore, the use of BoNTs for the treatment of the various forms of trunk dystonia is off-label in other countries.

### Level of Evidence

There are no published review articles on the topic of BoNT injections for the treatment of trunk muscle dystonia. The majority of the peer-reviewed studies published on this topic are case reports and case series. Using the search terms botulinum toxin A, botulinum toxin B, botulinum toxin, Botox, Dysport, Xeomin, Myobloc, NeuroBloc and trunk dystonia revealed a single placebo-controlled trial of ABTA (Dysport) for the treatment of axial trunk dystonia. A number of case reports and case series were also reviewed. The preceding search returned no peer-reviewed, published studies evaluating Myobloc or NeuroBloc for the treatment of trunk dystonia.

The currently available literature was reviewed using the American Academy of Neurology Classification of Quality of Evidence for Clinical Trials (138). The level of evidence for BoNT serotypes A and B currently supports a Level U (Data inadequate or conflicting: given current knowledge, treatment is unproven) recommendation. The single nonrandomized, placebo-controlled trial for ABTA did not meet the criteria for a Level C (Possibly effective, ineffective, or harmful for the given condition in the specified population) recommendation.

The majority of the published studies evaluated ABTA and OBTA for trunk dystonia (abdominal flexors, trunk extensors, and hip flexors). Clinicians should consider this when contemplating BoNT therapy for the treatment of trunk muscle dystonia. Additional studies for each of the available toxins are needed to determine the optimal starting dose per muscle, optimal effective dose per muscle(s), maximum dose, dilution, and optimal targeting technique(s) for the treatment of trunk muscle dystonia.

### Injection Pattern/Technique

Muscle selection for BoNT therapy is based on clinical presentation and evaluation of patients during functional tasks. Surface or fine-wire EMG, particularly when performed in conjunction with kinematic testing in a gait lab, may be helpful in patients with complex postures. Repeat testing may be useful in documenting clinical improvement.

Although some clinicians perform BoNT injections using only anatomic reference guides, surface anatomy, and palpation, many clinicians use adjunct localization methods. BoNT injections, particularly for the deep trunk or hip flexor muscles, are typically performed using either EMG or ultrasound (US) guidance or EMG and US in combination. US has the advantage of providing direct visual feedback of the muscle depth and location of target muscles, as well as nontargeted structures, including viscera, vessels, nerves, and nontargeted muscles. EMG provides auditory feedback of muscle activity, which may aid muscle selection (271, 273, 274).

## *Dosage*

The use of BoNTs as a class and of each individual commercial BoNT product remains off-label for the treatment of trunk dystonia. Therefore, there is no manufacturers' published data on starting dose. The maximum recommended dose for each product for labeled indications is available in the full prescribing information (34, 36, 38, 44). There are a limited number of controlled studies of BoNT therapy for the various forms of trunk muscle dystonia, most of which are case series or case studies. Therefore, the appropriate starting dose, optimal effective dose, and maximum dose of each of the BoNT products have yet to be established.

### *OnabotulinumtoxinA (OBTA, Botox®)*

The published dosage range for OBTA for the treatment of trunk dystonia is 10 to 600 units. Detailed information on the published dosage range and dose per muscle of OBTA for the treatment of trunk dystonia is presented in Table 12.1 (96, 272, 274–277).

### *AbobotulinumtoxinA (ABTA, Dysport®)*

The published dosage range for ABTA for the treatment of trunk dystonia is 20 to 3,000 units. Doses higher than 1,000 units were reported with a higher incidence of adverse events. Detailed information on the published dosage range and dose per muscle of ABTA for the treatment of trunk dystonia is presented in Table 12.1 (96, 271, 275, 278–280).

### *IncobotulinumtoxinA (IBTA, Xeomin®)*

The published dosage range for IBTA for the treatment of trunk dystonia is 10 to 300 units. Detailed information on the published dosage range and dose per muscle of IBTA for the treatment of trunk dystonia is presented in Table 12.1 (96, 273).

### *RimabotulinumtoxinB (RBTB, Myobloc®/NeuroBloc®)*

There is no published data on the use of RBTB specifically for the treatment of trunk muscle dystonia. The starting dose, dose per muscle, and dosage range for RBTB recommended by the first author (KEA) for the treatment of trunk dystonia are included in Table 12.1.

## *Toxin Dilution*

Dilution with preservative-free normal saline (PFNS, 0.9%) is recommended by the manufacturers of OBTA, ABTA, and IBTA (34, 36, 38).

#### OBTA

The most commonly reported dilution is 100 units with 1-mL PFNS.

#### ABTA

Dilutions of 300 units in 1.5-mL PFNS or 500 units in 2.5-mL PFNS result in a concentration of 200 units/mL or 20 units/0.1 mL. Dilution of 500 units in 4-mL PFNS is also reported, resulting in a concentration of 125 units/mL or 12.5 units/0.1 mL.

IBTA

The most commonly reported dilution is 100 units with 1-mL PFNS.

RBTB

RBTB is provided in solution and does not require reconstitution or dilution. If additional dilution is desired, PFNS can be added to the vial to arrive at the desired dilution.

## *Targeting Techniques*

The majority of published articles report the use of a supplementary localization technique (in addition to inspection/palpation). Reported techniques included EMG, B-mode US, and computed tomography (CT) imaging. EMG provides the advantage of auditory or visual feedback regarding the degree and intensity of muscle contraction. US and CT provide direct visual feedback of the location and depth of target muscles, as well as the proximity and location of nontargeted muscles or other structures. US has significant advantages over CT in that machines are portable, the procedure is less costly, and there is no ionizing radiation. Chapter 4 in this text provides a review of the various localization techniques used in BoNT injections. In addition, there are other published reviews of localization techniques (90, 281). Current data are conflicting whether any supplementary technique is superior to palpation/inspection and, if so, which technique is superior (271, 273, 274). Additional comparison studies are required to evaluate which technique is superior.

## *Clinical Effect*

Many, but not all, patients report improvement in symptoms or functional benefit following BoNT treatment of trunk dystonia. Up to 87% of patients treated for camptocormia report improvement in pain or posture (272). In studies evaluating the effect of BoNTs on trunk flexion in camptocormia, authors reported a greater benefit when abdominal muscles or abdominal muscles and hip flexors were injected than when the iliopsoas was injected in isolation (268, 271–274). In a placebo-controlled trial evaluating the effects of ABTA on lateral axial deviation (LAD), Bonanni et al. reported that 6 of 9 patients (67%) demonstrated benefits in LAD measures, pain, or function. They also reported that 1 of 9 patients reported subjective improvement and 2 of 9 had no improvement (279). In the same study, 7 of 9 patients (78%) reported a "remarkable" improvement in pain (279) and a mean reduction in pain of 31 points (measured on the visual analog scale), with a range of improvement from 19 to 55 points (279). Given the limited response to oral medications and reports of improvement with BoNTs, clinicians should consider this therapy for patients with symptomatic trunk dystonia who fail less invasive treatment.

## *Adverse Events/Side Effects*

The most commonly reported adverse events include pain at the injection site and weakness in both injected/targeted and nontargeted muscles. Abdominal wall prolapse has been reported with the treatment of abdominal muscles at doses exceeding 500 units of OBTA or 2,000 units of ABTA. Worsening of trunk flexion and systemic side effects have been reported when the iliopsoas is injected with ABTA doses higher than 1,000 units. Rare or less common adverse events will be listed in the boxed warning and in the full prescribing information of each of the commercially available preparations.

**TABLE 12.1 BoNTs for the Treatment of Trunk Muscle Dystonia: Dosage and Dilution Table (Adults ≥18 Years of Age)**

| BoNT Preparation | OBTA (Botox®) | ABTA (Dysport®) | IBTA (Xeomin®) | RBTB (Myobloc®) | Notes |
|---|---|---|---|---|---|
| **Rectus Abdominis** | | | | | |
| Starting dosage | 10–60 units/side | 40–240 units/side | 10–50 units/side | 250–750 units/side[2] | [1]Doses >500 units OBTA or >2,000 units ABTA in abdominal muscles have been associated with abdominal wall prolapse.<br>[2]First author's dosage range.<br>[3]Guidance with CT or US is recommended for proximal or trans-abdominal iliopsoas injections. US guidance is suggested for distal iliopsoas injections. |
| Dosage range | 100–300 units/side | 40–320 units/side | 10–300 units/side | 250–2,500 units/side[2] | |
| Mean dosage | Not reported | Not reported | 210 units | N/A | |
| Published dosage | 500–600 units[1] | 2,000 units[1] | 600 units<br>50 units/site | 5,000 units[2] | |
| Injection sites | 2–8 sites/side | 2–8 sites/side | 2–8 sites/side | 2–8 sites/side | |
| **External Oblique** | | | | | |
| Starting dosage | Not reported | Not reported | Not reported | 250–500 units/side[2] | |
| Published dosage range | 5–10 units/side | 20–40 units/side | 5–10 units/side | 250–1,500 units/side[2] | |
| Injection sites | 1–3 | 1–3 | 1–3 | 1–3 | |

*(continued)*

**TABLE 12.1 BoNTs for the Treatment of Trunk Muscle Dystonia: Dosage and Dilution Table (Adults ≥18 Years of Age) (*continued*)**

| BoNT Preparation | OBTA (Botox®) | ABTA (Dysport®) | IBTA (Xeomin®) | RBTB (Myobloc®) | Notes |
|---|---|---|---|---|---|
| **Internal Oblique** | | | | | |
| Starting dosage | Not reported | Not reported | Not reported | 250–500 units/side[2] | |
| Published dosage range | 5–10 units/side | 20–40 units/side | 5–10 units/side | 250–1,500 units/side[2] | |
| Injection sites | 1–3 | 1–3 | 1–3 | 1–3 | |
| **Transversus Abdominis** | | | | | |
| Starting dosage | Not reported | Not reported | Not reported | 250–500 units/side[2] | |
| Published dosage range | 5–10 units/side | 20–40 units/side | 5–10 units/side | 250–1,500 units/side[2] | |
| Injection sites | 1–3 | 1–3 | 1–3 | 1–3 | |
| **Iliopsoas[3]** | | | | | |
| Starting dosage | 25–80 units | 100–300 units/side | 25–80 units | 250–500 units/side[2] | |
| Published dosage range | 100–300 units/side | 100–700 units (100–1,500 units/side[1]) | 25–300 units | 250–1,500 units[2] | |
| Injection sites | 1–3 per muscle | 1–3 per muscle | 1–3 per muscle | 1–3 per muscle | |

(*continued*)

**TABLE 12.1 BoNTs for the Treatment of Trunk Muscle Dystonia: Dosage and Dilution Table (Adults ≥18 Years of Age) (*continued*)**

| BoNT Preparation | OBTA (Botox®) | ABTA (Dysport®) | IBTA (Xeomin®) | RBTB (Myobloc®) | Notes |
|---|---|---|---|---|---|
| **Paraspinal Muscles (Extension)** | | | | | |
| Starting dosage | 60–100 units/side | 240–500 units/side | 60–100 units/side[2] | 250–500 units/side[2] | |
| Dosage range | 60–150 units/side | 250–750 units/ side | 60–150 units/side[2] | 250–2,500 units/side[2] | |
| Maximum total dose | 300 units | 500–1,000 units | 200–300 units[2] | 5,000 units[2] | |
| Extension, lateral deviation | 75–150 units on side of deviation | 100–300 units on side of deviation[2] | 75–150 units on side of deviation[2] | 250–1,500 units on side of deviation[2] | |
| Injection sites | 1–6 per side | 1–6 per side | 1–6 per side | 1–6 per side | |
| Maximum units per injection site | 50 units | 75–100 units | 50 units | Not reported | |
| Total dosage per treatment session | 300–800 units[1] | 500–3,000 units[1] | 100–300 units | Not reported | |
| Dilution (concentration) | 100 units in 1-mL PFNS (100 units/mL), 100 units in 2-mL PFNS (50 units/mL), 200 units in 2-mL PFNS (100 units/mL), or 200 units in 4-mL PFNS (50 units/mL) | 300 units in 1.5-mL PFNS (200 units/mL), 500 units in 2.5-mL PFNS (200 units/mL), or 500 units in 4-mL PFNS (125 units/mL) | 100 units in 1-mL PFNS (100 units/mL) or 100 units in 2-mL PFNS (50 units/mL) | Provided in solution (5,000 units/mL) No dilution required PFNS may be added to the vial if a higher dilution is desired | |

*(continued)*

**TABLE 12.1 BoNTs for the Treatment of Trunk Muscle Dystonia: Dosage and Dilution Table (Adults ≥18 Years of Age) (*continued*)**

| BoNT Preparation | OBTA (Botox®) | ABTA (Dysport®) | IBTA (Xeomin®) | RBTB (Myobloc®) | Notes |
|---|---|---|---|---|---|
| Adverse events | Weakness, injection site pain (see full prescribing information boxed warning) | Weakness, injection site pain (see full prescribing information boxed warning) | Weakness, injection site pain (see full prescribing information boxed warning) | Weakness, injection site pain (see full prescribing information boxed warning) | |
| Reported Guidance Techniques | Palpation, EMG, E-stim, CT, US | | | | |

*Abbreviations:* ABTA, abobotulinumtoxinA; CT, computed tomography; EMG, electromyography; E-stim, electrical stimulation; IBTA, incobotulinumtoxinA; OBTA, onabotulinumtoxinA; PFNS, preservative-free normal saline (0.9%); RBTB, rimabotulinumtoxinB; US, ultrasound.

*Sources:* Refs. 34, 36, 38, 44, 268, 271, 272, 273, 274, 275, 276, 277, 278, 279, 280

# 13

# *Botulinum Neurotoxin Injections for the Treatment of Tremor*

*Katharine E. Alter, MD*
*Pritha Ghosh, MD*

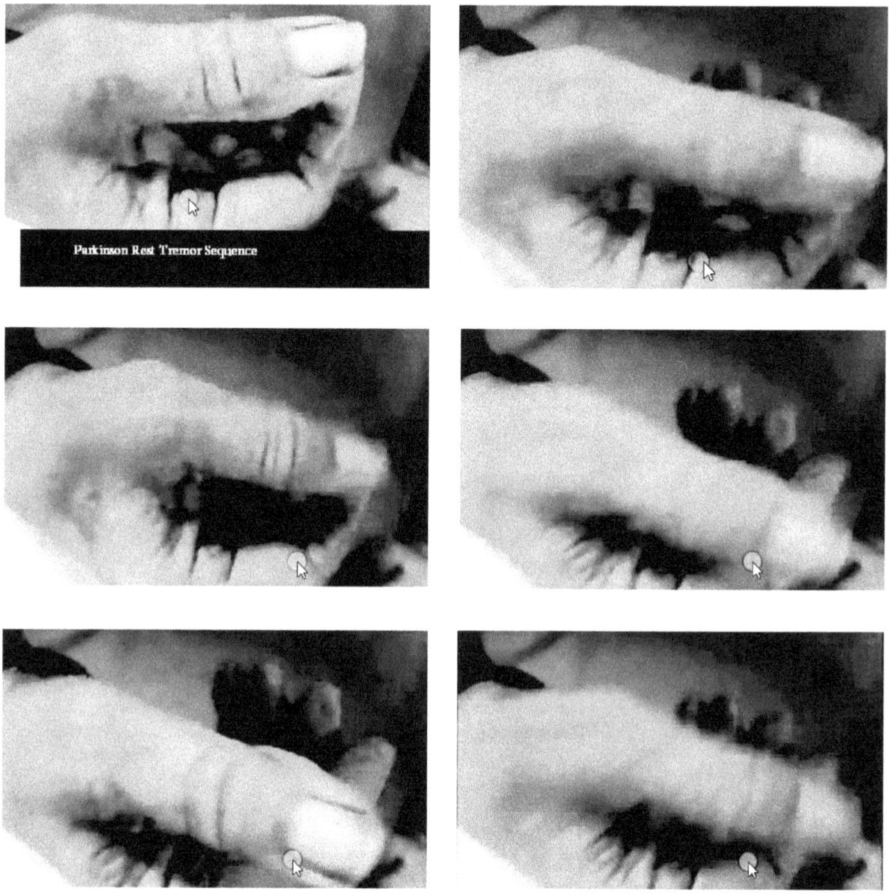

# Condition

Tremor is a hyperkinetic movement disorder characterized by rhythmic or semirhythmic oscillatory movements of one or more body parts and is due to involuntary contractions of agonist/antagonist muscle pairs. Some common forms of tremor include action tremor (AT), postural tremor (PT), the rest tremor associated with Parkinson disease (PD), dystonic tremor (DT), and occupational tremor. Tremor is also seen in association with various neurological disorders, including multiple sclerosis, peripheral nerve entrapment, and metabolic disorders (e.g., hyperthyroidism), and with psychogenic causes. Tremor may or may not limit function depending on its severity. In many cases, tremor can cause significant disability and/or emotional distress. A full discussion of the various types of tremor and their causes and treatments is beyond the scope of this chapter. This chapter provides a brief review of the more common types of tremor (essential tremor [ET], DT, PD) and the role of botulinum neurotoxin (BoNT) injections for the treatment of these types of tremor. Evidence supporting the use of BoNT injections for the treatment of tremor is also provided.

## *Essential Tremor*

ET is a clinical diagnosis and is the most commonly reported movement disorder in elderly adults. It is frequently familial but may also be seen in association with other neurological disorders (282). Patients with ET present with a kinetic tremor, a PT, or both. In some cases, ET may also be present at rest. ET most often affects the upper limbs and hands, but it may also affect (in decreasing order of incidence) the lower limbs, voice, tongue, face, and trunk. Key neurophysiologic studies of ET have established specific criteria for the diagnosis of ET (283, 284). For example, tremor frequency is classically >4 Hz (5–7Hz). If present at rest, the ET tremor is 1.5 Hz slower than an AT or PT. There is also a decrease in the dominant tremor frequency when a weight is applied to the affected body part. Although ET is generally considered a benign condition, it can cause significant functional disability, limit quality of life, and cause emotional distress. Readers are referred to several excellent reviews for detailed information related to the evaluation of ET (282, 285, 286).

## *Dystonic Tremor*

Tremor or tremor-like movements are fairly common in patients with dystonia affecting the upper limbs or head and neck. Tremor is particularly common in cervical dystonia (CD), affecting up to 68% of patients (282, 287, 288). Postural, action, or rest tremor can all be seen in patients with DT. In patients with writer's cramp or CD, it may be difficult to distinguish whether the observed tremor is due to dystonia or ET. Overall, however, the tremor associated with DT is less regular than that seen in ET. A consensus statement published in 1998 outlined definitions of the clinical features of DT, including tremor in the body part affected by dystonia, irregular amplitude, and variable frequency, and in some cases, task specificity (e.g., in writer's cramp). DT may also be an isolated finding in patients with a positive family history of a genetic dystonia (289).

### *Tremor Associated with Parkinson Disease*

PD is one of the most common neurodegenerative disorders in adults and includes many motor and cognitive symptoms. The motor features of PD include bradykinesia, rigidity, gait disturbance, and tremor (268). The typical tremor associated with PD includes the well-recognized, pill-rolling rest tremor that may also re-emerge with posture or during certain functional tasks. This re-emergent PT may have a significant impact on functional use of the hand, affecting activities of daily living (ADLs) such as holding a cup, tool, newspaper, or other objects.

### *Clinical/Functional Impact*

Head tremor associated with CD may limit a variety of ADLs including driving, reading, viewing TV/movies, computer work, and may cause social embarrassment/distress. Hand tremor associated with ET and DT (e.g., focal hand dystonia and writer's cramp) or PD may have a wide-ranging impact on ADLs, with both avocational and vocational tasks.

### *Pattern of Involvement*

As noted, ET may affect any part of the body, but most commonly affects the upper limbs, including distal and proximal muscle pairs. DT of the upper limb can also involve both proximal and distal muscles. Upper limb tremor in PD is often distal, involving forearm/wrist/hand muscles. Commonly affected agonist/antagonist muscle pairs include wrist and finger flexors/extensors, forearm supinator/pronators, and elbow flexor/extensors. Tremor of the head and neck is common in CD, often in a side-to-side direction, affecting various muscles including the sternocleidomastoid, splenius (capitis and/or cervicis), and deep occipital group (obliquus capitis inferioris). Tremor may also involve lower limb, facial, and axial muscles in PD (268).

### *Evaluation*

For evaluation of dystonia, see the chapters in this book specific to this topic. ET and PD are diagnosed clinically. Classic features of ET include a bilateral, often symmetric, postural and kinetic tremor that can occur with or without a rest tremor. Conversely, PD is characterized by a tremor that is most prominent at rest, but may re-emerge, after a brief pause, when maintaining a posture, or with targeted movements. Evaluation of tremor in these disorders first involves an assessment of the tremor with the affected body part in a supported, resting position (e.g., arms in lap). Mental distraction with tasks like counting backward may be used to enhance the rest tremor. The affected body part is then challenged by maintaining a posture against gravity (e.g., arms outstretched) and then with kinetic tasks, such as targeted finger-to-nose movements or nontargeted tasks, like pouring water between glasses. Further evaluation involves having the patient draw an Archimedes spiral, write, or draw a line between lines that are increasingly close together. Through all these tests, the examiner assesses the frequency, rhythmicity, amplitude, and axis of the tremor to determine which agonist/antagonist muscle pairs are contributing to the movements.

### *Treatment of Essential Tremor*

Treatment of ET is reserved for patients with symptomatic tremor that limits function or causes distress. Treatment options include nonpharmacologic, pharmacologic, BoNT injections, and surgical interventions. All patients should be counseled to avoid caffeine and other stimulants that may worsen tremor. The effects of ethyl alcohol in reducing ET are well known, but use is limited by the adverse effects of intoxication and social consequences of chronic use. In addition, tremor may increase temporarily when the effects of alcohol wear off. Treatment options include oral medications, specifically beta-blockers, gabapentin, primidone, topiramate, clonazepam, and combinations of these drugs. Widely accepted alternative treatment options for patients who fail to respond, or have an inadequate response to oral medications, include BoNT injections and deep brain stimulation (DBS) (282, 290, 291). Other treatment options, such as gamma knife surgery, are under investigation and are also not used routinely. Readers are referred to several excellent reviews for detailed information related to the evaluation and treatment of ET (282, 285, 286).

### *Treatment of Dystonic Tremor*

Like ET, treatment of DT is reserved for patients with symptomatic, distressing, or functionally limiting tremor. The treatment of DT largely focuses on treatment of the underlying dystonia. (See introduction and chapters on various subtypes of focal dystonia for a review of treatment options including oral medications and surgical treatment options.) BoNT injections in the agonist/antagonist muscles causing the tremor may be helpful in reducing the amplitude of the DT and thereby improving function (268, 292).

### *Treatment of Tremor Associated with Parkinson Disease*

Levodopa and dopamine agonists are the principal pharmacological treatments for the motor features of PD, including tremor. However, of the motor symptoms of PD, tremor is often most resistant to oral medications. BoNT injections or DBS may be options for patients whose symptoms are inadequately controlled with medications (268).

### *BoNTs Approved for the Treatment of Tremor in the United States*

None of the four BoNT products that are currently approved by the Food and Drug Administration (FDA; abobotulinumtoxinA [ABTA], incobotulinumtoxinA [IBTA], onabotulinumtoxinA [OBTA], and rimabotulinumtoxinB [RBTB]) carry approval specifically for the treatment of tremor. Therefore, the use of BoNT for the treatment of the various forms of tremor is an off-label use (34, 36, 38, 44).

### *BoNTs Approved for the Treatment of Tremor Outside the United States*

None of the four FDA-approved BoNT products (ABTA, IBTA, OBTA, and RBTB) are approved in countries outside the United States for the treatment of tremor. Therefore, the use of BoNT for the treatment of the various forms of tremor is off-label in other countries.

### *Level of Evidence*

There are a limited number of studies evaluating the effect of BoNT therapy for tremor including ET, DT, and PD-related tremor. Most published studies are case series and case studies.

### *Evidence for BoNT for Essential Tremor*

Hallett et al. reviewed the evidence for ET using the American Academy of Neurology Classification of Quality of Evidence (138, 197). Using these guidelines, the authors reviewed three Class II studies of OBTA for hand ET and one study of head ET. All studies reported modest benefit. The authors reported a Level B (Probably effective) recommendation for OBTA for the treatment of tremor and a Level U (Unproven) recommendation for ABTA, IBTA, and RBTB (197). Similarly, Zappia et al. conducted a systematic review of the literature for the treatment of ET that included nine articles related to the use of serotype A BoNTs for ET affecting the hand, head, and voice (286). Two randomized controlled trials, one crossover trial, and six case series were identified. All reported mild to moderate benefit. The authors concluded that serotype A BoNTs should be considered secondary treatments for ET involving the hand, head, or voice in patients refractory to other therapies. For ET of the hand and head, they reported a Level 1C (Strong recommendation/low quality of evidence) recommendation. For voice ET, they reported a 2D (Weak recommendation/very low quality of evidence) recommendation.

### *Evidence for BoNT for Dystonic Tremor*

In a 2013 article, Fasano et al. reported the results of a systematic review of BoNT for the treatment of various forms of DT (292). Their search revealed eight studies, involving 330 patients with primary writing tremor, dystonic head tremor, and spasmodic dysphonia. They concluded that the efficacy of BoNT for these conditions was "well documented" but did not report a specific recommendation using established evidence guidelines. Using AAN guidelines to evaluate the literature for tremor associated with CD, Hallett et al. concluded that there is high-quality Class I evidence to support a Level A (Established as effective) recommendation for all four of the BoNT products currently available in the United States (ABTA, IBTA, OBTA, and RBTB) (197). Studies evaluating BoNT for CD-related tremor showed at least modest improvements in tremor, as well as other CD-related symptoms (293, 294).

### *Evidence for BoNT for Tremor Associated with Parkinson Disease*

Using the currently available Class IV evidence from published studies (138), a Level U (Unproven) recommendation can be made for BoNT injections for the treatment of PD-related hand tremor. Published case series and case reports suggest modest benefit in tremor (295–298).

### *Injection Pattern/Technique*

When treating tremor with BoNT, muscle selection is based on the history of function problems, clinical examination, and/or surface or needle EMG activity of muscles during the clinical examination prior to, or during, the procedure. The clinician listens for rhythmic activity in potentially involved muscle groups and the most active muscles are generally selected for injection (268, 297). In addition to its use to identify muscle activity, EMG was also used as a targeting technique in almost all published studies.

### *Dosage*

As with all conditions in which BoNT is prescribed, the initial dosage and dosage range of BoNT for a given condition, muscle, and patient are specific to the individual BoNT product being used. The published dosage range per muscle for ET, DT, and tremor associated with PD is provided in Tables 13.1 to 13.3.

### *Toxin Dilution*

Serotype A BoNT products (ABTA, IBTA, and OBTA) should be reconstituted with preservative-free normal saline (PFNS, 0.9%). The published dilutions of OBTA when treating patients for tremor were 1 to 2 mL per 100-unit vial for a concentration of 100 units/mL or 10 units/0.1 mL and 50 units/mL or 5 units/0.1 mL, respectively. There is no published information on the dilution of ABTA or IBTA for the treatment of tremor. RBTA comes in solution and does not require reconstitution, but can be further diluted with PFNS, if desired.

### *Clinical Effect*

Both Hallett et al., in a 2013 review article on ET, and Zappia et al., in a 2013 review article on DT, reported modest or established benefit for BoNT in the treatment of ET and DT (197, 286). Trosch and Pullman reported a moderate benefit in 38% of patients with ET or PD-related tremor with a greater decrease in tremor amplitude in ET (297).

### *Adverse Events/Side Effects*

The most commonly reported adverse events when treating patients with BoNTs for tremor are weakness in the injected or adjacent muscles, injection site pain, and/or bruising (282, 290–292, 299, 300). Remote risks include all those listed in the FDA-mandated boxed warning and included in the full prescribing information for each toxin (34, 36, 38, 44).

**TABLE 13.1 BoNT for the Treatment of Essential Tremor: Dosage/Dilution Table (Adults ≥18 Years of Age)**

| BoNT Preparation | OBTA (Botox®) | ABTA (Dysport®) | IBTA (Xeomin®) | RBTB (Myobloc®) | Notes |
|---|---|---|---|---|---|
| U.S. FDA approval | Currently not FDA approved | Currently not FDA approved | Currently not FDA approved | Currently not FDA approved | |
| Approvals outside the United States | Currently not an approved indication | Currently not an approved indication | Currently not an approved indication | Currently not an approved indication | |
| **Essential Tremor Published Dosage Range: Adults (≥18 Years of Age)** | | | | | |
| **Arm Muscles** | | | | | |
| Biceps brachii<br>Dosage range | 5–75 units | 100–300 units | — | 1,000–3,000 units | |
| Triceps<br>Dosage range | 5–75 units | 100–300 units | — | 1,000–3,000 units | |
| Biceps brachii<br>Average dosage[1] | 66.7 ± 11.7 units[1] | — | — | — | [1](297)<br>[2](136) |
| Triceps<br>Average dosage[1] | 62.1 ± 20.8 units[1] | — | — | — | |
| **Forearm Muscles** | | | | | |
| Pronator teres<br>Dosage range | 25–75 units | 80–100 units | | 1,000–2,500 units | |
| Pronator quadratus<br>Dosage range | 10–50 units | 80–100 units | | 1,000–2,500 units | |

(continued)

**TABLE 13.1 BoNT for the Treatment of Essential Tremor: Dosage/Dilution Table (Adults ≥18 Years of Age) (*continued*)**

| BoNT Preparation | OBTA (Botox®) | ABTA (Dysport®) | IBTA (Xeomin®) | RBTB (Myobloc®) | Notes |
|---|---|---|---|---|---|
| **Forearm Muscles (*continued*)** | | | | | |
| Supinator<br>Starting dosage<br>Dosage range | <br>5–15 units<br>10–40 units | <br><br>50–100 units | | <br><br>1,000–2,500 units | [1](297)<br>[2](136) |
| FCR<br>Starting dosage<br>Dosage range | <br>10–30 units<br>5–100 units | <br><br>100–150 units | | <br><br>1,000–3,000 units | |
| FCU<br>Starting dosage<br>Dosage range | <br>10–30 units<br>5–70 units | | | <br><br>1,000–3,000 units | |
| FCR/FCU[1]<br>Average dose per muscle | 23.5 ± 6 units<br>25 ± 5 units[1] | | | | |
| FCR/FCU[2]<br>Initial dosage[2]<br>Repeat treatment dosage (at 4 weeks if no response and no weakness[2]) | <br><br>15 units/muscle[2]<br>30 units/muscle[2] | | | | |
| FDS<br>Dosage range | <br>20–60 units | <br>150–300 units | | <br>1,000–3,000 units | |
| FDP<br>Dosage range | <br>20–60 units | <br>150–200 units | | <br>1,000–3,000 units | |
| FPL<br>Dosage range | <br>10–30 units | <br>30–60 units | | <br>1,000–2,500 units | |
| ECR/ECU<br>Dosage range per muscle | <br>10–20 units | <br>30–100 units | | <br>500–1,000 units | |

(*continued*)

**TABLE 13.1 BoNT for the Treatment of Essential Tremor: Dosage/Dilution Table (Adults ≥18 Years of Age) (*continued*)**

| BoNT Preparation | OBTA (Botox®) | ABTA (Dysport®) | IBTA (Xeomin®) | RBTB (Myobloc®) | Notes |
|---|---|---|---|---|---|
| **Forearm Muscles (*continued*)** | | | | | |
| ECR/ECU[1]<br>Average dosage per muscle[1] | 14.8 ± 5.4 units[1]<br>14.3 ± 4.4 units[1] | | | | [1](297)<br>[2](136) |
| ECR longus/brevis[2]<br>Initial dose[2]<br>Repeat treatment dosage (at 4 weeks if no response and no weakness[2]) | 10 units[2]<br>20 units[2] | | | | |
| ECU[2]<br>Initial treatment<br>Repeat treatment dosage (at 4 weeks if no response and no weakness[2]) | 10 units[2]<br>20 units[2] | | | | |
| EDC<br>Dosage range | 10–25 units | | | | |
| **Essential Tremor: Proximal Upper Limb Muscle/Wing-Beating Tremor** | | | | | |
| Teres major | 18.3–48.6 units[3] | | | | [3](58), average dosage |
| Teres minor | 10–20 units[3] | | | | |
| Infraspinatus | 10 units[3] | | | | |
| Supraspinatus | 10 units[3] | | | | |
| Deltoid | 5–10 units | | | | |
| Pectoralis major | 5–10 units | | | | |
| Triceps | 5–20 units | | | | |
| Biceps | 5–20 units | | | | |

*(continued)*

**TABLE 13.1 BoNT for the Treatment of Essential Tremor: Dosage/Dilution Table (Adults ≥18 Years of Age) (*continued*)**

| BoNT Preparation | OBTA (Botox®) | ABTA (Dysport®) | IBTA (Xeomin®) | RBTB (Myobloc®) | Notes |
|---|---|---|---|---|---|
| **Limb Muscles: Published Total Dosage per Treatment Session** | | | | | |
| Proximal muscles<br>Initial dosage, divided<br>Retreatment dosage, divided | 25–80 units/side<br>100–300 units/side | 100–300 units/side<br>100–700 units per treatment session | 25–50 units/side[4]<br>100–300 units/side[4] | 250–500 units/side<br>250–1500 units[4] | [1](297)<br>[2](136)<br>[3](58), average dosage<br>[4]First author's dosage range<br>[5](299) |
| Forearm muscles<br>Total dosage, divided[5] | 50 or 100 units | | | | |
| Forearm muscles<br>Mean total dosage, divided[1]<br>Total dosage range, divided[1] | 108.8 ± 53.8 units[1]<br>50–225 units[1] | | | | |
| Forearm muscles<br>Initial total dosage[2]<br>Repeat treatment dosage (at 4 weeks if no response and no weakness[2]) | 50 units[2]<br>100 units[2] | | | | |
| **Essential Tremor Head/Neck** | | | | | |
| SCM<br>Published dose | 40 units per side[6] | 100 units per side[7] | | | [6](565)<br>[7](566)<br>[8]Muscles (1–3) Splenius Capitis, SCM (567) |
| Splenius capitis<br>Published dose | 60 units per side[6] | 150 units per side[7] | | | |
| Nondystonic head tremor[8]<br>Mean dosage<br>Dosage rangea | | 160 units[8]<br>320–560 units[8] | | | |

(*continued*)

**TABLE 13.1 BoNT for the Treatment of Essential Tremor: Dosage/Dilution Table (Adults ≥18 Years of Age) (*continued*)**

| BoNT Preparation | OBTA (Botox®) | ABTA (Dysport®) | IBTA (Xeomin®) | RBTB (Myobloc®) | Notes |
|---|---|---|---|---|---|
| **Essential Head Tremor: Published Total Dosage per Treatment Session** | | | | | |
| Nondystonic/ET head tremor<br>Total dose<br>Dosage range | 200 units[6] | 500 units[7]<br>160–720 units[8] | Not reported | Not reported | [6](565)<br>[7](566)<br>[8]Muscles (1–3) Splenius Capitis, SCM (567) |
| Dilution (concentration) | 100 units with 2-mL PFNS (50 units/mL, 5 units/0.1 mL) | 300 units in 0.6-mL PFNS or 500 units in 1-mL PFNS (50 units/0.1 mL) | Not reported | Not reported | |
| Guidance | EMG | EMG | Not reported | EMG | CT or US reported for some proximal muscles |
| Injection sites | 1–4 per muscle<br>Maximum 50 units per site | 1–4 per muscle | Not reported | 1–3 per muscle | |

*Abbreviations:* ABTA, abobotulinumtoxinA; ECR, extensor carpi radialis; ECU, extensor carpi ulnaris; EDC, extensor digitorum communis; EMG, electromyography; ET, essential tremor; FCR, flexor carpi radialis; FCU, flexor carpi ulnaris; FDS, flexor digitorum superficialis; FDP, flexor digitorum profundus; FPL, flexor pollicis longus; IBTA, incobotulinumtoxinA; OBTA, onabotulinumtoxinA; PFNS, preservative-free normal saline (0.9%); RBTB, rimabotulinumtoxinB; SCM, sternocleidomastoid.

*Sources:* Refs. 58, 136, 152, 199, 282, 286, 296, 297, 298, 299, 487, 565–568.

**TABLE 13.2 BoNT for the Treatment of Dystonic Tremors: Dystonic Tremor Published Dosage/Dilution Table (Adults ≥18 Years of Age)**

| BoNT Preparation | OBTA (Botox®) | ABTA (Dysport®) | IBTA (Xeomin®) | RBTB (Myobloc®) | Notes |
|---|---|---|---|---|---|
| U.S. FDA approval | Currently not FDA approved | Currently not FDA approved | Currently not FDA approved | Currently not FDA approved | |
| Approvals outside the United States | Currently not an approved indication | Currently not an approved indication | Currently not an approved indication | Currently not an approved indication | |
| **Cervical Dystonia (Head Tremor) Reported Dosage Range** | | | | | |
| SCM | 50–75 units[1]<br>25–100 units[2] | — | — | — | [1](293)<br>[2](294) |
| Splenius capitis | 50–75 units[1]<br>25–50 units[2]<br>≤250 units, divided bilaterally[2] | — | — | — | |
| Trapezius | 100 units[1]<br>25–75 units[2] | — | — | — | |
| Minimum dose<br>Maximum dose | 75 units[1]<br>280 units[1]<br>250 units[2] | — | — | — | |
| Levator scapulae | 25–100 units[2] | — | — | — | |
| Scalene, posterior | 25–75 units[2] | — | — | — | |

*(continued)*

**TABLE 13.2 BoNT for the Treatment of Dystonic Tremors: Dystonic Tremor Published Dosage/Dilution Table (Adults ≥18 Years of Age) (*continued*)**

| BoNT Preparation | OBTA (Botox®) | ABTA (Dysport®) | IBTA (Xeomin®) | RBTB (Myobloc®) | Notes |
|---|---|---|---|---|---|
| **Cervical Dystonia (Head Tremor) Reported Dosage Range (*continued*)** | | | | | |
| Tremulous CD[3] (SCM, splenius capitis)<br>Mean dosage<br>Dosage range | — | 500 units[4]<br>320–720 units[4] | — | — | [3]Muscles (2–4) Splenius capitis, SCM<br>[4](567) |
| Dilution | 100 units in 2-mL PFNS[1,2] | — | — | — | |
| Injection sites | 2–4 per muscle[1,2] | — | — | — | |
| **Dystonic Hand Tremor** | | | | | |
| Wrist flexors/ extensors | — | 200 units, divided[5] | — | — | [5](569)<br>[6](568) |
| FCU | 10–12.5 units[6] | — | — | — | |
| ECU | 10–12.5 units[6] | — | — | — | |
| EDC | 10 units[6] | — | — | — | |
| APL | 10 units[6] | — | — | — | |
| Dilution (concentration) | 100 units in 1-mL PFNS (100 units/mL, 10 units/0.1 mL) or 100 units in 2-mL PFNS (50 units/mL, 5 units/0.1 mL) | 300 units in 1.5-mL PFNS (200 units/mL), 500 units in 2.5-mL PFNS (200 units/mL) or 500 units in 4-mL PFNS (125 units/mL) | No published studies | No dilution required | |

(*continued*)

**TABLE 13.2 BoNT for the Treatment of Dystonic Tremors: Dystonic Tremor Published Dosage/Dilution Table (Adults ≥18 Years of Age) (*continued*)**

| BoNT Preparation | OBTA (Botox®) | ABTA (Dysport®) | IBTA (Xeomin®) | RBTB (Myobloc®) | Notes |
|---|---|---|---|---|---|
| Adverse events | Weakness, see full PI boxed warning | Weakness, see full PI boxed warning | No published studies | No published studies<br>See full PI boxed warning | |
| Guidance techniques | Palpation, EMG, CT, ultrasound | | | | |

*Abbreviations:* ABTA, abobotulinumtoxinA; APL, abductor pollicis longus; BoNT, botulinum neurotoxin; CD, cervical dystonia; CT, computed tomography; ECU, extensor carpi ulnaris; EDC, extensor digitorum communis; EMG, electromyography; FCU, flexor carpi ulnaris; IBTA, incobotulinumtoxinA; OBTA, onabotulinumtoxinA; PFNS, preservative-free normal saline (0.9%); PI, prescribing information; RBTB, rimabotulinumtoxinB; SCM, sternocleidomastoid.

*Sources:* Refs. 152, 199, 292–294, 567–569.

**TABLE 13.3 Botulinum Neurotoxin for the Treatment of Tremor Associated with Parkinson Disease: Dosage/Dilution Table (Adults ≥18 Years of Age)**

| BoNT Preparation | OBTA (Botox®) | ABTA (Dysport®) | IBTA (Xeomin®) | RBTB (Myobloc®) | Notes |
|---|---|---|---|---|---|
| U.S. FDA approval | Currently not FDA approved | Currently not FDA approved | Currently not FDA approved | Currently not FDA approved | |
| Approvals outside the United States | Currently not an approved indication | Currently not an approved indication | Currently not an approved indication | Currently not an approved indication | |
| **Published Dose Range: Forearm/Arm** | | | | | |
| Biceps brachii<br>Dosage range<br>Average dosage (±SD)<br>Sites per muscle | <br>30–75 units[1]<br>66.7 (±11.7) units[1]<br>96 (±32.7) units[3]<br>1–3 | | <br>50 units[2]<br>50 units[2] | | [1](297), open-label study of PD and ET<br>[2](295)<br>[3](199)<br>[4](296) |
| Triceps brachii<br>Dosage range<br>Average dosage (±SD)<br>Sites per muscle | <br>25–75 units<br>62.1 (±20.8) units[1]<br>58.6 (±15.7) units[3]<br>1–3 | | <br>50 units[2]<br>50 units[2] | | |

(*continued*)

**TABLE 13.3 Botulinum Neurotoxin for the Treatment of Tremor Associated with Parkinson Disease: Dosage/Dilution Table (Adults ≥18 Years of Age) (*continued*)**

| BoNT Preparation | OBTA (Botox®) | ABTA (Dysport®) | IBTA (Xeomin®) | RBTB (Myobloc®) | Notes |
|---|---|---|---|---|---|
| **Published Dose Range: Forearm/Arm (*continued*)** | | | | | |
| Pronators (PQ, PT)<br>Dosage range<br>Average dosage (±SD)<br>Sites per muscle | | | 20–25 units[2]<br>21 (± 3) units[2] | | |
| Supinator<br>Dosage range<br>Average dosage (±SD) | 32.5 ± 14.7 units[3] | | 15–20 units[2]<br>19 ± 3 units[2] | | |
| FCR/FCU<br>Dosage range<br>Average dosage (±SD)<br>Sites per muscle | 5–25 units[1]<br>FCR 23.5 (±6) units[1]<br>FCU 25 (±5) units[1]<br>FCR 25 (±13.2) units[3]<br>FCU 26 (±16.7) units[3]<br>1–2 | | 20–25 units[2]<br>22 ± 3 units[2] | | |

(*continued*)

**TABLE 13.3 Botulinum Neurotoxin for the Treatment of Tremor Associated with Parkinson Disease: Dosage/Dilution Table (Adults ≥18 Years of Age) (*continued*)**

| BoNT Preparation | OBTA (Botox®) | ABTA (Dysport®) | IBTA (Xeomin®) | RBTB (Myobloc®) | Notes |
|---|---|---|---|---|---|
| **Published Dose Range: Forearm/Arm (*continued*)** | | | | | |
| ECR/ECU<br>Dosage range<br>Average dosage (±SD)<br>Sites per muscle | <br>5–50 units[1]<br>ECR 14.8 (±5.4) units[1]<br>ECU 14.3 (±4.4) units[1]<br>ECR 20.4 (±14.2) units[3]<br>ECU 15.8 (±7) units[3]<br>1–2 | | <br>20–25 units[2]<br>22 ± 3 units[2] | | |
| EDC<br>Dosage range<br>Average dosage (±SD)<br>Sites per muscle | <br>5–50 units[1]<br>25 (±16) units[1]<br>16.3 (±5.5) units[3]<br>1–2 | | Not reported | | |
| FDP<br>Average dosage (±SD) | 30.6 (±7.8) units[3] | | Not reported | | |

(*continued*)

**TABLE 13.3 Botulinum Neurotoxin for the Treatment of Tremor Associated With Parkinson Disease: Dosage/Dilution Table (Adults ≥18 Years of Age) (*continued*)**

| BoNT Preparation | OBTA (Botox®) | ABTA (Dysport®) | IBTA (Xeomin®) | RBTB (Myobloc®) | Notes |
|---|---|---|---|---|---|
| **Published Dose Range: Forearm/Arm (*continued*)** | | | | | |
| FDS<br>Average dosage (±SD) | 17.6 (±9.4) units[3] | | 15 units[2] | | [1](297), open-label study of PD and ET<br>[2](295)<br>[3](199)<br>[4](296) |
| FPL<br>Average dosage (±SD) | 19.6 (±7.2) units[3] | | 10 units[2] | | |
| AbPL<br>Average dosage (±SD) | 8.3 (±2.9) units[3] | | Not reported | | |
| EDC, ECR, ECU, FCR, FCU, FDS | 50 units, divided[4] | | Not reported | | |
| EDC, ECR, ECU, EIP, EPL, FCR, FCU, FDS, FDP | 50 units, divided[4] | | Not reported | | |
| Total dosage | 50 units or 100 units[5] | | | | [5](297) |
| Mean total dosage<br>Total dose range | 107.5 ± 53.8 units[1]<br>25–205 units[1–4] | | | | |
| Localization | EMG | | | No published studies on maximum dose | |

(*continued*)

**TABLE 13.3 Botulinum Neurotoxin for the Treatment of Tremor Associated with Parkinson Disease: Dosage/Dilution Table (Adults ≥18 Years of Age) (*continued*)**

| BoNT Preparation | OBTA (Botox®) | ABTA (Dysport®) | IBTA (Xeomin®) | RBTB (Myobloc®) | Notes |
|---|---|---|---|---|---|
| Dilution (concentration) | 100 units in 1-mL PFNS (100 units/mL, 10 units/0.1 mL) or 100 units in 2-mL PFNS (50 units/mL, 5 units/0.1 mL) | 300 units in 1.5-mL PFNS (200 units/mL, 20 units/0.1 ml) or 500 units in 2.5-mL PFNS (200 units/mL, 20 units/0.1mL) or 500 units in 4-mL PFNS (125 units/mL, 1.25 units/mL) | 100 units in 1-mL PFNS (100 units/mL, 10 units/0.1 mL) | No dilution required | All dilutions with PFNS |
| Adverse events | Weakness, see full PI boxed warning | Weakness, see full PI boxed warning | Weakness, see full PI boxed warning | No published studies<br>See full PI boxed warning | |
| Guidance techniques | Palpation, EMG, CT, ultrasound | | | | |

*Abbreviations:* AbPL, abductor pollicis longus; AdPL, adductor pollicis longus; CT, computed tomography; ECR, extensor carpi radialis; ECU, extensor carpi ulnaris; EDC, extensor digitorum communis; EIP, extensor indices proprius; EPL, extensor pollicis longus; EMG, electromyography; FCR, flexor carpi radialis; FCU, flexor carpi ulnaris; FDS, flexor digitorum superficialis; FDP, flexor digitorum profundus; FPL, flexor pollicis longus; PFNS, preservative-free normal saline (0.9%); PI, prescribing information; PQ, pronator quadratus; PT, pronator teres; SCM, sternocleidomastoid; SD, standard deviation.

*Sources:* Refs. 152, 199, 268, 295–297.

# Illustrations for Upper Limb, Lower Limb, and Trunk Dystonia—Chapters 10–13

*FIGURE 1* *Thigh muscles, cross-sectional anatomy.*

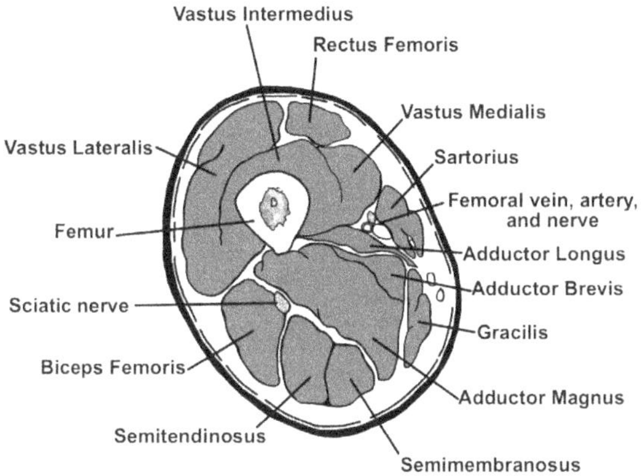


*FIGURE 2* *Calf muscles, cross-sectional anatomy.*

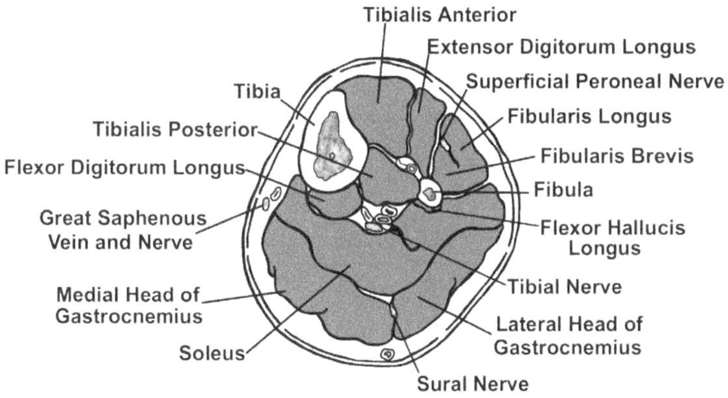


*FIGURE 3* *Arm muscles, cross-sectional anatomy.*

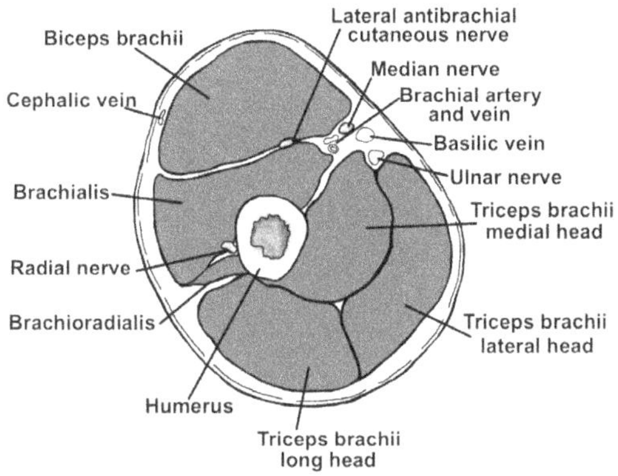

*FIGURE 4 Forearm muscles, cross-sectional anatomy.*

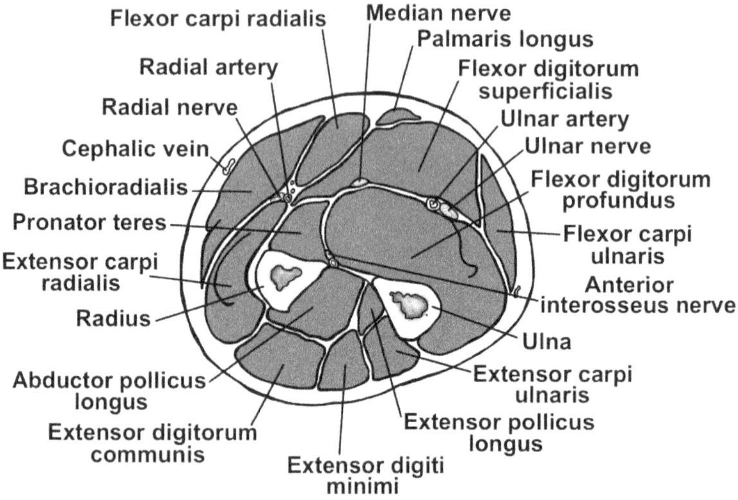


*FIGURE 5 Abdominal muscles.*

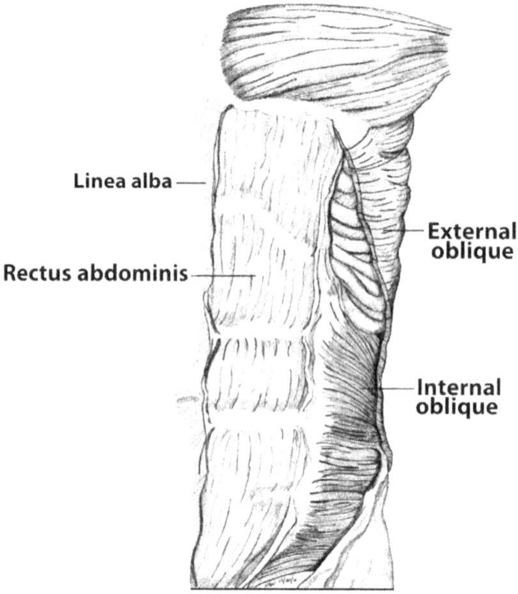

# Part II

## *Botulinum Neurotoxins for Neurosecretory Disorders*

# 14

# *Botulinum Neurotoxin Therapy for Problematic Sialorrhea*

*Katharine E. Alter, MD*

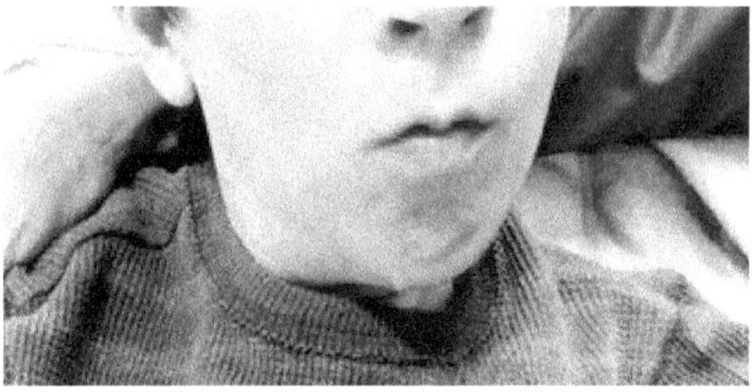

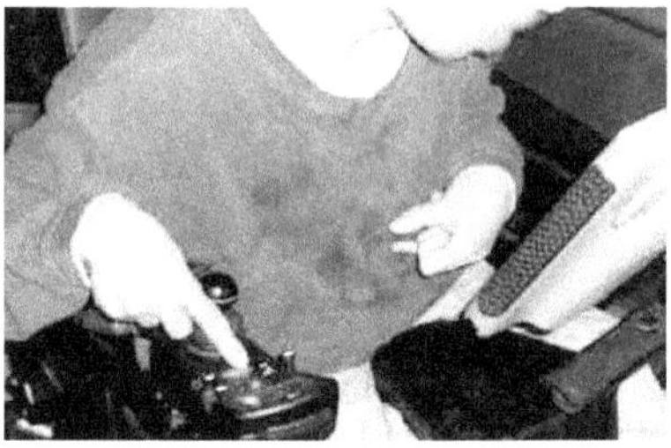

## Condition

On average, adults produce 750 mL of saliva per day. Of that, the submandibular glands reportedly produce upward of 70%, the parotid glands produce 25%, and the sublingual gland produces only 5% (301). The term sialorrhea (drooling, dribbling) refers to the involuntary loss of saliva from the mouth. Drooling is normal in infants and young children, but generally ends by school age. Beyond this age, sialorrhea is uncommon, except in patients with neurological conditions that affect head/trunk control, muscle tone, swallowing and the swallowing reflex, oromotor control, and/or combinations of these impairments (97, 302). In the vast majority of these patients, sialorrhea is caused by reduced or disordered swallowing, not by excessive saliva production.

Sialorrhea is reported in up to 38% of children with cerebral palsy and stroke, in 70% to 80% of patients with Parkinson disease, and also commonly in patients with amyotrophic lateral sclerosis [ALS], myasthenia gravis, and Lambert–Eaton syndrome (303–308). These conditions lead to a combination of sensory and motor impairments, including impaired sensation, lip closure, chewing, and swallowing.

### *Clinical/Functional Impact*

Sialorrhea often affects quality of life, causing emotional distress, embarrassment, and social isolation. Sialorrhea may also soil clothing and damage equipment, including computers, communication devices, and environmental controls. Immediate sequelae of sialorrhea and poor oral control of saliva include skin breakdown or maceration, aspiration of secretions with recurrent respiratory infections, and aspiration pneumonia (301, 302).

### *Pattern of Involvement*

Secretion of saliva occurs at a basal rate and increases with eating, chewing gum, or placing an object in the mouth. In patients with intact oromotor function, the saliva that is produced at rest and with eating/chewing is swallowed. Sialorrhea occurs when saliva escapes from the mouth due to poor lip closure, reduced or impaired swallowing, impaired sensation, and/or a flexed head position. After escaping the mouth, saliva runs over the chin, onto the neck, chest, and/or equipment for seating, positioning, and communication. Most patients with sialorrhea have disordered swallowing or dysphagia. Increased saliva in the mouth or pharynx may further compromise feeding and may lead to frequent coughing, choking, and/or aspiration.

### *Evaluation*

The first step in assessing the scope of the problem is to ask the patient how sialorrhea affects function, including activities of daily living, communication, and quality of life. More objective measures include a Visual Analog Scale to measure impact or clinical scales, such as the Teachers Drooling Scale, Drooling Rating Scale, the Drooling Severity and Frequency Scale, or portions of the Unified Parkinson's Disease Rating Scale (UPDRS) (301, 309). Quantitative measurement of saliva production can also be performed using cotton rolls or collection devices. These evaluations can be performed prior to and after an intervention (oral medications, botulinum neurotoxin [BoNT] therapy, or surgery) (309, 310).

### *Treatment*

Management of sialorrhea may include oral motor therapy, devices to remove saliva from the face or mouth, oral medications, transdermal medications, BoNT injections, and surgical procedures, such as salivary gland duct re-routing or ligation (302, 311–315). Oral and transdermal anticholinergic agents, such as glycopyrrolate, diphenhydramine, or scopolamine, may be trialed, although many patients report significant side effects, including diplopia, constipation, urinary retention, and sedation (301, 309). BoNT therapy is increasingly offered to patients for whom more conservative treatments do not provide adequate saliva control or for whom pharmacologic therapy causes intolerable side effects. Due to the low incidence of adverse effects and the potential to improve symptoms for several months, BoNT therapy is frequently recommended to patients prior to considering oral medications or surgery.

### *BoNTs Approved for the Treatment of Sialorrhea*

At the time of publication, the use of BoNT for the treatment of sialorrhea is considered off-label for all the Food and Drug Administration–approved BoNT products (abobotulinumtoxinA [ABTA], incobotulinumtoxinA [IBTA], onabotulinumtoxinA [OBTA], and rimabotulinumtoxinB [RBTB]).

### *Approvals Outside the United States*

At the time of publication, the use of BoNT for the treatment of sialorrhea is considered off-label.

### *Level of Evidence*

A 2013 article reviewed the evidence from published studies for neurosecretory disorders including sialorrhea (138, 303). The authors reported evidence supporting a Level B (Probably effective, ineffective, or harmful for the given condition in the specified population; Level B rating requires at least one Class I study or at least two consistent Class II studies) recommendation for ABTA, OBTA, and RBTB for the treatment of sialorrhea. They reported a Level U (Data inadequate or conflicting; given current knowledge, treatment is unproven) recommendation for IBTA. A 2008 review article reported the evidence for BoNTs for the treatment of sialorrhea and concluded that the evidence supported a Level A (Established as effective, ineffective, or harmful for the given condition in the specified population; Level A rating requires at least two consistent Class I studies) recommendation for the effectiveness of serotype A BoNTs for the treatment of sialorrhea and a Level B recommendation for serotype B BoNT (316).

### *Injection Pattern*

The majority of studies reported injection of the bilateral parotid and submandibular glands, with a higher reported dose in the larger parotid glands. Generally, a single injection site was reported in the submandibular gland and one to two sites in the parotid glands (see Figures 14.1 and 14.2).

### *Toxin Dilution*

Toxin dilution was not reported in many studies; therefore, optimal dilution of BoNT when treating patients with sialorrhea is unknown. For OBTA, most studies reported reconstituting 100 units of OBTA with 1 mL preservative-free normal saline (PFNS) (0.9%) and a 300-unit vial of ABTA was typically diluted or reconstituted with 0.6-mL PFNS. There is no published information on the reconstitution of IBTA for sialorrhea. The first author's practice is to reconstitute a 50-unit vial with 0.5 mL PFNS or a 100-unit vial with 1 mL PFNS. RBTB is provided in solution and does not require reconstitution. If desired, the RBTB vial can be further diluted with PFNS.

*FIGURE 14.1* *Parotid salivary gland and head/neck/facial muscles.*

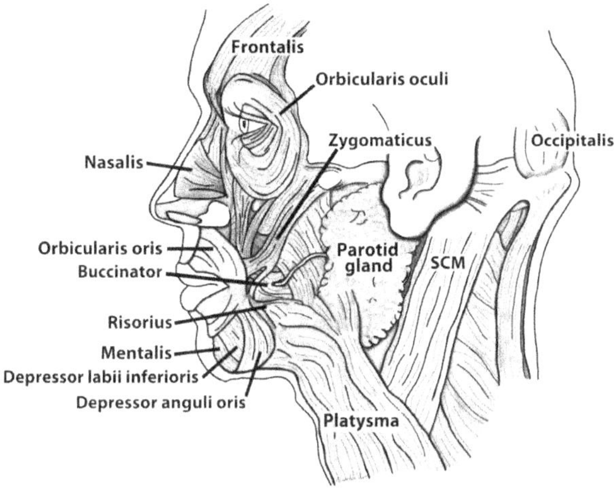


*FIGURE 14.2* *Submandibular and sublingual salivary glands.*

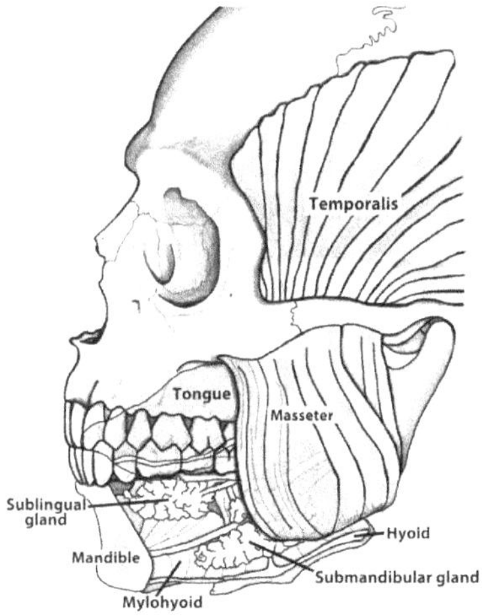


## *Dosage and Dilution*

There are limited data from controlled trials on the optimal starting dose, dose per gland, dose escalation, total dose, and dilution of the BoNT product for the treatment of sialorrhea. Available studies report a wide range of BoNT doses for a given BoNT product (301, 310, 317–320). When evaluating the current evidence on dosing, clinicians must recognize that the dose of each commercial BoNT product is unique due to each product's specific properties and relative potencies. This topic is discussed in detail in Chapter 2. Most expert clinicians recommend initiating treatment with a dose on the low side of the reported dose range. Based on the patient's response to therapy, the dose may then be increased at subsequent treatment sessions with a goal of optimizing the clinical response and avoiding adverse events. Conservative dosing is recommended for patients with reports of dysphagia, unless they have an existing feeding tube. Reduced dosing is also recommended in certain patient populations, such as those with motor neuron disease(s) (66, 321–323). Dose calculation in pediatric patients is generally based on total body weight (319, 324, 325).

### *Adult Patients*

SEROTYPE A BoNTS

The published mean total dose of OBTA ranged from 55 to 300 units and of ABTA was 250 to 450 units. The published starting dosage range of OBTA was 5 to 30 units for each submandibular gland and 5 to 75 units for individual parotid glands.

SEROTYPE B BoNT

The published total dosage range was 1,500 to 5,000 units. One study reported that 3,000 units of RBTB was equally effective to 5,000 units with fewer side effects. For RBTB, the reported dosage range for individual salivary glands is 250 to 1,000 units for the submandibular gland and 450 to 1,000 units for individual parotid glands. A comparison study reported similar efficacy between ABTA (250 units) and RBTB (2,500 units) (66).

### *Pediatric Patients*

In children, the dose of BoNT is typically calculated according to the patient's body weight in kilograms. Units per kilogram dosing is used until the child achieves a weight such that the weight-based dose would exceed the reported dose used in adult protocols. For OBTA, the published doses ranged from 2 to 22.5 units/kg/gland. The reported total dosage range for RBTB ranged from 1,500 to 5,000 units. In one study, comparing 1,500 to 5,000 units of RBTB, no added benefit was observed and increased adverse events were reported with the 5,000-unit dose (318, 319, 324, 325).

### *Injection Technique*

Palpation, anatomic landmarks, and B-mode ultrasound (US) can be used to guide BoNT injections in salivary glands (97, 301, 310, 316, 326–328). In older studies, palpation and landmarks were the most commonly reported localization techniques, whereas the majority of recent studies report using US guidance to localize the salivary glands. US guidance for BoNT injections has been reported to reveal abnormalities (dysplastic/atrophied glands), vessels, inflammatory changes, and has led to modification of the proposed BoNT injections (301). There are some reports that US guidance is reported to result in enhanced clinical benefit and reduced adverse events (328, 329). Additional studies are needed to make recommendations as to whether US should be recommended for these injections.

### *Clinical Effect*

BoNT therapy is reported to reduce the volume of saliva and the severity of sialorrhea, aspiration, infections, skin maceration, and social isolation (301, 303, 316).

### *Adverse Events/Side Effects*

Adverse events and side effects are relatively uncommon. The most commonly reported adverse event is viscous saliva or dry mouth. Rare events include dysphagia or respiratory failure (in patients with ALS) (303, 316). Some clinicians consider motor neuron disease to be a relative contraindication for BoNT injections, whereas others recommend using a lower dose of BoNT for these patients.

**TABLE 14.1 BoNT for the Treatment of Sialorrhea: Dosage/Dilution Table for Adults/Children**

| BoNT Preparation | OBTA (Botox®) | ABTA (Dysport®) | IBTA (Xeomin®) | RBTB (Myobloc®) | Notes |
|---|---|---|---|---|---|
| U.S. FDA approval | Currently not FDA approved | Currently not FDA approved | Currently not FDA approved | Currently not FDA approved | |
| Approvals outside the United States | Currently not an approved indication | Currently not an approved indication | Currently not an approved indication | Currently not an approved indication | |
| **Published Dosage Range: Adults (≥18 Years of Age)** | | | | | |
| Parotid Gland<br>Average dosage[1,2]<br>Dosage range[1,2] | 5–75 units<br>5–80 units | 30–75 units<br>10–145 units[3] | Not reported | 1,000 units<br>250–1,000 units | [1]Most studies report or advise using US guidance for salivary gland injections<br>[2]Lower dose reported for patients with ALS<br>[3]75 units/gland reported to decrease saliva by 50%<br>[4]3,000 units of RBTB reported to have equal efficacy and fewer adverse events when compared to 5,000 units |
| Submandibular gland<br>Starting dose[1,2]<br>Dosage range[1,2] | 5–30 units<br>10–50 units | 60 units<br>10–80 units | Not reported | 250 units<br>400–1,000 units | |
| Total dose per treatment session | 50–300 units, divided between parotid and submandibular glands | 250–450 units, divided between parotid and submandibular glands | Not reported | 2500–5000 units,[4] divided between bilateral parotid and submandibular glands | |

(*continued*)

**TABLE 14.1 BoNT for the Treatment of Sialorrhea: Dosage/Dilution Table for Adults/Children** *(continued)*

| BoNT Preparation | OBTA (Botox®) | ABTA (Dysport®) | IBTA (Xeomin®) | RBTB (Myobloc®) | Notes |
|---|---|---|---|---|---|
| **Published Dosage Range: Pediatric Patients (<18 Years of Age)** | | | | | |
| Parotid gland[1] | 15–25 units | 15–75 units per gland | Not reported | 150–250 units per gland | [1]Most studies report or advise using US guidance for salivary gland injections |
| Weight <15 kg[1]<br>Weight 15–25 kg[1]<br>Weight >25 kg[1] | 15 units per gland<br>20 units per gland<br>25 units per gland | | | | |
| Submandibular gland[1] | 5–15 units per gland<br>Range: 10–50 units | 15–75 units/gland | Not reported | 150–250 units per gland | |
| Total dose per treatment session | 30–100 units | 75–300 units | | 400–1000 units | |
| **Salivary Gland: Dilution/Guidance/Adverse Events** | | | | | |
| Dilution (concentration) | 100-unit vial diluted with 1-mL PFNS (100 units/1 mL, 10 units/0.1 mL) | 300-unit vial diluted with 1.5-mL PFNS (200 units/mL, 20 units/0.1 mL) | 50 units diluted with 0.5-mL PFNS or a 100-unit vial diluted with 1-mL PFNS (100 units/mL, 10 units/0.1 mL) | Not required, but can be further diluted<br>2,500-unit vial with 0.5 mL PFNS or a 5,000-unit vial with 1 mL PFNS (2,500 units/mL, 250 units/0.1 mL) | |

*(continued)*

**TABLE 14.1 BoNT for the Treatment of Sialorrhea: Dosage/Dilution Table for Adults/Children** (*continued*)

| BoNT Preparation | OBTA (Botox®) | ABTA (Dysport®) | IBTA (Xeomin®) | RBTB (Myobloc®) | Notes |
|---|---|---|---|---|---|
| Guidance techniques | B-mode US | B-mode US | B-mode US | B-mode US | |
| Adverse events and side effects | Hematoma, pain, ptosis, weakness in injected or adjacent muscle(s), diplopia | Hematoma, pain, ptosis, weakness in injected or adjacent muscle(s), diplopia | Hematoma, pain, ptosis, weakness in injected or adjacent muscle(s), diplopia | Viscous saliva, dry mouthUncommon: respiratory failure in ALS | |

*Note:* When treating sialorrhea, bilateral parotid and submandibular glands were injected in the majority of published studies. The sublingual glands are technically more difficult to inject as they require an intraoral injection. This may be difficult in patients with a tonic bite reflex, patients with intellectual disability, and in less-cooperative patients. When injecting BoNT in salivary glands, many, if not most, expert clinicians recommend ultrasound guidance (to avoid inadvertent injection of BoNT into adjacent muscles).

*Abbreviations:* ABTA, abobotulinumtoxinA; BoNT, botulinum neurotoxin; FDA, Food and Drug Administration; IBTA, incobotulinumtoxinA; OBTA, onabotulinumtoxinA; PFNS, preservative-free normal saline (0.9%); RBTB, rimabotulinumtoxinB; US, Ultrasound.

*Sources:* Refs. 21, 34–36, 38, 40, 44, 66, 97, 197, 243, 301, 302, 304, 305, 307–329, 470.

**TABLE 14.2 First Author's Suggested Dosage Table (Adults ≥18 Years of Age and Pediatric ≤ 18 Years of Age)**

| BoNT Preparation | OBTA (Botox®) | ABTA (Dysport®) | IBTA (Xeomin®) | RBTB (Myobloc®) | Notes |
|---|---|---|---|---|---|
| **Parotid Gland, Adults[1]** | | | | | |
| Mild<br>Moderate<br>Severe | 15–25 units/gland<br>25–40 units/gland<br>40–55 units/gland | 40–60 units/gland<br>60–80 units/gland<br>80–110 units/gland | 15–25 units/gland<br>25–40 units/gland<br>40–55 units/gland | 200–300 units/gland<br>300–400 units/gland<br>400–625 units/gland | [1]B-mode US used for guidance of all injections |
| **Submandibular Gland, Adults,[1] Initial Dose** | | | | | |
| Mild<br>Moderate<br>Severe | 5–15 units/gland<br>15–30 units/gland<br>30–50 units/gland | 20–40 units/gland<br>40–60 units/gland<br>60–110 units/gland | 5–15 units/gland<br>15–30 units/gland<br>30–50 units/gland | 100–200 units/gland<br>200–300 units/gland<br>300–500 units/gland | [1]B-mode US used for guidance of all injections |
| Maximum total dose | 200 units, divided bilaterally | 500 units, divided bilaterally | 200 units, divided bilaterally | 2,500–3,000 units, divided bilaterally | |
| Subsequent doses | Increase by 5%–10% | Increase by 5%–10% | Increase by 5%–10% | Increase by 5%–10% | |

(*continued*)

**TABLE 14.2 First Author's Suggested Dosage Table (Adults ≥18 Years of Age and Pediatric ≤ 18 Years of Age)** *(continued)*

| BoNT Preparation | OBTA (Botox®) | ABTA (Dysport®) | IBTA (Xeomin®) | RBTB (Myobloc®) | Notes |
|---|---|---|---|---|---|
| **Pediatric patients,[1] Initial Dose** | | | | | |
| **Parotid gland**<br>Weight 15–50 kg<br>Weight >50 kg | 0.5–1 units/kg<br>Follow adult protocol | 1.5–2.2 units/kg<br>Follow adult protocol | 0.5–1 units/kg<br>Follow adult protocol | 5–10 units/kg<br>Follow adult protocol | Patients stratified by symptoms: mild, moderate, severe<br>Initial dose: lower for patients with milder symptoms and higher for those with moderate or severe sialorrhea<br>[1]B-mode US used for guidance of all injections |
| **Submandibular gland**<br>Weight 15–50 kg<br>Weight >50 kg | 0.5–1 unit/kg<br>Follow adult protocol | 1.5–2.2 units/kg<br>Follow adult protocol | 0.5–1 units/kg<br>Follow adult protocol | 5–10 units/kg<br>Follow adult protocol | |
| Subsequent doses | Increase by 5%–10% | Increase by 5%–10% | Increase by 5%–10% | Increase by 5%–10% | |
| Maximum total dose per treatment session | 150 units | 300 units | 150 units | 2,500 units | |

*Abbreviations:* ABTA, abobotulinumtoxinA; BoNT, botulinum neurotoxin; IBTA, incobotulinumtoxinA; OBTA, onabotulinumtoxinA; RBTB, rimabotulinumtoxinB; US, ultrasound.

# 15

# *Botulinum Neurotoxin Therapy for Hyperhidrosis*

*Katharine E. Alter, MD*
*Codrin Lungu, MD*

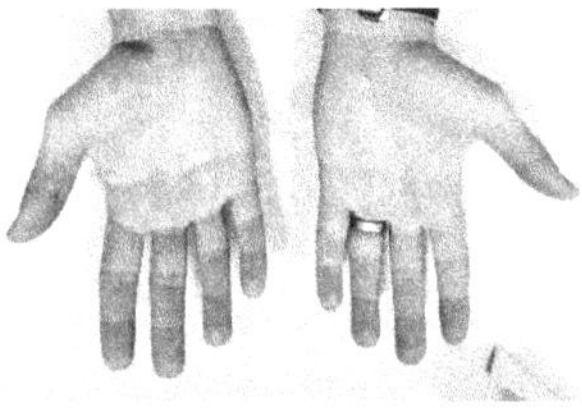

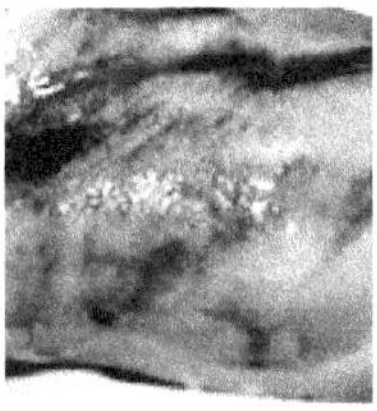

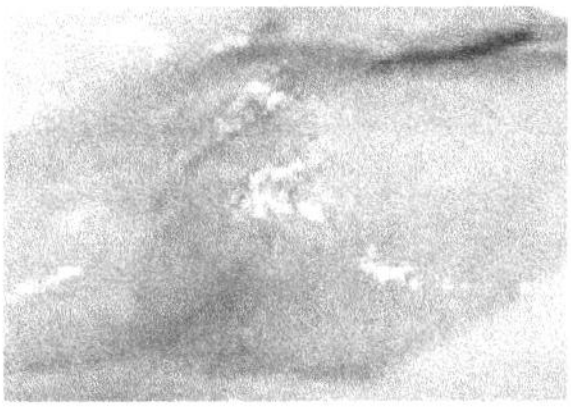

## Condition

Hyperhidrosis (HH) or excessive sweating can be a debilitating condition that may affect quality of life, cause social embarrassment, hygiene issues, and may interfere with an individual's ability to socialize and work. Sweating is controlled by the autonomic (sympathetic) nervous system. Normally sweating helps regulate body temperature by evaporative cooling. HH is an autonomic disorder leading to production of sweat in excess of that needed to maintain body temperature (330) and is broadly divided into primary and secondary subtypes.

### *Primary Hyperhidrosis*

Primary HH (PHH) is further subdivided into idiopathic PHH (IPHH) and a rare familial subtype. IPHH is the most common subtype of PHH with a reported incidence of 0.6% to 1% in the general population. The autosomal dominant familial subtype of PHH is much less common and, in some families, is linked to a chromosomal abnormality at 14q (331). When evaluating a patient with PHH, a detailed family history is required to rule out a potential inherited or familial cause of this condition (332).

### *Idiopathic Primary Hyperhidrosis*

In many patients with IPHH, symptoms begin in childhood and may worsen in adolescence. When workup fails to elicit a cause, the diagnosis of IPHH is established (331, 333). The diagnostic criteria for PHH include excessive sweating lasting ≥6 months with no apparent cause for the sweating and must include a minimum of two of the following features: excessive sweating that impairs daily activities, bilateral and fairly symmetric sweating, excessive sweating occurring at least once per week, onset of symptoms at younger than 25 years, excessive sweating not present during sleep, and a positive family history of HH, which may be elicited in a subset of patients (333).

Gustatory sweating (Frey syndrome) is a distinctive form of HH and may be primary (familial) or secondary to trauma. Patients report sweating of the face, scalp, and/or neck during or immediately following drinking or eating (331, 334).

### *Secondary Hyperhidrosis*

The causes of secondary HH (SHH) include a wide variety of systemic illnesses (tumors, metabolic, and endocrine disorders), spinal cord injury, and/or drug or toxin-induced HH. Other potential causes of SHH include familial dysautonomia (Riley–Day syndrome), posttraumatic/surgical SHH, and compensatory SHH. Compensatory SHH may occur following trauma, surgery, and postsympathectomy. Compensatory SHH is characterized by HH occurring in a part of the body unrelated to the location of surgery, trauma, or other treatment. As noted, gustatory sweating is also a form of SHH and may be either posttraumatic or from other local insults (331). When the cause for SHH can be identified, this problem should be addressed or treated prior to considering botulinum neurotoxin (BoNT) injections.

### *Clinical/Functional Impact*

As noted, PHH and SHH may have a significant impact on a patient's function and quality of life and may be socially debilitating. Patients often resort to wearing underarm pads, carrying towels, and may avoid social interactions such as shaking hands.

### *Pattern of Involvement*

Any eccrine sweat gland may be affected. In PHH, the involvement is generally bilateral and symmetric. Most commonly, complaints are of excessive sweating of the axilla and palms or soles of the feet. In SHH, excessive sweating may be symmetric and bilateral. However, in postsurgical or traumatic cases, it may be unilateral, asymmetric, and/or focal or localized.

### *Evaluation*

Evaluation of PHH and SHH should include a detailed history to determine the scope, pattern, and severity of the problem, as well as the impact of the excessive sweating on the patient's function and quality of life.

Clinicians should consider administering the Minor's iodine starch test (MIST) prior to and after injections to document the pattern and severity of sweating both pre- and postinjection (34). Patients should be instructed to shave their underarms the night before the appointment and to avoid over-the-counter or prescription deodorants or antiperspirants on the affected area for ≥24 hours prior to the MIST. Patients should also be instructed to avoid exercising or consuming hot drinks for at least 30 minutes prior to the test. The area to be tested (underarm, palm, or sole) should be patted dry with a towel and then immediately painted with iodine solution. Allow the area to dry completely and then lightly sprinkle the painted area with starch powder. Remove any excess starch powder by gently blowing on the area. Within 10 minutes, areas of HH will develop a deep blue or black color (34, 335).

### *Treatment of Hyperhidrosis*

Various treatments for HH include topical agents, enteral medications, injections, and surgery. Topical agents include over-the-counter or prescription antiperspirants or deodorants, other agents (glycopyrrolate), and iontophoretic therapy. Although some patients may benefit from enteral medications (anticholinergic agents or beta-blockers), many patients discontinue these drugs due to side effects or minimal clinical benefit. Surgical options for HH include sympathectomy and/or surgical resection of sweat glands. In addition to the risks of surgery, these treatments may also lead to compensatory HH in previously unaffected areas (331, 336). For patients who fail conservative treatment, BoNT therapy may provide significant long-lasting symptomatic relief, reduced disability, and improved function/quality of life (303, 331, 337). Acetylcholine (Ach) is the main neurotransmitter at the neuroglandular junction of the eccrine glands, and the effective blockage of Ach release is the basis for the efficacy of BoNT.

### *BoNTs Approved for the Treatment of Hyperhidrosis*

OnabotulinumtoxinA (OBTA [Botox®]) is approved for the treatment of primary axillary HH that is unresponsive or underresponsive to conventional treatment (34). Currently, none of the other Food and Drug Administration (FDA)-approved BoNT products (abobotulinumtoxinA [ABTA; Dysport®], incobotulinumtoxinA [IBTA; Xeomin®], and rimabotulinumtoxinB [RBTB; Myobloc®]) have FDA-approved indications for treatment of HH (36, 38, 44). The use of these products in the United States to treat axillary HH is currently off-label. None of the BoNT products available in the United States carry an indication for palmar or plantar HH, and treatment of these conditions is also considered off-label.

### *Approvals Outside of the United States*

OBTA is approved in the United Kingdom for the treatment of axillary HH. The use of other BoNT products for the treatment of axillary HH and the use of any of the currently available BoNT products for the treatment of palmar or plantar HH is considered off-label.

## *Level of Evidence*

A 2013 article reviewed the levels of evidence supporting or refuting the use of BoNT for the treatment of neurosecretory disorders including HH (303).

### AXILLARY HYPERHIDROSIS

The authors reported that current evidence supports a Level A (Established as effective) recommendation for the use of OBTA and a Level B (Probably effective) recommendation for the use of ABTA for the treatment of axillary HH (303). Due to a limited number of studies using IBTA and RBTB, a Level U (Unknown or unproven efficacy) recommendation was reported for these BoNT formulations. Another 2013 review article also reviewed the evidence from studies evaluating the efficacy and safety of BoNTs for the treatment of axillary and palmar HH and reported that current evidence supported a Level B recommendation for OBTA and ABTA, a Level C (Possibly effective) recommendation for IBTA, and Level U recommendation for RBTB (331).

### PALMAR HYPERHIDROSIS

The authors reported that the current level of evidence supports a Level B recommendation for the use of serotype A BoNTs and a Level C recommendation for serotype B BoNT for the treatment of palmar HH (303). Lakraj et al. reported a Level B recommendation for OBTA and ABTA, Level C recommendation for RBTB, and a Level U recommendation for IBTA (331).

### GUSTATORY SWEATING

Due to the limited number of studies and patients, the authors report a Level U recommendation for using BoNTs for the treatment of gustatory sweating (303).

## *Dosage (303, 331)*

### AXILLARY HYPERHIDROSIS

The manufacturer's recommended dose for the treatment of axillary HH with OBTA is 50 units per axilla (34). The published/reported effective dosage range of BoNT for the treatment of axillary HH is 50 to 75 units per side for OBTA, 100 to 200 units per side for ABTA, 50 units per side for IBTA, and 2,500 units per side for RBTB.

### PALMAR HYPERHIDROSIS

The published therapeutic dosage range for palmar HH for the various BoNT products is 50 to 100 units per palm for OBTA, 284 units per palm for ABTA, and 5,000 units per palm for RBTB.

## *Toxin Dilution*

For OBTA, the manufacturer's recommended dilution is 100 units with 4 mL of preservative-free sterile normal saline (PFNS; 0.9%) for injection. There is limited information on the optimal dilution for ABTA and IBTA. RBTB is provided in solution and does not require reconstitution. If desired, RBTB can be diluted with normal saline.

### *Injection Pattern and Technique*

The diluted BoNT (2 mL) should be evenly distributed within the hyperhidrotic region of the axilla (as identified by MIST) and should be divided into 10 to 15 equal aliquots of 0.1 to 0.2 mL (Figure 15.1). Palmar injections should be distributed at 1-cm intervals, a grid may be drawn on the palm if desired (Figure 15.2). Injections are performed intradermally using a 30-gauge needle. The needle should be inserted to a depth of approximately 2 mm, at a 45° angle to the surface of the skin (Figure 15.3). The bevel side of the needle should point to the surface of the skin to minimize leakage and to make certain that the injected BoNT remains intradermal. If injection sites are marked in ink, do not inject the BoNT directly through the ink mark to avoid creating a permanent tattoo effect. No adjunctive localization technique (electromyography, e-stim, or ultrasound) is required for these intradermal injections (34, 331).

*FIGURE 15.1 Hyperhidrosis, axilla injection grid.*

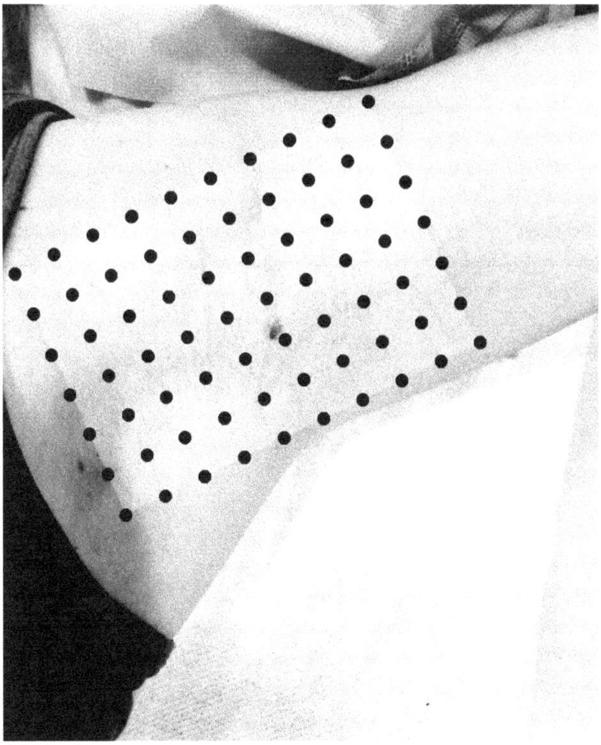

*FIGURE 15.2 Hyperhidrosis, palmar injection grid.*

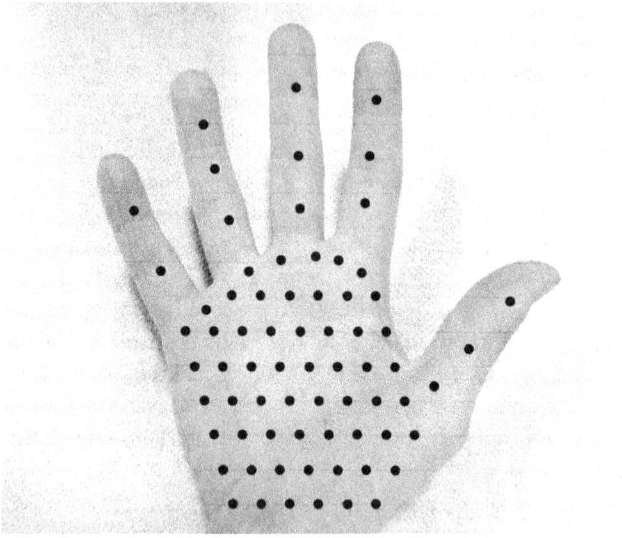

*FIGURE 15.3 Technique for intradermal botulinum neurotoxin injections.*

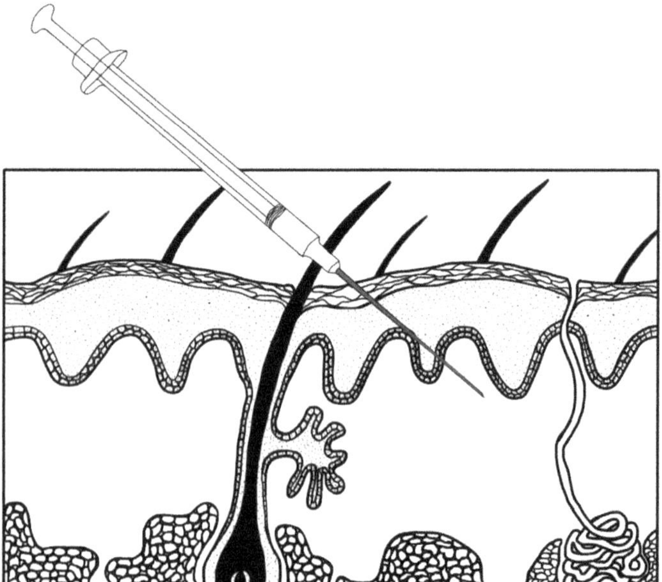

### *Clinical Effect*

The clinical effect is generally apparent within 5 to 7 days, with an average duration of effect ranging from 3 to 7 months. Re-injection should be performed as clinically indicated, based on the return of symptoms.

### *Adverse Events/Side Effects*

The most common adverse events following BoNT injections for HH include pain following injection, headache, nausea, flu-like symptoms, and dry mouth. Compensatory HH in untreated areas is also reported (303, 338).There is a single case report of systemic adverse effects (blurred vision and dysphagia) following treatment of palmar HH with 2,500 units RBTB (339). Skin irritation is sometimes reported when using topical anesthetic agents. Patients should receive information on the general risks associated with BoNT therapy, which is provided in the risk evaluation and management information product insert included with each vial of BoNT.

**TABLE 15.1 BoNT for the Treatment of Hyperhidrosis Dosage/Dilution Table**

| BoNT Preparation | OBTA (Botox®) | ABTA (Dysport®) | IBTA (Xeomin®) | RBTB (Myobloc®) | Notes |
|---|---|---|---|---|---|
| U.S. FDA approval | Primary axillary and palmar hyperhidrosis | Currently not FDA approved | Currently not FDA approved | Currently not FDA approved | |
| **Axillary Hyperhidrosis, Manufacturer Recommended Dosage* (Adults ≥18 Years of Age)** | | | | | |
| Dose per side<br>Total dosage | 50 units<br>100 units | N/A | N/A | N/A | Use a 30-gauge, 0.5-inch needle. |
| Dilution | 100 units diluted with 4-mL PFNS* | N/A | N/A | N/A | |
| Injection technique | Intradermal injections, needle bevel pointed up (to the surface of the skin) | N/A | N/A | N/A | If injection sites are marked with a pen, do not insert needle through the ink to avoid creating a permanent ink tattoo. |
| Injection pattern | Draw a 1-cm square grid on the axilla. One injection site per square | N/A | N/A | N/A | |
| Treatment interval | Minimum 12 weeks<br>May last 4–7 months | | | | |
| **Hyperhidrosis, Published Dosage Range: Adults (≥18 Years of Age)** | | | | | |
| Axillary | 50–165 units per side | 125–200 units per side[1] | 50–100 units per side | 375–2,500 units per side | [1]For ABTA, 200 units per side is most commonly reported. |
| Palmar[2] | 25–165 units per hand, divided bilaterally | 120–200 units per side | 100–150 units per hand | 250–5,000 units per side | [2]Prior to the procedure, topical anesthesia and/or anesthetic nerve blocks may be considered. |

*(continued)*

**TABLE 15.1 BoNT for the Treatment of Hyperhidrosis Dosage/Dilution Table (*continued*)**

| BoNT Preparation | OBTA (Botox®) | ABTA (Dysport®) | IBTA (Xeomin®) | RBTB (Myobloc®) | Notes |
|---|---|---|---|---|---|
| **Hyperhidrosis, Published Dosage Range: Adults (≥18 Years of Age) (*continued*)** | | | | | |
| Gustatory sweating | 20–30 units, divided | 40–60 units, divided | 20–30 units, divided | 250–600 units, divided | |
| Recommended dilution for hyperhidrosis and gustatory sweating[3] (concentration) | 100 units in 4-mL PFNS (2.5 units/0.1 mL) or 100 units in 5 mL (2 units/0.1 mL) | 300 units in 1.5-mL PFNS (200 units/mL, 10 units/0.05 mL) or 300 units in 3-mL PFNS (100 units/mL, 10 units/0.1 mL) or 500 units in 5- mL PFNS (100units/mL, 10 units/0.1mL) | 50 units in 2–2.5 mL or 100 units in 4–5 mL | No reconstitution required | [3]Reconstitute with PFNS (0.9%). |
| Units per injection site | 1.5–5 units per cm | 5–20 units per cm | 2.5–5 units per cm | 7.5–200 units per cm | |
| Injection pattern | Intradermal injection every 1–2 cm | Intradermal injection every 1–2 cm | Intradermal injection every 1–2 cm | Intradermal injection every 1–2 cm | Note: If injection sites are marked with a pen, do not insert needle through the ink to avoid creating a permanent ink tattoo. |
| Axilla | 20–40 sites | 18–40 sites | 18–40 sites | 20–40 sites | |
| Palm | 20–30 sites | 20–30 sites | 20–30 sites | 20–30 sites | |
| Gustatory sweating | Multiple sites in the affected area, number not specified | Multiple sites in the affected area, number not specified | Multiple sites in the affected area, number not specified | Multiple sites in the affected area, number not specified | |

(*continued*)

**TABLE 15.1 BoNT for the Treatment of Hyperhidrosis Dosage/Dilution Table (*continued*)**

| BoNT Preparation | OBTA (Botox®) | ABTA (Dysport®) | IBTA (Xeomin®) | RBTB (Myobloc®) | Notes |
|---|---|---|---|---|---|
| **Hyperhidrosis, Published Dosage Range: Adults (≥18 Years of Age) (*continued*)** | | | | | |
| Re-injection interval | 3–7 months | 3–7 months | 3–7 months | 3–7 months | |
| Adverse events | Injection site pain, dry mouth, flu-like symptoms | Injection site pain, dry mouth, flu-like symptoms | Injection site pain, dry mouth, flu-like symptoms | Injection site pain, dry mouth, flu-like symptoms, dysphagia, blurred vision | |

*Abbreviations*: ABTA, abobotulinumtoxinA; BoNT, botulinum neurotoxin; FDA, Food and Drug Administration; IBTA, incobotulinumtoxinA; OBTA, onabotulinumtoxinA; PFNS, preservative-free normal saline (0.9%); RBTB, rimabotulinumtoxinB.

*Sources*: Refs. 34, 36, 38, 44, 57, 96, 303, 331, 334, 335–339, 570–587.

# Part III

## *Botulinum Neurotoxins for Urologic Disorders*

# 16

# *Botulinum Neurotoxin for Urologic Conditions*

*Katharine E. Alter, MD*
*Dallas A. Lea II, MD*

## Condition

Disorders of voiding, or micturition, are common clinical problems for a large portion of the population worldwide, including individuals with and without physical impairments or disabilities. Detrusor overactivity (DO) from idiopathic overactive bladder (IOAB), neurogenic detrusor overactivity (NDO), detrusor dyssynergia (DD), and outflow obstruction due to benign prostatic hyperplasia (BPH) may affect all bladder functions, including urine storage, voiding, and urinary continence (230, 340, 341).

### *Detrusor Overactivity*

DO is characterized by involuntary contractions of the detrusor muscle during bladder filling. Involuntary detrusor contractions cause symptoms of urgency, urge incontinence, and may cause pain. The majority of patients presenting with DO have IOAB (342). DO may be idiopathic or may be found in association with neurological disorders affecting bladder innervation or control, for example, when it is attributed to neurogenic DO or detrusor dysfunction associated with neurological conditions (NDO) (343, 344).

### *IOAB*

IOAB is defined by the International Continence Society as urinary urgency, usually accompanied by frequency and nocturia, with or without urgency urinary incontinence (UUI) in the absence of urinary tract infection (UTI) or other obvious pathology (343). The incidence of IOAB in the general population is reported to be 11.8% to 16.8% (342, 344).

### *NDO*

NDO, like IOAB, is a form of DO characterized by involuntary bladder contractions during filling/storage phases. This may lead to a noncompliant bladder with increased bladder pressure and incontinence. NDO may also be associated with sphincter-DD with a loss of coordination between detrusor and sphincter function leading to upper urinary tract dysfunction and other symptoms. NDO is commonly seen in patients with Parkinson disease, multiple sclerosis, spinal cord injury, cerebral palsy, spina bifida, and other upper motor neuron syndromes. Mobility impairments in patients with NDO may also contribute to the problem of incontinence due to difficulty getting to the toilet, performing a transfer, and then removing items of clothing. Bladder symptoms and incontinence may adversely affect hygiene and quality of life (QOL) and may cause isolation (340).

### *DD*

Detrusor-external sphincter dyssynergia (DD) is caused by involuntary contraction of the detrusor and the external urethral sphincter muscles. DD is caused by various neurological lesions between the brainstem and the sacral spinal cord. DD is most commonly seen in patients with spinal cord injuries (SCI), transverse myelitis, multiple sclerosis (MS), and myelodysplasia or spina bifida. Various treatments are prescribed including enteral medications, BoNTs, and surgical interventions (351, 593).

### *BPH*

Prostatic hyperplasia, or enlargement, may lead to lower urinary tract obstruction with incomplete bladder emptying, nocturia, and frequency. BPH is common, with a reported incidence of up to 50% in men over 40 years of age (345).

### *Clinical/Functional Impact*

Urgency, frequency, incomplete bladder emptying, nocturia, and incontinence may affect QOL, including maintenance of hygiene and socialization. In addition, this constellation of symptoms, either individually or in combination, can lead to upper urinary tract pathology in some patients (generally those with DD).

### *Pattern of Involvement*

In DO, the most common symptoms are frequency, urgency, urge incontinence, and nocturia. In BPH, outflow tract obstruction produces the most common symptoms, causing frequency, urgency, nocturia, and incontinence.

### *Evaluation*

A detailed clinical history will often point to the probable diagnosis. While a presumed diagnosis of overactive bladder (OAB) or NDO can be made based on a patient's clinical symptoms, a confirmed diagnosis requires urologic/urodynamic testing (230).

All patients should be screened for the presence of a UTI, which can be a contributing factor to the patient's symptoms. A diagnosis of BPH is established based on clinical symptoms, physical examination, imaging (ultrasound and/or MRI), or urologic testing, as deemed appropriate. A full discussion of the workup of DO/IOAB/NDO/DD/BPH is beyond the scope of this chapter. Readers are referred to relevant review articles (341, 346–349). Prior to proceeding with treatment, including oral medications and other treatments, a clear diagnosis of the type of bladder dysfunction should be established.

### *Treatment*

Treatment of DO includes behavioral techniques, physical therapy, catheterization, oral medications, injectable agents, and surgery. Behavioral techniques include avoidance of caffeine and other bladder irritants as well as timed voiding. Physical therapy includes bladder training, pelvic floor exercises (e.g., Kegel exercises), and electrical stimulation. Pharmacologic management includes enteral medications, specifically anticholinergic and antimuscarinic agents (344, 346, 350). Surgical options are available but are limited (344). While many patients may be treated effectively with one or more of these treatments, many patients are incompletely treated or have undesirable side effects with these traditional treatment options. For these patients, botulinum neurotoxin (BoNT) injections should be considered as a potential therapy (344).

BoNT may be a useful therapy for patients affected by a number of urologic conditions that affect voiding or micturition, such as OAB, DD, and benign prostatic hyperplasia. BoNT is an approved treatment (for IOAB, NDO) or an investigational treatment (for DD, BPH) for a number of urological conditions (16, 34, 230). While BoNT injections in the bladder are most commonly performed by urologists, other specialists who prescribe/inject BoNT must also be familiar with the use of BoNT for these conditions. This is particularly important as a patient may be receiving BoNT therapy for different indications and from multiple specialists. For example, a patient with a spinal cord injury may be a candidate for BoNT to treat spasticity and to treat DD or a patient with a brain injury or stroke may require BoNT injections for treatment of chronic migraine headache and OAB. To avoid an excessive total dose and/or an inadequate injection interval, it is imperative that physicians ask patients whether they have received or plan to receive BoNT injections performed by another physician for a separate condition.

### *BoNTs Approved for the Treatment of Urologic Conditions*

OnabotulinumtoxinA (OBTA) is approved by the Food and Drug Administration (FDA) for the treatment of adult patients (≥18 years of age) with OAB that impairs QOL and is unresponsive to anticholinergic medications. OBTA is also approved for the treatment of adult patients (≥18 years of age) with NDO that impairs QOL and upper urinary tract function.

Neither of the other FDA-approved serotype A BoNT products (abobotulinumtoxinA [ABTA] and incobotulinumtoxinA [IBTA]) nor the single serotype B BoNT (rimabotulinumtoxinB [RBTB]) is approved for OAB or NDO. None of the BoNT products available in the United States are currently approved for DD, BPH, or for the treatment of urologic conditions in children.

### *Approvals Outside of the United States*

None were discovered in a review of the literature and/or government agency publications related to the approved indications of BoNTs.

### *Duration of Effect*

The reported duration of action of BoNTs in smooth muscle is significantly longer than that observed in skeletal muscle. For OBTA, the typical duration of effect is reported to be 6 months for IOAB and 9.5 months for NDO (16, 346).

### *Level of Evidence*

Chancellor et al. performed an evidence-based review of BoNT for the treatment of urologic disorders including IOAB, NDO, DD, and BPH (230).

#### IOAB

The authors concluded that evidence from existing trials supports a Level A (Established as effective) recommendation for the use of OBTA for the treatment of IOAB. Due to limited evidence for IOAB, a Level U (Unproven) recommendation was reported for the other serotype A BoNTs (ABTA and IBTA) and for RBTB (230).

#### NDO

A Level A recommendation was reported for OBTA and ABTA. Due to a lack of studies evaluating the efficacy of IBTA and RBTB, a Level U recommendation was reported for these BoNT products (230).

#### BPH

A Level B (Probably effective) recommendation was reported for BoNT (specifically, OBTA) for the treatment of BPH. Due to the lack of sufficient evidence, the authors reported a Level U recommendation for ABTA, IBTA, and RBTB for the treatment of BPH (230).

A 2011 evidence-based review of BoNT therapy for the treatment of DO (IOAB, NDO, and DD), bladder outflow obstruction (BOO), and painful bladder (PB) reported Level I evidence supporting the use of OBTA and ABTA for the treatment of NDO in adult patients (2011). The review also concluded that there was Level I evidence for ABTA in the treatment of NDO in children. Level 1 evidence was also reported for OBTA for the treatment of IOAB, DD, BOO, and PB associated with interstitial cystitis (351).

#### DD

A review of the literature revealed a limited number of studies of BoNT. In 2014, the existing evidence is insufficient to make a recommendation for the use of BoNTs in the treatment of DD (230, 351).

## *Dosage*

IOAB AND NDO

OBTA is approved for the treatment of IOAB and NDO in the United States. For the treatment of IOAB, the manufacturer's recommended dose of OBTA is 100 units. For NDO, the manufacturer's recommended dose of OBTA is 200 units. For DO, the duration of efficacy is reported to be longer in smooth muscle than in skeletal muscle, with a reported duration of 6 months for OAB and 9.5 months for NDO (16).

OBTA

The published dose range for the treatment of IOAB is 50 to 300 units. A higher incidence of adverse events (e.g., urinary retention and infection) is reported with doses exceeding 100 units (16, 230). The published dose range for NDO is 200 to 300 units.

ABTA

For the treatment of NDO and IOAB, the reported dose of ABTA is 500 to 1,000 units (352–355).

IBTA

PubMed and Medline searches returned no studies or reports related to IBTA in the treatment of DO (IOAB, NDO).

RBTB

Evidence and studies using RBTB for IOAB and NDO are limited. The optimal dose for RBTB for DO (IOAB, NDO) is not well defined. Currently available studies reported a dose of 5,000 units RBTB for these conditions (356).

DD

There are a limited number of studies evaluating the efficacy of BoNTs for the treatment of DD and the use of BoNT to treat DD remains off-label. The published dose range for OBTA for DD is 100 to 240 for adult patients. A 2014 article reported a dose of 300 units ABTA for the treatment DD in adults (357). In pediatric patients with myelodysplasia, Safari et al. reported a dose of 8 units/kg of ABTA injected into the detrusor and 2 units/kg injected into the external sphincter muscle (358). PubMed and Medline searches returned no articles reporting on the use of IBTA or RBTB for the management of DD.

BPH

As noted, there are a limited number of studies evaluating the optimal dose of the various BoNT products for the treatment of BPH (230). The published dose range of OBTA for the treatment of BPH is 100 to 600 units. Nikoobakht et al. reported using 300 to 600 units ABTA for BPH (359). There are no published reports on the dose of IBTA or RBTB for the treatment of BPH.

## *Toxin Dilution*

OBTA, ABTA, and IBTA should only be reconstituted or diluted with preservative-free normal saline (PFNS, 0.9%). RBTB is provided in solution and does not require dilution. If desired, RBTB can be diluted with normal saline.

### OBTA FOR IOAB

For treatment of IOAB, a 100-unit vial of OBTA is diluted with 10 mL of PFNS, which results in a concentration of 10 units/mL or 1 unit/0.1 mL.

### OBTA FOR NDO

The recommended dose is 200-units. To achieve the correct dilution for a 200-unit dose, either two 100-unit vials or one 200-unit vial of OBTA can be used.

When using two 100-unit vials of OBTA, each vial is diluted with 6 mL PFNS. Following this initial reconstitution, draw up 4 mL into three 10-mL syringes. To complete the dilution/reconstitution, draw up an additional 6 mL of PFNS into each of the 10-mL syringes for a total volume of 30 mL.

For a 200-unit vial of OBTA, first dilute/reconstitute the 200-unit vial with 6 mL PFNS. Following this initial reconstitution/dilution, draw up 2 mL into three 10-mL syringes. Then draw up an additional 8 mL PFNS into each syringe for a total volume of 30 mL. Using either of these reconstitution techniques results in a concentration of approximately 67 units/10 mL or 0.67 units/0.1 mL (34).

## *Injection Pattern*

For IOAB and NDO, BoNT is injected into the detrusor muscle (see Figure 16.1). For DD, BoNT is injected into the detrusor and/or external sphincter. For BPH, BoNT is injected into the transurethral portion of the prostate gland (see Figure 16.2).

***FIGURE 16.1*** *Botulinum neurotoxin injection pattern for detrusor muscle and prostate.*

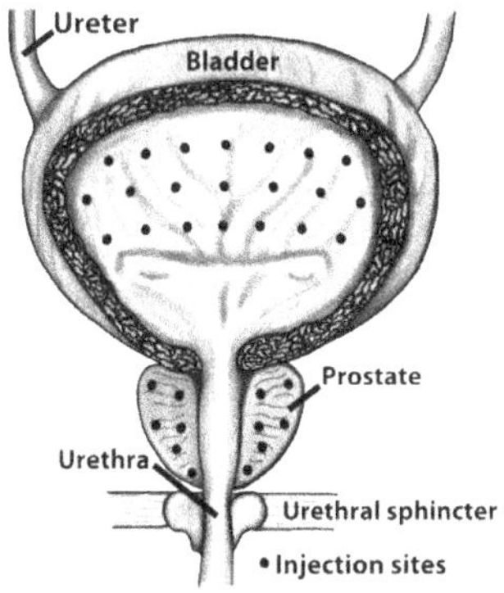

*FIGURE 16.2 Bladder filling.*

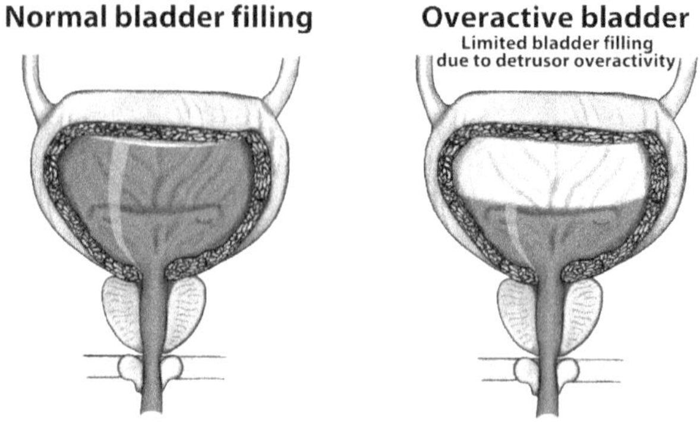


### *Injection Technique*

Bladder injections are performed using a flexible or rigid cystoscope (230). The needle is inserted to a depth of approximately 2 mm and the dose of BoNT is injected into the detrusor muscle. The total dose is divided into 20 or 30 equal aliquots or injection sites, depending on the dose. Following the injection of the final aliquot of BoNT, 1 mL PFNS should be injected so that the BoNT remaining in the needle is flushed from the needle and injected into the bladder (34). For the treatment of NDO, injections are performed in the detrusor and/or external sphincter using a cystoscope. The most common techniques for prostate injections are the transperineal or transrectal approach using ultrasound guidance (359, 360).

### *Clinical Effect*

The reported benefits following BoNT injections when treating IOAB and NDO include improved bladder function (i.e., filling/storage, decreased frequency, and urge incontinence) (346). Injections of BoNT are reported to reduce bladder and upper urinary tract pressures when treating patients with DD. OBTA has been shown to reduce lower urinary tract obstructive symptoms and nocturia in patients with BPH (34, 230).

### *Adverse Events/Side Effects*

The most commonly reported adverse events following BoNT injections for DO, IOAB, NDO, and DD are urinary retention and UTIs. Remote risks include the risks listed in the full prescribing information for each BoNT product (34, 36, 38, 44, 346, 351). The most commonly reported adverse events following BoNT therapy for BPH include postinjection hematuria, prostatitis, and exacerbation of pre-existing incontinence (351).

**TABLE 16.1 BoNT for Urologic Disorders Dosage/Dilution Table. Manufacturer's Published/Approved Dosage (Adults ≥18 Years of Age)**

| BoNT Preparation | OBTA (Botox®) | ABTA (Dysport®) | IBTA (Xeomin®) | RBTB (Myobloc®) | Notes |
|---|---|---|---|---|---|
| U.S. FDA approval | IOAB and DDANC | Currently not FDA approved | Currently not FDA approved | Currently not FDA approved | |
| UK MHRA | Currently not an approved indication | Currently not an approved indication | Currently not an approved indication | Currently not an approved indication | |
| IOAB | 100 units | — | — | — | >100 units associated with UTI and urinary retention |
| DO associated with neurological conditions (NDO) | 200 units | — | — | — | |
| Dilution | 100 units in 10 mL PFNS or 200 units in 30 mL PFNS | — | — | — | |
| **Typical Injection Interval** | | | | | |
| IOAB | 6 months | — | — | — | |
| NDO | 9 months | — | — | — | |
| Injection pattern | See chapter | See chapter | See chapter | See chapter | |

*(continued)*

**TABLE 16.1 BoNT for Urologic Disorders Dosage/Dilution Table. Manufacturer's Published/Approved Dosage (Adults ≥18 Years of Age) (*continued*)**

| BoNT Preparation | OBTA (Botox®) | ABTA (Dysport®) | IBTA (Xeomin®) | RBTB (Myobloc®) | Notes |
|---|---|---|---|---|---|
| **Published Dosage Range: Adults (≥18 Years of Age)** | | | | | |
| IOAB | 100–300 units | 500 units | — | 5,000 units | |
| NDO | 50–300 units | 500–1,000 units | — | 5,000 units | |
| DD | 100–240 units | 300 units | — | — | |
| BPH | 100–200 units | 300–600 units | — | — | |
| **Published Dosage Range: Pediatric Patients (<18 Years of Age)** | | | | | |
| IOAB | 10 units/kg | 400–500 units (13–14 units/kg) 6–16 years of age | — | — | |
| NDO | 10 units/kg | 10–20 units/kg | — | — | |
| DD | Detrusor: 10 units/kg or 8 units/kg (detrusor) + 2 units/kg (external sphincter) | — | — | — | |

*Abbreviations:* ABTA, abobotulinumtoxinA; BPH, benign prostatic hyperplasia; DD, detrusor dyssynergia; DDANC, detrusor dysfunction associated with neurologic conditions; FDA, Food and Drug Administration; IBTA, incobotulinumtoxinA; IOAB, idiopathic overactive bladder; NDO, neurogenic detrusor overactivity; OBTA, onabotulinumtoxinA; PFNS, preservative-free normal saline (0.9%); RBTB, rimabotulinumtoxinB; UTI, urinary tract infection.

*Sources:* Refs. Adapted from Refs. 16, 34, 36, 38, 44, 230, 340–342, 344, 345, 348, 349, 351–360, 373, 588–603.

# Part IV

# *Botulinum Neurotoxins for Pain Conditions*

While the efficacy and safety of botulinum neurotoxins (BoNTs) for treating pain associated with cervical dystonia and chronic migraine are well recognized, the precise mechanism of action (MOA) by which BoNTs exert antinociceptive effects is not entirely understood (11, 628, 638).

BoNTs may indirectly reduce pain by reducing muscle spasm or muscle overactivity. However, there is an increasing body of literature suggesting that BoNTs also have a direct antinociceptive effect that is likely responsible for the reduced pain seen in patients with pain syndromes or conditions. For example, BoNTs block vesicle-mediated exocytosis at the neuromuscular junction and at pain signaling synapses, thereby blocking the release of neurotransmitters (e.g., acetylcholine), nociceptive neurotransmitters, and other pain peptides (11). BoNTs may also modify afferent input from muscles spindles and pain from inflammation (11, 371, 397). A full description of the BoNT MOA for pain reduction is beyond the scope of this text and readers are referred to several review articles (450, 416, 11, 371, 397).

All four of the BoNT products currently available in the United States are approved by the Food and Drug Administration (FDA) for the treatment of pain and muscle overactivity associated with cervical dystonia (Botox PI®, Dysport PI®, Myobloc PI®, Xeomin PI®). OnabotulinumtoxinA (OBTA, Botox) is also approved for the treatment of pain associated with chronic migraine and for the treatment of upper limb spasticity in adult patients. There are also reports of decreased pain and spasms in addition to decreased spasticity with the use of OBTA injections in these conditions (Botox PI). Currently none of the BoNT products available in the United States is approved for the treatment of other pain conditions. Therefore, their use for treatment of pain disorders remains off-label.

There is an increasing body of literature on the use of BoNT injections to reduce the pain associated with a wide variety of musculoskeletal and neurologic disorders including:

- Myofascial pain (Göbel et al., 2006 [396]; Porta, 2000 [383])
- Trigger points (Singh, 2013 [416])

- Piriformis syndrome (Al-Al-Shaikh et al., 2014 [611])
- Thoracic outlet syndrome (TOS) (Foley et al., 2012 [443])
- Epicondylitis/epicondylosis (Singh, 2013 [416])
- Plantar fasciitis (Chou et al., 2011 [385])
- Arthritis-related joint pain (Singh et al., 2009 [422])
- Shoulder pain, including poststroke shoulder pain (Baker and Pereira, 2013 [612])
- Hip pain and perioperative pain in children and adults with cerebral palsy (Baker and Pereira, 2013 [612]; Barwood et al., 2000 [251])
- Spasms and pain from spasticity (Brown et al., 2014 [450]; Singh, 2013 [416]; Baker and Pereira, 2013 [612]; Barwood et al., 2000 [251])
- Neuropathic pain (Brown et al., 2014 [450])

Although the use of BoNTs to treat musculoskeletal pain remains off-label, BoNT therapy may be offered to patients who have failed other treatment modalities. This section of the text includes chapters on the use of BoNT injections for the treatment of chronic migraine and a review of BoNT injections for various musculoskeletal pain syndromes.

# 17

# *Botulinum Neurotoxins for the Treatment of Headache*

*Katharine E. Alter, MD*
*Pritha Ghosh, MD*

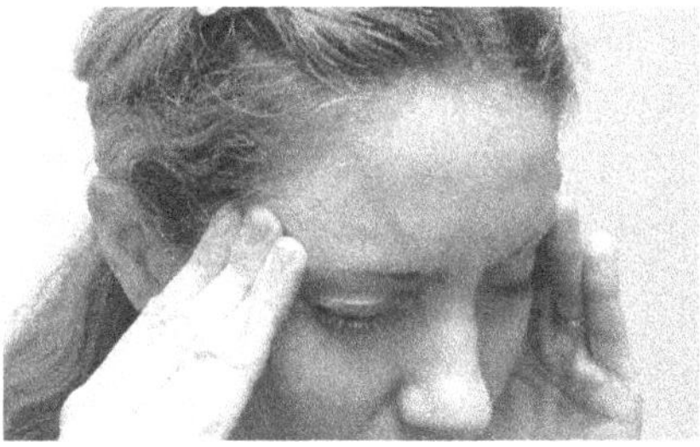

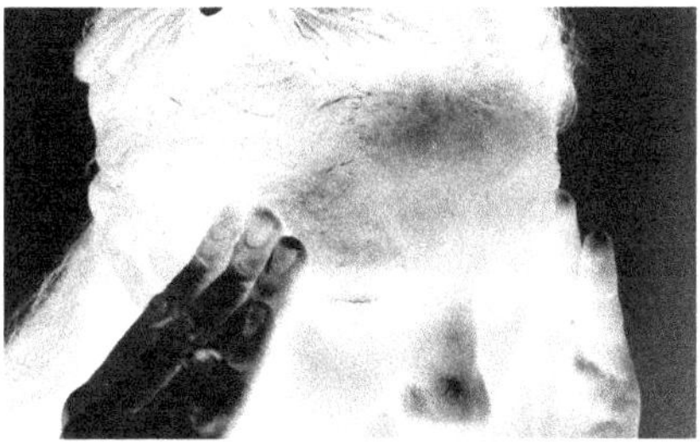

## Condition

Pain associated with headache (HA) is a common clinical complaint, affecting 45 million individuals annually in the United States and being the fifth most common cause of presentation to an emergency department. In the United States, the prevalence of severe HA in adults (≥18 years of age) is reported to be between 16% and 26%, with a reported worldwide incidence of 8% to 18% (361, 362). The International Headache Society (IHS) has specific diagnostic criteria for various HA subtypes including migraine HA (MHA), chronic migraine HA (CMHA), and tension type HA (TTH) (363, 364). A full discussion of this classification is beyond the scope of this chapter and for details readers are referred to the IHS. In brief, HAs are first divided into two categories, primary and secondary HA. In primary HA, the HA is the primary condition (e.g., MHA and TTH), whereas in secondary HAs, the HA symptoms can be attributed to another primary condition (e.g., posttraumatic HA or low pressure/post-lumbar puncture HA). HA is further subdivided into episodic (≤15 days/month) and chronic HA (≥15 days/month for longer than 3 months) (365).

### *Migraine*

MHA is a primary HA disorder that is often accompanied by other symptoms including photophobia, phonophobia, nausea, and vomiting. Although the pathophysiology of MHA is incompletely understood, it is attributed at least in part to activation of nociceptors on the meninges and surrounding blood vessels leading to stimulation of intracranial pain signaling pathways and dysfunction of endogenous pain control pathways (366, 367). This process includes stimulation of trigeminal neurons and perivascular nerve endings, resulting in the release of vasoactive peptides and peptide mediators involved with pain signaling. Chronic migraine is a HA disorder with a frequency of greater than or equal to 15 days with MHA per month for at least 3 months.

### *Tension Type Headache*

TTH is the most common primary HA subtype and is associated with both disability and reduced quality of life (364, 368). The pathophysiology of TTH is not well understood, in part because TTH likely has a variety of causes. Current opinion on the pathophysiology of TTH includes central and peripheral mechanisms of pain. Pain can be mild or moderate and is most often described as bilateral, band-like tightening, or aching pain. It is not typically associated with nausea or vomiting, but photophobia may be described.

### *Chronic Daily HA*

Chronic daily HA (CDA) is a group of HA disorders that includes both CMHA and TTH. Patients typically report having daily HAs. They have higher use/overuse of medications and report a higher incidence of disability (365).

### *Clinical/Functional Impact*

HA, particularly chronic HA, has a significant impact on quality of life, participation in family life, and may lead to frequent absences from work. Chronic pain associated with HA may lead to medication overuse and other adverse events.

### *Pattern of Involvement*

The pain of MHA is often unilateral and is typically described as moderate to severe pain that is pulsating or stabbing in character. Pain is increased by lights, sound, physical activity, and, as noted, patients often report nausea and/or vomiting. The pain of TTH is typically bilateral, band-like, and mild to moderate in severity.

### *Evaluation*

The diagnosis of migraine, migraine variants, and TTH is largely based on a thorough clinical history and physical examination to rule out potential causes of secondary HA. Evaluation should include a HA diary, which helps establish the frequency, severity, chronicity, and impact of HA on a patient's function. Establishing the frequency of

HAs in terms of days per month is critical when considering botulinum neurotoxin (BoNT) therapy, as many insurers require preauthorization with documentation of this information prior to approving treatment.

# Treatment of Headache

## *Migraine*

The treatment of migraine is subdivided into abortive and preventive treatments. Treatment is also divided into oral medication, injectable agents, neurostimulation, and surgery (366, 367). Patients use a variety of over-the-counter (OTC) medications for acute treatment of both MHA and TTH, including acetaminophen, nonsteroidal anti-inflammatory drugs (NSAIDs), and caffeine-containing drugs. Migraine-specific prescription abortive agents include tryptans, ergot-containing drugs, and analgesics (367). Preventive treatments are used to reduce the frequency, duration, and/or severity of MHA and options include anticonvulsants (e.g., topiramate and valproate), beta-adrenergic blockers, calcium channel blockers, and selective serotonin reuptake inhibitors (SSRIs).

## *Tension Type Headache*

The treatment of TTH includes OTC analgesics (e.g., acetaminophen and NSAIDs), antidepressants (e.g., SSRIs and tricyclic antidepressants), and occasionally injections of local anesthetics or steroids. Behavioral techniques include behavioral modification, relaxation techniques, and massage therapy (369, 370).

## *BoNT Therapy for HA*

BoNT injections have been effective in reducing the frequency and severity of CMHAs that occur 15 days or more per month. BoNT may also be useful in some patients with CDA, episodic migraine (≤15 HA days per month), and TTH (362, 371, 372). The BoNT mechanism of action (MOA) at presynaptic cholinergic nerve terminals involves blocking the release of acetylcholine. There is also evidence that BoNTs block the release of vasoactive and neuropeptides involved in pain signaling. Although the precise MOA for how BoNTs reduce the frequency, duration, and severity of pain associated with CMHA, CDHA, and TTH is not fully described, it is likely related to reduced afferent pain signaling and central sensitization, rather than from a direct neuromuscular effect (362, 365).

## *BoNTs Approved for the Treatment of HA*

OnabotulinumtoxinA (OBTA or Botox®) was approved by the FDA in 2010 for HA treatment in adult patients with chronic migraine (>15 HA days per month, lasting ≥4 hours per day). None of the other FDA-approved BoNTs are currently approved for the treatment of HA (abobotulinumtoxinA [ABTA/Dysport®], incobotulinumtoxinA

[IBTA/Xeomin®], or rimabotulinumtoxinB [RBTB/Myobloc®/NeuroBloc®]), (36, 38, 44). Therefore, the use of BoNTs other than OBTA and/or the use of BoNTs for prevention/treatment of episodic migraine (<15 days per months) and for treatment of TTH is currently off-label.

### *Approvals Outside the United States*

OBTA or Botox was approved in 2010 by regulatory agencies in Canada and the United Kingdom for the treatment of chronic migraine.

### *Level of Evidence*

There is high-quality evidence to support the use of serotype A BoNT (OBTA) for the treatment of chronic migraine. BoNTs for the treatment of other HA subtypes may be effective, but this has not yet been established (369–371, 373). In a recent review, Jabbari and Machado evaluated the evidence supporting the use of BoNTs for the treatment of refractory pain including MHA, CMHA, and TTH (138, 371). The authors concluded that that there is sufficient evidence from Level 1 studies to support a Level A (Established as effective) recommendation for use of OBTA for the treatment of CMHA (≥15 HA days per month, >4 hours per day, and ≥3 months duration). The same authors concluded that there is sufficient evidence to support a Level B (Insufficient evidence to support or refute efficacy/safety, but established as probably effective) recommendation for use of OBTA for the treatment of CDHA and TTH. The authors recommended additional studies for chronic TTH and CDHA to evaluate efficacy in these patients as the currently available studies were limited by their design and inclusion criteria.

## *Injection Pattern*

The three most commonly used injection patterns when injecting BoNT for CMHA are a "fixed dose protocol" (FDP), a "follow the pain protocol" (FTPP), and a "combined approach." In the FDP, a prescribed dose of BoNT is injected into a predetermined set of muscles at a fixed number of injection sites. This injection paradigm is used regardless of the patient's symptoms. When using the FTPP, physicians alter/adjust the injection pattern and toxin dosage based on the patient's symptoms. The combined approach utilizes fixed injection sites and doses in some muscles along with asymmetric injections from the FTPP in other muscles.

#### FIXED DOSE PROTOCOL

BoNT is injected bilaterally in a total of 31 sites (corrugator: 2 sites, procerus: 1 site, frontalis: 4 sites, temporalis: 8 sites, occipitalis: 6 sites, cervical paraspinal: 4 sites, and trapezius: 6 sites) (see Figure 17.1).

*FIGURE 17.1 Fixed dose injection pattern.*

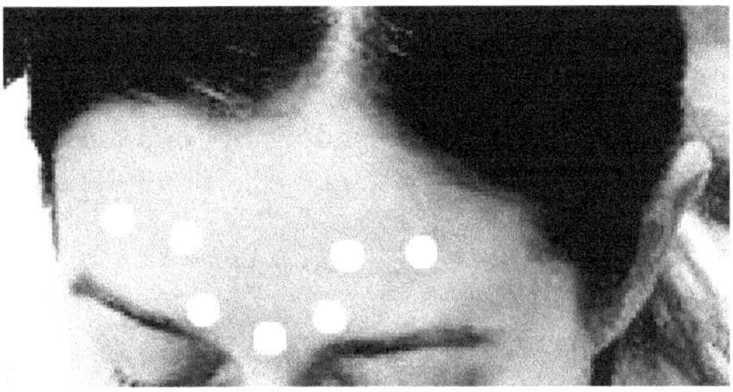

## *Follow the Pain Protocol*

The sites of injection and dose per site are adjusted based on the patient's symptoms and/or where the clinician elicits pain or tenderness with palpation. The muscles that may be targeted in this approach include the muscles listed previously in the FDP as well as the masseter, splenius capitis, and sternocleidomastoid.

## *Combined Approach*

In this approach, a fixed injection pattern is performed in the facial/frontal muscles with additional injections performed at posterior sites (Figure 17.2) (365).

*FIGURE 17.2 Combined approach injection pattern (fixed and follow the pain).*

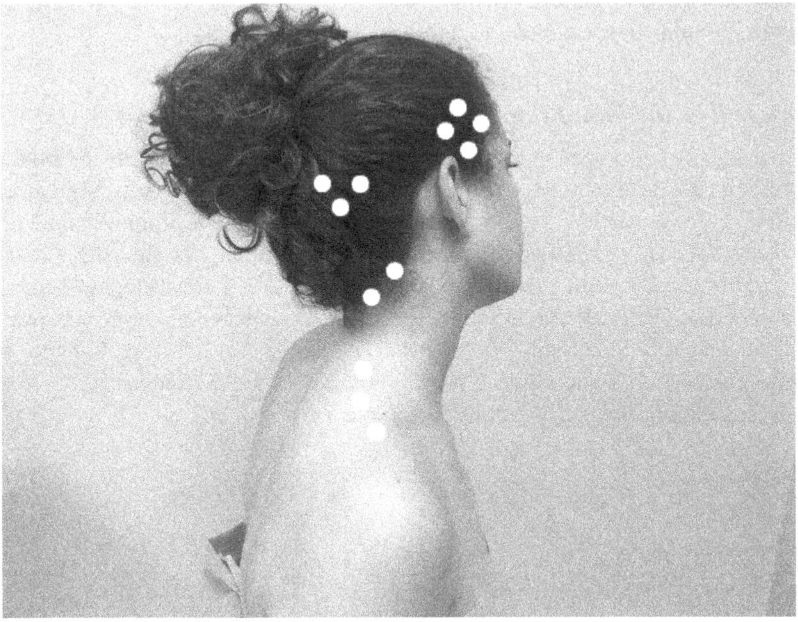

## Toxin Dilution

### *OnabotulinumtoxinA*

A 100-unit vial of OBTA is diluted with 2 mL preservative free normal saline (PFNS, 0.9%) or a 200-unit vial is diluted with 4 mL PFNS for a concentration of 50 units/mL or 5 units/0.1 mL (see BoNT dosage/dilution tables for full information on dilution).

### *Dosage*

For the treatment of CDHA, MHA, and TTH, information on the starting dose and/or optimal dose for all of the available BoNT products is limited. There is more information on dosing of serotype A BoNT (OBTA) for the treatment of CMHA (34). Additional studies are required to determine the efficacy, dosage, and safety of ABTA, IBTA, and RBTB for the treatment of CMHA. Additional studies are also required to establish the efficacy, optimal dosage, and safety of OBTA, ABTA, IBTA, and RBTB for the treatment of other migraine subtypes and other types of HA. The following section summarizes doses of FDA-approved BoNT products, as available for the treatment of CMHA.

### *OBTA Fixed Dose Protocol*

The manufacturer's recommended dose for CMHA is 155 units divided into 31 sites (5 units at each injection site) using a fixed injection site pattern as follows: corrugators, 10 units (2 sites; 1 on the right and 1 on the left); procerus, 5 units (single site); frontalis, 20 units (4 sites; 2 on the right and 2 on the left); temporalis, 40 units (8 sites, 4 on the right and 4 on the left); occipitalis, 30 units (6 sites; 3 on the right and 3 on the left); cervical paraspinals, 20 units (4 sites; 2 on the right and 2 on the left); and trapezius, 30 units (6 sites; 3 on the right and 3 on the left) (34).

### *OBTA Follow the Pain Protocol*

When using this protocol, injections may be performed unilaterally or bilaterally and the injected dose may be asymmetric. A total of 155 to 200 units is divided into 39 sites or fewer with 2.5 to 5 units per injection site as follows: corrugators (2.5 units/site, 1–2 sites/side); procerus (2.5–5 units, single site); frontalis (2.5–5 units/site, 2–4 sites, 1–2 sites/side); temporalis (2.5–5 units/site, 8–10 sites/side, 4–5 sites/side); occipitalis (2.5–5 units/site, 2 sites, 1 site/side); cervical paraspinals (2.5–5 units/site, 1–3 sites/side); trapezius (2.5–5 units/site, 2–8 sites, 1–4 sites/side); splenius capitis (2.5–5 units/site, 2 sites/side); masseter (2.5–5 units/site, 1–2 sites); and sternocleidomastoid (2.5–5 units/site, 2 sites) (365).

### *AbobotulinumtoxinA*

Studies have evaluated the efficacy of various doses of ABTA for the treatment of migraine and chronic TTH. In migraine studies, the reported dosage ranged from 80 to 350 units of ABTA. Injection patterns included up to 15 sites in facial/frontal muscles and posterior neck muscles (374–376). In chronic TTH studies, 200 to 500 units were studied. Injections were described as targeting the following muscles: frontalis, corrugator, temporalis, sternocleidomastoid, auricularis, occipitalis, splenius capitis, semispinalis capitis, and trapezius (370, 377, 378).

### *IncobotulinumtoxinA*

PubMed and Medline search for IBTA and HA, MHA, CDA, and TTH revealed no English language studies or reports on the dose of IBTA dosage or pattern of injection.

### *RimabotulinumtoxinB*

Studies on the use of RBTB for chronic migraine are limited. In several studies of CDHA, the dosage of RBTA ranged from 5,000 to 7,500 units, with 5,000 units being the most common dose. Injection patterns and dose per muscle are not well described (379).

### *Injection Technique*

Injections are performed with 30-gauge, ½- or 1-inch needles. To date no studies have evaluated the benefit of using guidance techniques other than palpation.

### *Clinical Effect*

The expected effect is reduced frequency, duration, and severity of HA attacks.

### *Reinjection Interval*

The minimum recommended interval between injections is 12 weeks.

### *Adverse Events/Side Effects*

The primary adverse events are pain postinjection and weakness in injected muscles. Less frequent adverse events/side effects include ptosis, diplopia, and respiratory infections. Generalized weakness, anaphylaxis, and death are theoretical risks.

**TABLE 17.1 BoNT for Chronic Migraine Manufacturer Recommended Dosage and Recommended Dilution**

| BoNT Preparation | OBTA (Botox®) | ABTA (Dysport®) | IBTA (Xeomin®) | RBTB (Myobloc®) |
|---|---|---|---|---|
| U.S. FDA approval | Approved for chronic migraine | Currently not an FDA-approved indication | Currently not an FDA-approved indication | Currently not an FDA-approved indication |
| UK Medicines and Healthcare products Regulatory Agency (MHRA) | Approved for chronic migraine (≥15 HA days per month, ≥8 migraine days) | Currently not an approved indication | Currently not an approved indication | Currently not an approved indication |
| Total dose | 155 units | N/A | N/A | N/A |
| Corrugator | 10 units divided into 2 sites (1 site per side, 5 units per site) | N/A | N/A | N/A |
| Frontalis | 20 units divided into 4 sites (2 sites per side, 5 units per site) | N/A | N/A | N/A |
| Occipitalis | 30 units, divided into 6 sites (3 sites per side, 5 units per site) | N/A | N/A | N/A |
| Cervical paraspinals | 20 units divided into 4 sites (2 sites per side, 5 units per site) | N/A | N/A | N/A |
| Procerus | 5 units, 1 site | N/A | N/A | N/A |
| Temporalis | 40 units divided into 8 sites (4 site per side, 5 units per site) | N/A | N/A | N/A |
| Trapezius | 30 units divided into 6 sites (3 sites per side, 5 units per site | N/A | N/A | N/A |

*(continued)*

**TABLE 17.1 BoNT for Chronic Migraine Manufacturer Recommended Dosage and Recommended Dilution (*continued*)**

| BoNT Preparation | OBTA (Botox®) | ABTA (Dysport®) | IBTA (Xeomin®) | RBTB (Myobloc®) |
|---|---|---|---|---|
| Dilution (concentration) | 200 units in 4 mL PFNS or 100 units in 2 mL PFNS[a] (50 units/mL or 5 units/0.1 mL) | N/A | N/A | N/A |
| Minimum recommended dosage interval | 12 Weeks | N/A | N/A | N/A |
| **Migraine Treatment Outside the United States** | | | | |
| Total dose: fixed dose injection pattern | 155 units, 31 sites (see chapter for details) | N/A | N/A | N/A |
| Total dose: follow the pain injection pattern | 155–195 units, 31–39 sites in 7 head and neck regions[b] | N/A | N/A | N/A |
| Corrugator | 10 units divided into 2 sites (1 site per side, 5 units per site) | N/A | N/A | N/A |
| Frontalis | 20 units divided into 4 sites (2 sites per side, 5 units per site) | N/A | N/A | N/A |
| Procerus | 5 units, 1 site | N/A | N/A | N/A |
| Temporalis | 40 units divided into 8 sites (4 sites per side, 5 units per site) or 50 units divided into 10 sites (5 sites per side, 5 units per site) | N/A | N/A | N/A |
| Cervical paraspinals | 20 units divided into 4 sites (2 sites per side, 5 units per site) | N/A | N/A | N/A |
| Occipitalis | 30–40 units divided into 6–8 sites (3–4 sites per side, 5 units per site) | N/A | N/A | N/A |

(*continued*)

**TABLE 17.1 BoNT for Chronic Migraine Manufacturer Recommended Dosage and Recommended Dilution** (*continued*)

| BoNT Preparation | OBTA (Botox®) | ABTA (Dysport®) | IBTA (Xeomin®) | RBTB (Myobloc®) |
|---|---|---|---|---|
| **Migraine Treatment Outside the United States (*continued*)** | | | | |
| Trapezius | 30–50 units divided into 6–10 sites (3–5 sites per side, 5 units per site) | N/A | N/A | N/A |
| Dilution (concentration) | 200 units in 4 mL PFNS or 100 units in 2 mL PFNS[a] (50 units/mL or 5 units/0.1 mL) | N/A | N/A | N/A |
| Minimum recommended dosage interval | 12 Weeks | N/A | N/A | N/A |

[a]Reconstitute only with PFNS.

[b]All injections are bilateral except the procerus.

*Abbreviations:* ABTA, abobotulinumtoxinA; HA, headache; IBTA, incobotulinumtoxinA; OBTA, onabotulinumtoxinA; PFNS, preservative-free normal saline (0.9%); RBTB, rimabotulinumtoxinB.

*Sources:* Adapted from Refs. 34, 36, 38, 44.

**TABLE 17.2 BoNT for Headache Conditions, Published Dosage Range and Recommended Dilution (*continued*)**

| BoNT Preparation | OBTA (Botox®) | ABTA (Dysport®) | IBTA (Xeomin®) | RBTB (Myobloc®) |
|---|---|---|---|---|
| **Migraine Published Dosage Range: Adults (≥18 Years of Age)** | | | | |
| Dosage range per treatment session | 65–260 units | 80–350 units | Not reported[a]<br>50–200 units[b] | 5,000–8,000 units |
| Corrugators | 10 units divided into 2 sites (1 site per side, 5 units per site) | 20–40 units divided into 2 sites (1 site per side, 10–20 units per site) | Not reported[a] | 250–1000 units, divided into 1–2 sites per side |
| Frontalis | 20 units divided bilaterally into 4 sites (2 sites per side, 5 units per site) | 20–40 units divided bilaterally (1–2 sites per side, 10–20 units per site) | Not reported[a]<br>20 units divided bilaterally into 4 sites (2 sites per side, 5 units per site)[b] | 500–2,000 units, divided bilaterally (1–2 sites per side, 250–500 units per site) |
| Masseter (optional) | 0–5 units per side divided into 1–2 sites (0–1 site per side, 0–2.5 units per side, 2.5–5 units per site) | Not reported[a]<br>0–15 units per side divided into 2 sites (5–7.5 units per site)[b] | Not reported[a]<br>0–5 units per side divided into 1–2 sites (0–1 site per side, 0–2.5 units per side, 2.5–5 units per site)[b] | Not reported[a] |

*(continued)*

**TABLE 17.2 BoNT for Headache Conditions, Published Dosage Range and Recommended Dilution** (*continued*)

| BoNT Preparation | OBTA (Botox®) | ABTA (Dysport®) | IBTA (Xeomin®) | RBTB (Myobloc®) |
|---|---|---|---|---|
| **Migraine Published Dosage Range: Adults (≥18 Years of Age) (*continued*)** | | | | |
| Procerus | 5 units, 1 site | 10–15 units, 1 site[b] | 5 units, 1 site[b] | 250–500 units, 1 site |
| Temporalis | 40–50 units divided bilaterally into 8–10 sites (4–5 sites per side, 5 units per site) | 20–40 units divided bilaterally (1 site per side, 10–20 units per site) | Not reported[a]<br>40–50 units divided bilaterally into 8–10 sites (4–5 sites per side, 5 units per site)[b] | 500–6,000 units divided bilaterally (1–3 sites per side, 250–1,000 units per site) |
| Sternocleidomastoid | Not reported[a]<br>5–30 units per side, 1–2 sites[b] | Not reported[a]<br>10–60 units per side, divided (1–2 sites per side)[b] | Not reported[a]<br>5–30 units per side, divided (1–2 sites per side)[b] | 500–1,250 Units per muscle (1–2 sites per side) |
| Splenius capitis | 10–20 units divided bilaterally (2 sites per side, 2.5–5 units per site) | 40 units divided bilaterally (20 units per side, 2 sites per side, 10 units per site) | Not reported[a]<br>10–20 units divided bilaterally (2 sites per side, 2.5–5 units per site)[b] | Reported as "cervical muscles and trapezius" 750–1,250 units per side for cervical muscles (4 sites per side, 250–500 units per side), trapezius (1–6 sites per side, 250–1,000 units per side) |

(*continued*)

**TABLE 17.2 BoNT for Headache Conditions, Published Dosage Range and Recommended Dilution (*continued*)**

| BoNT Preparation | OBTA (Botox®) | ABTA (Dysport®) | IBTA (Xeomin®) | RBTB (Myobloc®) |
|---|---|---|---|---|
| **Migraine Published Dosage Range: Adults (≥18 Years of Age) (*continued*)** | | | | |
| Semispinalis capitis | 10–20 units divided (2 sites per side, 2.5–5 units per site) | Not reported[a]<br>50–75 units per side (1–2 sites, 25–37.5 units per site)[b] | Not reported[a]<br>10–20 units divided bilaterally (2 sites per side, 1.5–5 units per site)[b] | |
| Occipital region | 30–40 units divided bilaterally (6–8 sites, 3–4 sites per side, 5 units per site) | 20–40 units per side (1–4 sites per side, 5–10 units per site) | Not reported[a]<br>30–40 units divided bilaterally, 6–8 sites (3–4 sites per side, 5 units per site)[b] | |
| Trapezius | 20–50 units per side (2–3 sites per side, 10–15 units per site) | 20–80 units per side (1–4 sites per side, 10–20 units per site)[b] | Not reported[a]<br>20–40 units per side (2–3 sites per side, 10–15 units per site)[b] | |
| Dilution (concentration) | 200 units in 4 mL PFNS or 100 units in 2 mL PFNS (50 units/mL or 5 units/0.1 mL) | For <300 units: 300 units diluted in 3 mL PFNS (100 units/mL, 10 units/0.1 mL)<br>For >300 units: 500 units diluted in 2.5 mL PFNS or 300 units in 1.5 mL PFNS (200 units/mL, 20 units/0.1 mL) | Not reported[a]<br>200 units in 4 mL PFNS or 100 units in 2 mL PFNS (50 units/mL or 5 units/0.1 mL)[b] | Not required, provided in solution, 5,000 units/mL[c] |

(*continued*)

**TABLE 17.2 BoNT for Headache Conditions, Published Dosage Range and Recommended Dilution (*continued*)**

| BoNT Preparation | OBTA (Botox®) | ABTA (Dysport®) | IBTA (Xeomin®) | RBTB (Myobloc®) |
|---|---|---|---|---|
| **Other Headache Conditions** | | | | |
| Tension type HA total dosage | 7.5–240 units | 210–500 units | Not reported[a]<br>50–100 units[b] | 5,000–7500 units |
| Muscle injection pattern | Divided, up to 24 sites | Divided bilaterally, up to 18 sites | | |
| Auricularis | Not reported[a] | 20 units per side (1 site per side, 20 units per site) | Not reported[a] | Not reported[b] |
| Corrugator | 2.5–5 units per side (1–2 sites, 1.2–2.5 units per site) | 10–20 units divided into 2 sites (1 site per side, 5–10 units per site) | Not reported[a]<br>2.5–5 units per side, 1–2 sites (1.2–2.5 units per site)[b] | Similar to migraine pattern, as above |
| Frontalis | 5–20 units per side (2–4 sites per side, 1.25–5 units per site) | 10–30 units per side (2 sites per side, 12.5–25 units per site) | Not reported[a]<br>5–20 units per side (2–4 site per side, 1.25–5 units per site)[b] | Similar to migraine pattern, as above |
| Occipitalis | 10–20 units (1–2 sites per side, 5–10 units per site) | Up to 20 units per side (1–2 sites per side, 5–10 units per site) | Not reported[a]<br>10–20 units (1–2 sites per side, 5–10 units per site)[b] | Not reported[a] |

(*continued*)

**TABLE 17.2 BoNT for Headache Conditions, Published Dosage Range and Recommended Dilution** *(continued)*

| BoNT Preparation | OBTA (Botox®) | ABTA (Dysport®) | IBTA (Xeomin®) | RBTB (Myobloc®) |
|---|---|---|---|---|
| **Other Headache Conditions (*continued*)** | | | | |
| Procerus | 2.5–5 units, 1 site | 5–10 units, 1 site | Not reported[a]<br>2.5–5 units, 1 site[b] | Similar to migraine pattern, as above |
| Semispinalis capitis | 10–20 units per side (2–4 sites per side, 2.5–5 units per site) | Up to 25 units per side (1–2 sites per side, 2.5–25 units per site) | Not reported[a]<br>10–20 units per side (2–4 sites per side, 2.5–5 units per site)[b] | Similar to migraine pattern, as above |
| Splenius capitis | 20–30 units per side (1–2 sites per side, 10–15 units per site) | 20–40 units per side (4 sites per side, 5–10 units per site) | Not reported[a]<br>20–30 units per side (1–2 sites per side, 10–15 units per site)[b] | Similar to migraine pattern, as above |
| Sternocleidomastoid | 2.5–10 units per side (1–2 sites per side, 2.5–5 units per site) | 20–30 units per side (1 site per side, 20–30 units per site) | Not reported[a]<br>2.5–10 units per side (1–2 sites per side, 2.5–5 units per site)[b] | Similar to migraine pattern, as above |
| Temporalis | 10–40 units per side (1–8 sites per side, 5 units per site) | 25–50 units per side (2–4 sites, 12.5–25 units per site) | 10–40 units per side (1–8 sites per side, 5 units per site) | Similar to migraine pattern, as above |
| Trapezius | 20–50 units per side (4–10 sites per side, 4–5 units per site) | 25–90 units per side (3–6 sites, 10–15 units per site) | Not reported[a]<br>20–50 units per side (4–10 sites per side, 4–5 units per site)[b] | Similar to migraine pattern, as above |

*(continued)*

**TABLE 17.2 BoNT for Headache Conditions, Published Dosage Range and Recommended Dilution** *(continued)*

| BoNT Preparation | OBTA (Botox®) | ABTA (Dysport®) | IBTA (Xeomin®) | RBTB (Myobloc®) |
|---|---|---|---|---|
| **Other Headache Conditions (*continued*)** | | | | |
| Chronic daily HA | 20–240 units divided bilaterally, injection pattern not specified | 200–500 units divided bilaterally, injection pattern not specified | Not reported[a]<br>50–200 units divided bilaterally, similar to tension HA[b] | 5,000–7,500 units<br>Injection pattern similar to migraine, as above |
| Dilution (concentration) | 200 units with 4 mL PFNS or 100 units with 2 mL PFNS (50 units/mL or 5 units/0.1 mL) | For doses <300 units: 300 units diluted in 3 mL PFNS (100 units/mL or 10 units/0.1 mL)<br>For doses 300–400 units: 500 units with 2.5 mL PFNS or 300 units in 1.5 mL PFNS (200 units/mL, 20 units/0.1 mL) | 200 units with 4 mL PFNS or 100 units with 2 mL PFNS (50 units/mL or 5 units/0.1 mL)[b] | |

[a]No published information on dose/dosage.

[b]First author's dosage range.

[c]If desired, may be diluted with normal saline for injection.

*Abbreviations:* ABTA, abobotulinumtoxinA; HA, headache; IBTA, incobotulinumtoxinA; OBTA, onabotulinumtoxinA; PFNS, preservative-free normal saline (0.9%); RBTB, rimabotulinumtoxinB.

*Source:* Adapted from Refs. 34, 36, 38, 44, 362, 366, 371, 374–376, 379, 604–609.

# Illustrations for Migraine Injection Patterns—Chapter 17

*FIGURE 1* *Botulinum neurotoxin injection pattern for migraine, facial muscle injection sites.*

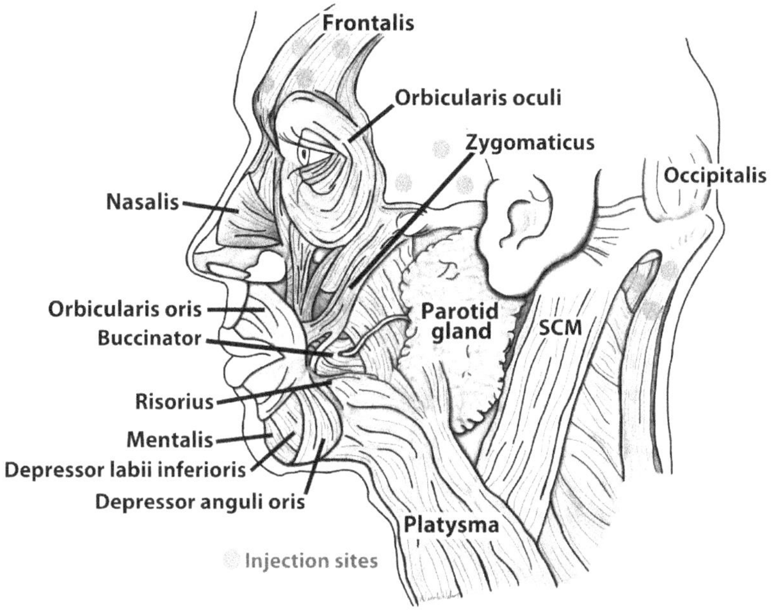


*FIGURE 2* *Botulinum neurotoxin injection pattern for migraine, facial and neck muscle injection sites.*

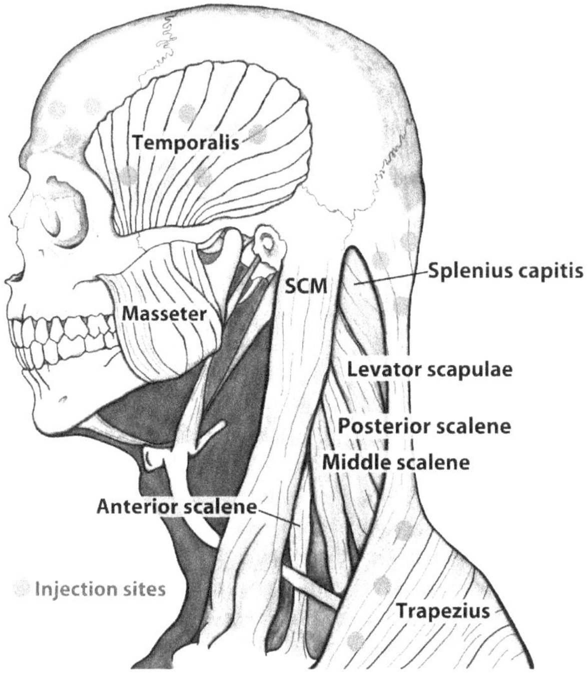

# 18

# *Botulinum Neurotoxin for Musculoskeletal Pain Conditions*

*Katharine E. Alter, MD*
*Nicole A. Wilson, PhD, MD*

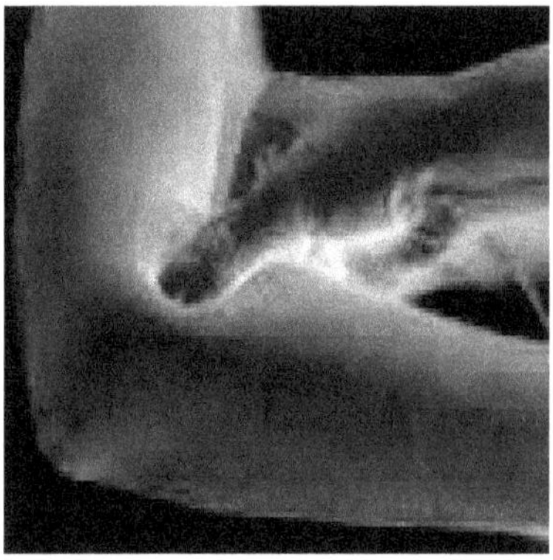

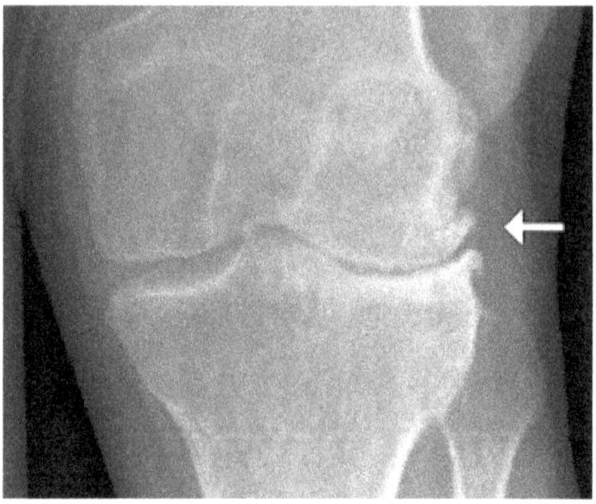

## Condition

The biological theory that forms the rationale for the use of botulinum neurotoxins (BoNTs) to treat pain is discussed in the Introduction to Part IV of this text "Botulinum Neurotoxins for Pain Conditions." Because of the well-recognized effects of BoNTs for reduction of pain and muscle contraction, BoNTs have been used to treat a wide variety of conditions associated with intractable pain. These conditions include myofascial pain syndromes (MPS), cervical dystonia, chronic migraine, osteoarticular conditions, various musculoskeletal pain syndromes, thoracic outlet syndrome (TOS), pain associated with spasticity, herpetic neuralgia, diabetic neuropathy, and other conditions. These conditions are associated with pain from a variety of causes and the treatments are also varied. Therefore, proven efficacy and/or safety for one pain condition (e.g., cervical dystonia or chronic migraine) do not necessarily provide evidence that BoNTs are safe and effective for all pain conditions. This chapter and the table that follows focus on the musculoskeletal (MSK)-related pain syndromes for which BoNTs are frequently recommended. A brief summary of each condition is presented, as a full discussion of each condition is beyond the scope of this chapter.

## Myofascial Pain/Trigger Points

MPS is a chronic condition characterized by muscle pain and associated with taut bands or "trigger points." The origin of taut bands, trigger points, and the associated pain is not completely understood (11, 380).

### *Pattern of Involvement*

The most commonly affected muscles include upper limb and neck muscles, including the trapezius, levator scapulae, infraspinatus, and scalene muscles (381, 382).

### *Clinical/Functional Impact*

The chronic pain associated with MPS may limit several aspects of daily life, including activities of daily living (ADLs), avocational/vocational tasks and participation, and quality of life (382).

### *Evaluation*

MPS is a clinical diagnosis that is established through a detailed history and physical exam. The presence of pain and trigger points or taut bands is required to establish a diagnosis of MPS.

### *Treatment Options*

A wide variety of nonpharmacologic treatments are used including physical therapy, massage, and dry needling. Pharmacologic treatments for MPS include various analgesics, antidepressants, trigger-point injections with steroids, and/or local anesthetics (383). Despite the wide variety of treatment options available for patients with MPS, many patients are incompletely treated or undertreated and continue to report chronic pain.

#### BoNTS FOR MPS

For patients who fail to respond to traditional treatment modalities, BoNT injections may be considered and/or recommended as a treatment option. Some patients report significant relief with BoNT therapy, whereas others report limited or no reduction in pain (381).

#### BoNTS APPROVED FOR THE TREATMENT OF MPS

None of the BoNT products currently available in the United States are approved for treatment of MPS. The use of BoNTs for the treatment of MPS is considered off-label therapy.

### *Level of Evidence*

In a 2011 article, Jabbari and Machado reviewed the evidence for BoNT in the treatment of intractable pain, including MPS (371). The authors reviewed available studies of BoNT for MPS using American Academy of Neurology (AAN) guidelines for the classification of quality of evidence from clinical trials (138). They concluded that despite the positive response to BoNT in a number of studies, the diverse nature of these studies made it difficult to formulate a clear recommendation to clinicians. As a result, the authors reported a Level U (Unestablished or unknown) level of evidence for BoNT for MPS and recommended additional rigorous clinical trials for this condition.

### *Pattern and Technique*

When performing BoNT injections in MPS, clinicians typically target trigger points. Most physicians report using a "follow the pain" approach in which palpation is used to identify the most symptomatic tender points, trigger points, and/or taut bands. To guide injections, most physicians report using palpation alone, while some report using B-mode ultrasound, and a few clinicians report using EMG.

### *Dosage*

The dose of BoNT is product specific; therefore, a wide variety of doses are reported in the literature and in clinical practice for the treatment of MPS (384). Clinical trials have investigated the efficacy, safety, and dose of onabotulinumtoxinA (OBTA), abobotulinumtoxinA (ABTA), and rimabotulinumtoxinB (RBTB) for MPS. As noted, the recommended or reported dose per trigger point is, in part, determined by the particular BoNT product being used.

#### OBTA

The reported dose of OBTA is 20 to 50 units per trigger point with the majority of authors reporting a total dose per treatment session of 100 to 300 units (380, 385–392). In a 2001 retrospective chart review, Lang reported using up to 600 units of OBTA per treatment session (393).

#### ABTA

For ABTA, the reported dose for MPS is 40 to 120 units per trigger point with a reported total dose of 250 to 400 units per treatment session (394–396).

#### RBTB

In a retrospective chart review, Lang reported a mean dose of 9,000 units and a dose range of 3,000 to 20,000 units per treatment session. The dose per site was not reported, but multiple injection sites per muscle were described (393). In a 2003 article, Royal reported a maximum dose of 25,000 units RBTB with most patients requiring a lower dose. Royal also reported using OBTA and RBTA in MPS patients with a dose per muscle that was extrapolated from the literature for cervical dystonia and spasticity

(380). No dosing data were found for incobotulinumtoxinA (IBTA) in the treatment of MPS (see Table 18.1: BoNT Dosage Table at the end of this chapter for detailed information on dosing BoNT for MPS).

### *Dilution*

The most commonly reported dilution for OBTA was 100 units in 1 mL preservative-free normal saline (PFNS) and 500 units in 2.5 mL PFNS for ABTA. RBTB is supplied in solution and does not require reconstitution. If desired, RBTB can be further diluted with PFNS.

### *Adverse Events*

Flu-like symptoms, muscle spasm, and injection-site pain are the most commonly reported adverse events. For a complete list of potential adverse events, the full prescribing information and boxed warning provided by the manufacturers of each of the commercial BoNT products should be consulted.

## Piriformis Syndrome

From its origin on the interior surface of the sacrum, the piriformis muscle exits the pelvis through the greater sciatic foramen and runs across the buttock to its insertion on the greater trochanter of the femur (397, 398). Typically, the sciatic nerve lies deep to the piriformis, but in some patients, the sciatic nerve may pierce or pass through the piriformis muscles. Trauma in the buttock region, spasm or hypertrophy of the piriformis muscle, and entrapment or compression of the sciatic nerve may cause a constellation of symptoms that can be labeled piriformis syndrome (398, 399).

### *Pattern of Involvement*

Patients present with varied complaints, including aching buttock pain, trigger points, and/or sciatica.

### *Clinical/Functional Impact*

Pain is often disabling and can limit standing, walking, and sleep. Pain may affect quality of life and participation in work and avocational tasks.

### *Evaluation*

The diagnosis of piriformis syndrome is largely based on the history and clinical examination. Palpation along the course of the piriformis as it crosses the buttock often elicits pain and/or an involuntary twitch response. X-rays and/or MRI of the spine may be considered to rule out spine or hip pathology and electrodiagnostic testing may be necessary to rule out a lumbar radiculopathy or sciatic nerve compromise.

## *BoNTs Approved for the Treatment of Piriformis Syndrome*

Piriformis syndrome-related pain and sciatica are not approved indications for any of the FDA-approved BoNT products. Therefore, the use of BoNTs for the treatment of piriformis syndrome remains off-label.

## *Level of Evidence*

In a 2011 article, Jabbari and Machado reviewed the evidence for BoNT in the treatment of intractable pain conditions, including piriformis syndrome. The authors reviewed available studies of BoNT for piriformis syndrome using AAN guidelines for the classification of quality of evidence from clinical trials (138). On the basis of current evidence, they reported Level B (Probably effective, should be considered) evidence for BoNT in the management of piriformis syndrome (371).

## *Injection Pattern and Technique*

When injecting the piriformis, the majority of clinicians use palpation in addition to another guidance technique, such as EMG, ultrasound, fluoroscopy, or CT (156, 398, 400). In most centers and practices, ultrasound has largely replaced fluoroscopy and CT due to comparable accuracy and outcomes when compared to fluoroscopy. Ultrasound had additional advantages, including lower cost, portability, and lack of ionizing radiation. Depending on dose of BoNT injected, 1 to 4 injection sites are reported (156, 401).

## *Dosage*

The dose of BoNT is product specific, leading to a wide variety of reported doses for the treatment of piriformis syndrome found both in the literature and in clinical practice.

OBTA

A dose range of 50 to 200 units has been reported, with the most common doses between 50 and 100 units (398, 399, 402).

ABTA

Yoon et al. reported a 50% decrease in pain postinjection after a "low dose" of ABTA (150 units) was used along with stretching (403).

RBTB

A dose of 5,000 to 12,500 units has been reported in clinical case series (400, 404).

IBTA

There is no information in the literature on the use of IBTA for the treatment of piriformis syndrome.

### *Dilution*

OBTA

One-hundred units of OBTA is typically reconstituted with 1 mL PFNS for a concentration of 100 units/mL or 10 units/0.1 mL. A maximum dose of 50 units at a single site is recommended.

ATBA

Only a single case series was identified and dilution was not reported (400).

RBTB

RBTB is provided in solution and does not require reconstitution. If desired, RBTB can be diluted with PFNS.

### *Adverse Events*

Flu-like symptoms, muscle spasm, and injection-site pain are the most commonly reported adverse events. For a complete list of potential adverse events, the full prescribing information and boxed warning provided by the manufacturers of each of the commercial BoNT products should be consulted.

## Plantar Fasciitis

Plantar fasciitis (PF) is the most common cause of acute and chronic heel pain. The etiology is generally from inflammation following repeated injury and microtears in the plantar fascia (385).

### *Pattern of Involvement*

Patients present with unilateral or bilateral heel pain that worsens with weight bearing and/or walking.

### *Clinical/Functional Impact*

Pain can limit weight bearing and, therefore, may limit functional tasks requiring standing and/or walking, including avocational and occupational tasks.

### *Evaluation*

The history and clinical examination frequently establish the diagnosis. Ultrasound evaluation may show thickening of the plantar fascia with hypoechoic areas suggesting edema. X-rays may also be useful to rule out boney pathology as a cause of pain.

### *Treatment Options*

Treatment options include orthotics, physical therapy modalities (e.g., therapeutic ultrasound and extracorporeal shockwave therapy), oral anti-inflammatory agents, dry needling, injections of steroids and/or local anesthetics, prolotherapy, and/or platelet-rich plasma (PRP) therapy (371, 405, 406). BoNT injections are often recommended when other interventions fail to relieve pain.

### *BoNTs Approved for the Treatment of PF*

PF is not an approved indication for any of the FDA-approved BoNT products. Therefore, the use of BoNTs for the treatment of PF remains off-label.

### *Level of Evidence*

Jabbari and Machado reviewed the evidence for BoNT in the treatment of intractable pain conditions, including PF (371). As noted, the authors reviewed available studies of BoNT for PF using AAN guidelines for the classification of quality of evidence from clinical trials (138). On the basis of current evidence, they reported Level B (Probably effective, should be considered) evidence for BoNT for PF (371).

### *Injection Pattern and Technique*

When performing BoNT injections for PF most physicians use palpation alone or palpation with B-mode ultrasound to guide PF injections (385). EMG is not typically used.

### *Dosage*

As mentioned, dosage is in part determined by the specific BoNT product used, as the recommended dose of a BoNT is product specific. The majority of studies to date have used either OBTA or ABTA for PF injections.

#### OBTA

The reported dose range of OBTA for PF is 30 to 70 units per heel divided among 1 to 3 injection sites (385, 407, 408).

#### ABTA

The reported dose of ABTA is 100 to 200 units per heel in divided doses (409, 410).

### *Dilution*

#### OBTA

One-hundred units of OBTA is typically reconstituted with 1 mL PFNS for a concentration of 100 units/mL (10 units/0.1 mL). A maximum dose of 50 units may be injected into a single site.

ABTA
The typical dilutions for ABTA is 500 units in either 1 mL or 2.5 mL PFNS for a dilution of 500 units/mL (50 units/0.1 mL) or 200 units/mL (20 units/0.1 mL), respectively.

### *Adverse Events*

Flu-like symptoms, muscle spasm, and injection-site pain are the most commonly reported adverse events. For a complete list of potential adverse events, the full prescribing information and boxed warning provided by the manufacturers of each of the commercial BoNT products should be consulted.

## Osteoarticular Pain Syndromes

### *Arthritis/Articular Pain*

Arthritis can be either acute or chronic. The two most common causes of chronic arthritis are osteoarthritis (OA), a degenerative joint disease (DJD), and rheumatoid arthritis, an autoimmune process. OA is more common than rheumatoid arthritis, but both conditions cause significant pain, limitations in joint range of motion and/or function, affect quality of life and participation, and may lead to disability (411). Studies related to BoNT therapy for arthritis have primarily focused on OA-/DJD-related pain and this section is limited to a discussion of BoNT for this condition.

### *Clinical Impact*

Arthritis affects up to 28% of adults in the United States and is one of the leading causes of disability in adults (412). Total knee arthroplasty (TKA) is a primary treatment option, but pain is common following TKA for OA, occurring in up to 18% of patients (411, 413).

### *Evaluation*

The evaluation of a patient with suspected OA starts with a detailed history and physical examination. Laboratory and radiologic studies are often recommended to establish the correct diagnosis.

### *Treatment*

The treatment of OA is primarily focused on reducing inflammation. Oral nonsteroidal anti-inflammatory drugs (NSAIDs) are a mainstay of treatment. Topical NSAIDs, intra-articular steroid injections, and viscoelastic agents, such as hyaluronic acid, may also be effective treatments (414, 415). Unfortunately, many patients experience side effects from oral NSAID therapy and/or their pain is incompletely controlled with these drugs and with other traditional treatments. Because of the well-recognized effects of BoNTs for reduction of pain, the use of BoNTs for OA-related pain has been evaluated in clinical trials and may be recommended as a treatment option to patients (411, 416–418).

### *BoNTs Approved for the Treatment of Arthritis-Related Pain*

Articular joint pain is not an approved indication for any of the FDA-approved BoNT products. Therefore, the use of BoNTs for the treatment of articular joint pain remains off-label. Clinical trials evaluating the efficacy and safety of BoNTs for the treatment of joint pain have primarily focused on the knee and shoulder joints (417, 419, 420). A limited number of trials have explored the use of BoNT in other joints (421–423).

### *Level of Evidence*

Jabbari and Machado reviewed the evidence for BoNT in the treatment of intractable pain conditions, including refractory knee pain following TKA and painful knee arthritis from OA/DJD (371). As mentioned, the authors reviewed available studies of BoNT for articular pain using AAN guidelines for the classification of quality of evidence from clinical trials (138). On the basis of current evidence, they reported Level B (Probably effective, should be considered) evidence for the use of BoNT in the treatment of refractory knee pain following TKA. The authors also reported Level C (Possibly effective, may be used at the discretion of the clinician) evidence for OA-related knee pain (371). These authors did not review data for BoNT injections in OA affecting the ankle, hip, shoulder, or other joints.

### *Injection Technique*

Knee joint injections are generally performed "blind," using only palpation or with ultrasound guidance. Fluoroscopy or CT guidance is infrequently used. EMG and e-stim are not useful for guiding joint injections (18, 156).

### *Dosage: OA-Related Knee Pain*

OBTA

The reported dose for OBTA in the treatment of OA-related knee pain is 25 to 150 units per joint, with 100 units per joint as the most commonly reported dose (418, 419).

OBTA FOR REFRACTORY TKA-RELATED KNEE PAIN

In a 2010 study, Singh et al. reported a dose of 100 units OBTA per joint for this indication (417).

DILUTION

One-hundred units of OBTA is typically reconstituted with 1 mL PFNS resulting in a concentration of 100 units/mL (10 units/0.1 mL).

ADVERSE EVENTS

Flu-like symptoms, muscle spasm, and injection-site pain are the most commonly reported adverse events. For a complete list of potential adverse events, the full prescribing information and boxed warning provided by the manufacturers of each of the commercial BoNT products should be consulted.

## Shoulder and Ankle Joints

In a 2009 double-blind placebo-controlled study, Singh et al. reported the effects of OBTA for refractory shoulder pain. Using a dose of 100 units OBTA injected into the shoulder joint using a blind posterior approach, statistically significant improvements were reported in pain (418). In a 2006 open label study, Mahowald et al. reported the effects of OBTA for chronic arthritis-related pain including OA in the ankle, knee, and shoulder (419).

### *Evidence for BoNT Injections for Joints other than the Knee*

On the basis of one Class I study and one Class III study, there is sufficient evidence to support a Level B or C (Probably effective or possibly effective, respectively) recommendation for the use of BoNT injections for shoulder pain associated with arthritis (411). The current evidence supports only a Level U recommendation (Unproven) for other joints (411).

### *Dosage*

OBTA

Published studies report doses between 25 and 50 units per ankle and 50 and 100 units per knee or per shoulder (418, 419, 424).

ABTA

The reported dose of ABTA for treatment of adhesive capsulitis in the shoulder is 200 units per joint (425).

### *Dilution*

OBTA

One-hundred units of OBTA should be reconstituted with 1 mL PFNS resulting in a concentration of 100 units/mL (10 units/0.1 mL).

ABTA

No information was identified on dilution/reconstitution of ABTA.

### *Adverse Events*

Flu-like symptoms, muscle spasm, and injection-site pain are the most commonly reported adverse events. For a complete list of potential adverse events, the full prescribing information and boxed warning provided by the manufacturers of each of the commercial BoNT products should be consulted.

## BoNT Injections for Axial Skeletal Joints

In a 2007 case series, Dykstra et al. reported on the efficacy of OBTA and RBTB for axial skeletal joint pain (cervical/lumbar facet joints, sacroiliac joint, and sternoclavicular joints) (423). They reported a longer duration of pain relief with either BoNT A or BoNT B than with corticosteroid injections.

### *Dosage*

Reported dose ranges were 25 to 100 units of OBTA or a dose of 5,000 units of RBTB was injected, divided between the various joints listed previously (423).

### *Adverse Events*

Flu-like symptoms, muscle spasm, and injection-site pain are the most commonly reported adverse events. For a complete list of potential adverse events, the full prescribing information and boxed warning provided by the manufacturers of each of the commercial BoNT products should be consulted.

## Anterior Knee Pain Associated with Patellar Maltracking

The proposed mechanism for knee pain associated with patellofemoral pain (PFP) syndrome is that imbalance in the quadriceps extensor mechanism (426), potentially related to weakness in the vastus medialis (VM) and/or the vastus medialis obliquus (VMO) muscles, leads to lateral patellar maltracking and anterior knee pain.

### *Clinical/Functional Impact*

Patients report significant knee pain and functional problems.

### *Treatment*

Initial conservative management has focused on strengthening the VM and/or VMO muscles. After failing conservative management, some advocate surgery to release the vastus lateralis (VL) tendon and correct maltracking (427, 428).

### *BoNTs Approved for Treatment of PFP Syndrome/Patellar Maltracking*

PFP is not an approved indication for any of the FDA-approved BoNT products. Therefore, the use of BoNTs for the treatment of PFP/patellar maltracking is currently considered off-label therapy.

### *Level of Evidence*

Using AAN guidelines for the evaluation of the quality of evidence from clinical trials, Jabbari and Machado reported Level C (Possibly effective, may be used at the discretion of the clinician) evidence for the use of BoNT in the treatment of anterior knee pain associated with PFP syndrome and VM muscle dysfunction (371).

### *Injection Pattern and Technique*

Injections were reported at multiple sites (up to eight) in the distal 1/3 of the VL muscle. EMG guidance is the most common adjunct, but the use of US guidance has also been reported (156, 420, 429).

### *Dosage*

The dose of BoNT is specific to the product used. When treating PFP, the following dose ranges were reported in the literature:

OBTA
The mean reported dose was 161 units, with a range of 120 to 210 units (429).

ABTA
The mean reported dose was 526 units, with a range of 300 to 700 units (429). Typically, 300 to 500 units are injected into the VL (generally, the distal 1/3 of the muscle) in divided doses (420, 429).

### *Dilution*

OBTA
The dilution of OBTA for the treatment of PFP syndrome was not reported. However, the typical dilution is 100 units of OTBA diluted in 1 mL of PFNS resulting in a concentration of 100 units/mL (10 units/0.1 mL).

ABTA
Five-hundred units of ABTA are diluted with 1 mL PFNS resulting in a concentration of 500 units/mL (50 units/0.1 mL) (420).

### *Adverse Events*

Flu-like symptoms, muscle spasm, and injection-site pain are the most commonly reported adverse events. For a complete list of potential adverse events, the full prescribing information and boxed warning provided by the manufacturers of each of the commercial BoNT products should be consulted.

## Lateral "Epicondylitis" (or Epicondylosis)

Lateral epicondylitis (LE), or tennis elbow, is a chronic tendinopathy involving the common extensor tendons at or near their insertion on the lateral epicondyle. LE is not an inflammatory process; rather, it is a tendinosis or tendinopathy, and is characterized by degenerative changes in the common tendons of the extensor muscle group (extensor carpi ulnaris [ECU], extensor capri radialis brevis [ERCB] and longus [ECRL], extensor digitorum [ED], and extensor digiti minimi [EDM]) (430). LE is primarily an idiopathic syndrome; however, some patients will present with a clear precipitating cause.

### *Pattern of Involvement*

LE typically occurs in middle age and affects males and females equally. Patients present with pain in the lateral elbow that is exacerbated by grasping movements and wrist extension.

### *Evaluation*

The diagnosis is most often established by history and physical examination. X-rays may be useful to rule out boney pathology. US examination may show a thickened (or thinned) tendon that is typically hypoechoic, although it may be hyperechoic/calcified in some patients.

### *Treatment*

For most patients, the condition is self-limited and no treatment is required other than rest. Some patients may require referral to physical therapy for massage, stretching, or other treatment modalities. Pharmacologic treatments include oral or topical NSAIDs. Injections of steroids and local anesthetics were common in the past because LE was originally thought to be an inflammatory process. In recent years, with the recognition that LE is a degenerative tendinopathy, other procedures (e.g., tendon fenestration, prolotherapy, and PRP) have replaced steroid injections in many practices (431). BoNT injections have also been used to treat pain refractory to other treatments.

### *BoNTs Approved for Treatment of LE-Related Pain*

LE is not currently an approved indication for any of the FDA-approved BoNT products. Therefore, the use of BoNTs for the treatment of this indication remains off-label therapy. However, while BoNTs are off-label for LE, there is ample evidence from Class I clinical trials that BoNT injections are effective for treating LE (371).

### *Level of Evidence*

In a 2011 article, Jabbari and Machado reviewed the evidence for BoNT in the treatment of intractable pain conditions, including pain from LE (371). The authors reviewed available studies of BoNT for LE-related pain using AAN guidelines for the classification of quality of evidence from clinical trials (138). On the basis of current evidence, they reported Level A (Established as effective, recommended) evidence for the use of BoNT in the treatment of LE.

### *Injection Pattern*

BoNT may be injected with or without ultrasound guidance just distal to/near the origin of the common extensor tendon on the lateral epicondyle of the humerus. Intramuscular injections, greater than 5-cm distal to the tendon origin (i.e., intramuscular injections), were not found to be effective (432).

### *Dosage*

There was no information from clinical trials on the dose of either IBTA or RBTB for the treatment of LE.

OBTA

A single Class I trial reported a dose of 50 units of OBTA injected into the extensor carpi radialis brevis near the origin of the common extensor tendons (433, 434).

ABTA

Three Class I trials of BoNT injections for LE used ABTA. The reported dose of ABTA in all three studies was 60 units (432, 435, 436).

### *Dilution*

OBTA

The typical dilution for OBTA is 100 units in 1 mL of PFNS resulting in a concentration of 100 units/mL (10 units/0.1 mL).

ABTA

The typical dilution for ABTA is 500 units in 1.5 mL of PFNS resulting in a concentration of 333.33 units/mL (33.33 units/0.1 mL).

### *Adverse Events*

Weakness in wrist and finger extension is the most commonly reported adverse event following injections of BoNT for LE. For a complete list of potential adverse events, the full prescribing information and boxed warning provided by the manufacturers of each of the commercial BoNT products should be consulted.

## Other Musculoskeletal Pain Syndromes

### *Chronic Low Back Pain*

Low back pain (LBP) is a common complaint or symptom with up to 24% of adults reporting at least one episode of LBP per year. Although in most patients LBP is self-limited and resolves, in up to 10% of patients low back pain becomes chronic (CLBP) (437).

### *Clinical/Functional Impact*

Many patients report significant functional limitations with pain that limits work, avocational interests, family life, and participation in a variety of activities. The cost in lost wages and health care expenditures is substantial. A full discussion of the many potential causes of CLBP and treatments for CLBP is beyond the scope of this text. Physicians have prescribed BoNT injections for CLBP and researchers have investigated the efficacy of BoNT for reducing pain and improving function in patients with CLBP (416, 437–439).

### *BoNTs Approved for Treatment of CLBP*

Currently none of the FDA-approved BoNT products are approved for the treatment of CLBP. Therefore, the use of BoNTs for the treatment of this indication remains off-label therapy.

### *Level of Evidence*

The age range of patients, distribution of pain, injection patterns, and doses have varied in published clinical studies (437). In their 2011 review, Jabbari and Machado reported Level C (Possibly effective, may be considered at the discretion of the clinician) evidence for BoNT therapy for CLBP based on a single Class I study (371).

### *Injection Patterns*

Various injection patterns are described, including a fixed-dose per site paradigm. Injection patterns generally follow the distribution of the pain.

### *Dosage*

The published dose of BoNT varied with the specific BoNT product used, the number and size of muscles involved, and whether the injections were unilateral or bilateral (399, 404, 438–440).

#### OBTA

Doses of 200 to 500 units have been reported with multiple injection sites in the "paraspinal" muscles, piriformis, and other muscle groups (399, 438–440).

ABTA
A published dose of 100 units of ABTA was reported for LBP related to sacroiliac pain (441).

RBTB
For piriformis muscle injections, a dose of 5,000 to 12,500 units was reported (404).

IBTA
There is no published information on the dose of IBTA for CLBP.

### *Adverse Events*

Flu-like symptoms, muscle spasm, and injection-site pain were the most commonly reported adverse events. For a complete list of potential adverse events, the full prescribing information and boxed warning provided by the manufacturers of each of the commercial BoNT products should be consulted.

## Thoracic Outlet Syndrome

TOS is an uncommon, sometimes confounding, group of disorders caused by compression of various neurovascular structures in the neck/thoracic outlet. This compression leads to cervicogenic–brachial pain and/or symptoms in the lower neck and upper limb.

### *Clinical/Functional Impact*

Symptoms vary depending on the cause of TOS and the structures that are compressed or entrapped. Patients may present with a wide variety of signs and symptoms, including neck pain, shoulder pain, neuropathic pain, vascular symptoms, or combinations thereof. The wide range of symptoms and signs in TOS may puzzle clinicians unfamiliar with this condition (390, 442, 443).

### *Evaluation*

Because TOS has many causes, there is no "gold standard" for establishing the diagnosis. An extensive clinical evaluation and ancillary testing may be required to irrefutably establish a diagnosis of TOS. This work up is frequently required to avoid misdiagnosis in patients whose symptoms suggest TOS, but arise from another cause (444). Testing may include x-rays, MRI, vascular studies, electrodiagnostic testing, and others. It is imperative that physicians correctly establish the cause of TOS before proceeding to invasive interventions for a presumed diagnosis of TOS, including BoNT injections.

### *Treatment of TOS*

The treatment of TOS is partly determined by the cause of the pain. For example, a patient with clear compression of the lower trunk of the brachial plexus by a bone callus or accessory rib would be unlikely to benefit from BoNT therapy. Treatment for TOS includes physical therapy, postural exercises, manipulation, acupuncture (445), BoNT injections, and surgical procedures. The reader is referred to several reviews for a full discussion of the various proposed treatments for TOS (390, 443, 446).

### *BoNTs Approved for the Treatment of TOS*

TOS is not an approved indication for any of the FDA-approved BoNT products. Therefore, the use of BoNT injections for the treatment of TOS remains off-label therapy.

### *Evidence*

BoNT injections for the treatment of TOS are supported only by anecdotal case reports or case series. Clinicians must recognize that BoNT has no role in the treatment of patients in whom the diagnosis of TOS is not clearly established or where neurovascular compression is caused by boney structures, such as an accessory rib or bone callus.

### *Dosage*

There is limited information on the use of BoNT injections for the treatment of TOS, with only a single randomized controlled trial in the literature (447). A literature search revealed no information on the dose of ABTA, IBTA, or RBTB for the treatment of TOS. Given the lack of specific information on dose for these products when used to treat TOS, a recommendation on dose range cannot be provided. When using these BoNT products for treating TOS, clinicians could consider starting with the manufacturers' recommended dose range per muscle approved for the treatment of cervical dystonia.

OBTA

A range of 50 to 100 units has been reported for the total dose. The total dose is divided among various muscles, depending on the patient's symptoms and the cause of the TOS. The most commonly targeted muscles are the anterior and middle scalenes, ipsilateral trapezius, pectoralis minor, and/or subclavius muscles (93, 446–449). For detailed information, see the TOS section of Table 18.1.

### *Adverse Events*

Flu-like symptoms, muscle spasm, and injection-site pain are the most commonly reported adverse events. For a complete list of potential adverse events, the full prescribing information and boxed warning provided by the manufacturers of each of the commercial BoNT products should be consulted.

## Musculoskeletal Pain Associated with Upper Motor Neuron Syndromes (UMNS)

Pain is a commonly reported symptom in patients with UMNS, including stroke and cerebral palsy (CP). The role of BoNT for treating muscle hypertonia associated with UMNS is covered in detail in Chapter 11 ("Upper Motor Neuron Syndrome" section). A number of studies have evaluated the analgesic effects of BoNTs in various UMNS for preoperative muscle lengthening and for muscle and joint pain (251, 434, 450–456).

### *Preoperative BoNT*

In a randomized controlled trial, Barwood et al. reported reduced length of stay and analgesic use in children treated preoperatively with BoNT (OBTA) 5 to 10 days before undergoing a muscle lengthening procedure (251).

### *Poststroke Shoulder Pain*

Several double-blind randomized controlled trials and randomized controlled trials have been conducted evaluating shoulder pain in adults with poststroke spasticity (PSS) and have reported conflicting results (434, 454–458). Some studies have reported significant improvement in pain and function, whereas others report improvement in pain, but not in function, and still others report no benefit.

### *Level of Evidence*

Several authors have reviewed the clinical trial evidence for BoNT injections for treatment of PSS and shoulder pain. In a 2012 review, Viana et al. concluded that there was conflicting evidence from current trials on PSS-related shoulder pain in adult patients (451). In a 2011 Cochrane review of BoNT injections for shoulder pain, including PSS, Singh and Fitzgerald concluded that BoNTs were effective in reducing shoulder pain in patients with PSS and for OA-related pain (459). Conversely, in a systematic review of interventions for PSS shoulder pain, Koog et al. concluded that there was insufficient evidence to support the use of BoNT for hemiplegic shoulder pain (460).

### *Dosage*

In PSS, injections of BoNT are described in the muscles of the shoulder girdle, trapezius, and biceps, as well as into the glenohumeral joint.

OBTA

A dose of 100 to 200 units may be divided between shoulder girdle muscles or the glenohumeral joint with 100 units being the most commonly reported dose injected into the glenohumeral joint (see Table 18.1) (453, 457).

ABTA

Doses of 200 units were injected in various pectoral/shoulder muscles or into the glenohumeral joint (453).

IBTA

A dose of 100 units may be injected into the glenohumeral joint (453).

RBTB

There is no published information on the dose of RBTB for the treatment of PSS shoulder pain.

### *Dosage*

There were no studies evaluating RBTB for use in CP/preoperative indications.

OBTA

The total dose used was 8 units/kg, divided between the bilateral adductor muscles (251).

### *Dilution*

OBTA

The most commonly reported dilution is either 100 units of OBTA in 1 mL or 2 mL PFNS resulting in a concentration of 100 units/mL (10 units/0.1 mL) or 50 units/mL (5 units/0.1mL), respectively. Alternatively, a 200-unit vial is diluted with 2 mL PFNS or 4 mL PFNS for a dilution of 100 units/mL or 50 units/mL.

ABTA

Dilutions of 500 units in 1 mL (50 units/0.1 mL), 1.5 mL (333 units/mL, 33.3 units/0.1mL), and 2.5 mL (200 units/mL, 20 units/0.1mL) have been described.

IBTA

Dilution of 100 units in 1 mL (10 units/0.1 mL) has been described for glenohumeral injections.

### *Adverse Events*

Flu-like symptoms, muscle spasm, and injection-site pain are the most commonly reported adverse events. For a complete list of potential adverse events, the full prescribing information and boxed warning provided by the manufacturers of each of the commercial BoNT products should be consulted.

**TABLE 18.1 Musculoskeletal/Myofascial Pain Conditions Dosage/Dilution Table**

| BoNT Preparation | OBTA (Botox®) | ABTA (Dysport®) | IBTA (Xeomin®) | RBTB (Myobloc®) |
|---|---|---|---|---|
| U.S. FDA approval | Currently not FDA approved | Currently not FDA approved | Currently not FDA approved | Currently not FDA approved |
| UK MHRA | Currently not an approved indication | Currently not an approved indication | Currently not an approved indication | Currently not an approved indication |
| **Published Dosage Range: Adults (≥18 Years of Age)** | | | | |
| **Myofascial Pain Syndromes** | | | | |
| Myofascial pain syndrome/trigger points | 5–10 units/small muscle, 10–30 units/medium muscle, 50 units/large muscle | 40–80 units/trigger point, up to 120 units/trigger point reported in larger muscles | No published studies of IBTA for MPS[a] | 250 units/small muscles × 1 site, 250–500 units/medium muscle × 1 site, 500–750 units/trigger point in large muscles × 1–2 sites |
| MPS: total dose/treatment session | 100–400 units (dosages up to 600 units have been reported) (393) | 240–500 units | No published data on dosage | Mean dose 9,000 units (393), dosage range 2,500–10,000 units (393); doses of 22–25,000 units have been reported (393, 380) |
| MPS: localization | Palpation, US | Palpation, US | — | Palpation, US |
| Piriformis syndrome | 80–200 units | 150 units (403) (reported as "low dose") | No published data on dosage | 5,000–12,500 units (404) |

(continued)

**TABLE 18.1 Musculoskeletal/Myofascial Pain Conditions Dosage/Dilution Table** *(continued)*

| BoNT Preparation | OBTA (Botox®) | ABTA (Dysport®) | IBTA (Xeomin®) | RBTB (Myobloc®) |
|---|---|---|---|---|
| **Myofascial Pain Syndromes (*continued*)** | | | | |
| Localization | EMG, US, fluoroscopy | EMG | — | EMG, US, fluoroscopy |
| CLBP | 100–500 units divided, 40–50 units/site | 100 units, sacroiliac joint (441) | No published data on dosage | See piriformis syndrome |
| **Osteoarticular Pain Syndromes** | | | | |
| Hip OA | No published data on dosage | 250 units adductor longus (421), 150 units adductor magnus (421) | No published data on dosage | No published data on dosage |
| Knee pain, OA | 25–150 units/joint, 100 units, most commonly reported dose | No published data on dosage | No published data on dosage | No published data on dosage |
| Knee pain, post-TKA | 100 units | No published data on dosage | No published data on dosage | No published data on dosage |
| Shoulder pain, OA related | 100 units | No published data on dosage | No published data on dosage | No published data on dosage |
| Shoulder, adhesive capsulitis | | 200 units (425) | No published data on dosage | No published data on dosage |
| Axial skeletal joints: sacroiliac, sternoclavicular, C2/lumbar facet joints | 25–100 units, divided (423) | No published data on dosage | No published data on dosage | 5,000 units, divided (423) |

*(continued)*

**TABLE 18.1 Musculoskeletal/Myofascial Pain Conditions Dosage/Dilution Table (*continued*)**

| BoNT Preparation | OBTA (Botox®) | ABTA (Dysport®) | IBTA (Xeomin®) | RBTB (Myobloc®) |
|---|---|---|---|---|
| **Osteoarticular Pain Syndromes (*continued*)** | | | | |
| Temporo-mandibular joint | | 200 units, divided | No published data on dosage | No published data on dosage |
| Lateral epicondylosis, "epicondylitis" | 20–40 units | 60 units | No published data on dosage | No published data on dosage |
| PFP/knee pain | | 300–500 units, divided dose, distal 1/3 of VL (420) | No published data on dosage | No published data on dosage |
| | Mean dose: 161 units (429), range: 120–210 units (429) | Mean dose: 526 units (429), range 300–700 units (429) | | |
| PFP: Number of injection sites | 8 | 8 | — | — |
| PF | 30–70 units/heel, 1–3 injection sites | 100–200 units/heel, 1–3 injection sites | No published data on dosage | No published data on dosage |
| **Thoracic Outlet Syndrome** | | | | |
| TOS | 50–100 units, divided | No published data on dosage | No published data on dosage | No published data on dosage |

(*continued*)

**TABLE 18.1 Musculoskeletal/Myofascial Pain Conditions Dosage/Dilution Table** *(continued)*

| BoNT Preparation | OBTA (Botox®) | ABTA (Dysport®) | IBTA (Xeomin®) | RBTB (Myobloc®) |
|---|---|---|---|---|
| **Thoracic Outlet Syndrome (*continued*)** | | | | |
| Scalenes | 12–15 units/muscle, (up to 37.5 units/muscle has been reported) | No published data on dosage | No published data on dosage | No published data on dosage |
| Pectoralis minor | 15 units (449) | No published data on dosage | No published data on dosage | No published data on dosage |
| Subclavius | 12 units (449) | No published data on dosage | No published data on dosage | No published data on dosage |
| Trapezius | 50–76 units | No published data on dosage | No published data on dosage | No published data on dosage |
| **Localization MSK Conditions** | | | | |
| Localization | Palpation, EMG, US, fluoroscopy, CT | Palpation, US, EMG, fluoroscopy, CT | Palpation, US, EMG, fluoroscopy, CT | EMG, palpation |
| Dilution | 100 units with 1 mL PFNS | 500 units in 1 mL or 2.5 mL PFNS | 100 units in 1 mL | Not required, RBTB can be diluted with PFNS if desired |
| Injection interval | 12–16 Weeks | 12–14 Weeks | 12–16 Weeks | 12–14 Weeks |

*(continued)*

**TABLE 18.1 Musculoskeletal/Myofascial Pain Conditions Dosage/Dilution Table** (*continued*)

| Injected Muscle or Structure | OBTA (Botox®) | ABTA (Dysport®) | IBTA (Xeomin®) | RBTB (Myobloc®) |
|---|---|---|---|---|
| **Pediatric Patients ≤18 Years of Age** | | | | |
| CP: adductor BoNT injections prior to muscle lengthening | 4 units/kg/leg divided into 2 injection sites, 2 units/kg/site, total dose: 8 units/kg (251) | No published data on dosage | No published data on dosage | No published data on dosage |
| **Poststroke Shoulder Pain, Intra-articular Injection (Adult Patients ≥18 Years of Age)** | | | | |
| Glenohumeral joint | 100 units (453) | 500 units (453)<br>Poststroke Shoulder Pain, Muscle injections | 100 units (453) | |
| Pectoralis major, teres major | 100–150 units (457), 40–60 units (457), dilution: 100 units in 1 mL PFNS | | | |
| Subscapularis | 100 units, 2 sites, dilution: 100 units in 1–2 mL PFNS (455) | 500 units (456), dilution not reported | | |

(*continued*)

TABLE 18.1 Musculoskeletal/Myofascial Pain Conditions Dosage/Dilution Table (*continued*)

| Injected Muscle or Structure | OBTA (Botox®) | ABTA (Dysport®) | IBTA (Xeomin®) | RBTB (Myobloc®) |
|---|---|---|---|---|
| **Poststroke Shoulder Pain, Intra-articular Injection (Adult Patients ≥18 Years of Age) (*continued*)** | | | | |
| Pectoralis major | | 500 units, 4 injection sites, dilution not reported (458) | | |
| Pectoralis major biceps | | 250 units/muscle, 500 units total dose, dilution: 500 units in 2.5 mL PFNS (454) | | |
| Infraspinatus, pectoralis major, subscapularis | 100 units, divided, dilution: 100 units in 4 mL PFNS (610) | | | |

[a]Studies using IBTA in adults for cervical dystonia and blepharospasm suggest dose equivalency to OBTA. The use of conversion ratios is not recommended by manufacturers (see full prescribing information).

*Abbreviations:* ABTA, abobotulinumtoxinA; IBTA, incobotulinumtoxinA; OBTA, onabotulinumtoxinA; RBTB, rimabotulinumtoxinB; PFNS, preservative-free normal saline (0.9%).

*Sources:* Adapted from Refs. 34, 36, 38, 44, 93, 251, 371, 380, 383–390, 392–396, 398–400, 402–411, 416–423, 425, 429, 432–436, 438–441, 443, 446–450, 453–459, 610–615.

# *Appendices*

# A

# *Ashworth and Modified Ashworth Scale for Grading Muscle Hypertonia*

## Ashworth Scale for Grading Muscle Hypertonia

*Grade Description*

1 No increase in muscle tone

2 Slight increase giving a catch when part is moved in flexion or extension

3 More marked increase in tone but only after part is easily flexed

4 Considerable increase in tone

5 Passive movement is difficult and affected part is rigid in flexion or extension

## Modified Ashworth Scale for Grading Muscle Hypertonia

*Grade Description*

0 No increase in muscle tone

1 Slight increase in muscle tone, manifested by a catch and release or by minimal resistance at the end of the range of motion when the affected part(s) is moved in flexion or extension

1+ Slight increase in muscle tone, manifested by a catch, followed by minimal resistance throughout the remainder (less than half) of the ROM

2 More marked increase in muscle tone through most of the ROM, but affected part(s) easily moved

3 Considerable increase in muscle tone, passive movement difficult

4 Affected part(s) rigid in flexion or extension

*Source:* Ref. 217. Ansari NN, Naghdi S, Arab TK, Jalaie S. The interrater and intrarater reliability of the Modified Ashworth Scale in the assessment of muscle spasticity: limb and muscle group effect. *NeuroRehabilitation*. 2008a;23(3):231–237.

# B

# *Blepharospasm Disability Index Scale*

| Items |
| --- |
| Reading<br>Driving a vehicle<br>Watching television<br>Shopping<br>Doing everyday activities<br>Getting about on foot (walking) |
| **Rating** |
| 0 = No impairment<br>1 = Mild impairment<br>2 = Moderate impairment<br>3 = Severe impairment<br>4 = Not possible because of disease<br>Not applicable |

*Sources:* Refs. 620, 621.

# C

# *Blepharospasm Disability Scale*

| Sunglasses (check one or both if these apply) | Score (Maximum 2) |
|---|---|
| 1. Need to wear sunglasses outdoors | 1 |
| 2. Usually need sunglasses indoors | 1 |
| **Driving (check those that apply)** | **Score (Maximum 5)** |
| 1. Uncomfortable but no limitation | 1 |
| 2. Cannot drive at night because of blepharospasm | 2 |
| 3. Can drive in daytime, needs to prop eyelids open | 2 |
| 4. Can drive only short distances | 3 |
| 5. Cannot drive at all because of blepharospasm | 4 |
| 6. Usually cannot ride in a car | 5 |
| **Reading (check one if affected)** | **Score (Maximum 3)** |
| 1. Uncomfortable but no limitation | 1 |
| 2. Mild to moderate limitation of reading | 2 |
| 3. Marked limitation of reading | 3 |
| **Television (check one if affected)** | **Score (Maximum 3)** |
| 1. Uncomfortable but no limitation | 1 |
| 2. Mild to moderate limitation of viewing TV | 2 |
| 3. Marked limitation of viewing TV | 3 |
| **Movies (check one if affected)** | **Score (Maximum 3)** |
| 1. Uncomfortable but no limitation | 1 |
| 2. Mild to moderate limitation of watching movies | 2 |
| 3. Marked limitation of watching movies | 3 |
| **Shopping (check one if affected)** | **Score (Maximum 3)** |
| 1. Uncomfortable but no limitation | 1 |
| 2. Not able to shop alone | 2 |
| 3. Not able to shop, even when accompanied | 3 |

| Walking about (check one if affected) | Score (Maximum 4) |
|---|---|
| 1. Uncomfortable but no limitation | 1 |
| 2. Difficulty walking in crowds | 2 |
| 3. Not able to walk alone outside | 3 |
| 4. Not able to walk unassisted indoors | 4 |
| **Housework or outside job (check one if affected)** | **Score (Maximum 3)** |
| 1. Uncomfortable but no limitation | 1 |
| 2. Difficulty working because of blepharospasm | 2 |
| 3. Not able to work, housework or outside job, because of blepharospasm | 3 |

Total Score: **(Maximum 26).**

Percentage of Normal Activity = **90% - 90** (score ÷ maximum possible).

100% = Unaware of any difficulty.

95% = Aware of some blepharospasm; some annoyance but no limitations of activities.

90% = Completely independent; socially affected, but otherwise no limitations of activities because of the blepharospasm; if there are any limitations of functional activities, the patient should check the ones listed in the table that apply.

*Source:* Ref. 622. Fahn S, List T, Moslowitz C, et al. Double-blind controlled study of botulinum toxin for blepharospasm. *Neurology*. 1985;35(suppl 1):271–272.

# D

# *Burke–Fahn–Marsden Dystonia Scale*

Movement scale, scored by clinician. This scale consists of provoking factors (scored 0–4) and severity factors (scored 0–4). Scores are given a weight of either 0.5 or 1. The three are multiplied to give the adjusted score. All scores are summed to give an overall score from 0 to 120.

## Provoking Factors

### *General*

0 No dystonia at rest or with action

1 Dystonia on particular action

2 Dystonia on many actions

3 Dystonia on action of distant part of body, or intermittently at rest

4 Dystonia present at rest

### *Speech and Swallowing*

0 None

1 Occasional, either or both

2 Frequent, either

3 Frequent one, occasional other

### *Severity Factors*

EYES

0 None

1 Slight: Occasional blinking

2 Mild: Frequent blinking without prolonged spasms of eye closure

3 Moderate: Prolonged spasms of eyelid closure, but eyes open most of the time

4 Severe: Prolonged spasms of eyelid closure, with eyes closed at least 30% of the time

MOUTH

0 No dystonia present

1 Slight: Occasional grimacing or other mouth movements (e.g., jaw open or clenched, tongue movement)

2 Mild: Movement present less than 50% of the time

3 Moderate: Dystonic movement or contractions present most of the time

4 Severe: Dystonic movement or contractions present most of the time

SPEECH AND SWALLOWING

0 Normal

1 Slightly involved; speech easily understood or occasional choking

2 Some difficulty in understanding speech or frequent choking

3 Marked difficulty in understanding speech or inability to swallow firm foods

4 Complete or almost complete anarthria or marked difficulty in swallowing soft foods or liquids

NECK

0 No dystonia present

1 Slight: Occasional pulling

2 Obvious torticollis, but mild

3 Moderate: Pulling

4 Extreme: Pulling

ARM

0 No dystonia present

1 Slight: Dystonia; clinically insignificant

2 Mild: Obvious dystonia but not disabling

3 Moderate: Able to grasp, with some manual function

4 Severe: No useful grasp

TRUNK

0 No dystonia present

1 Slight: Bending; clinically insignificant

2 Definite: Bending but not interfering with standing or walking

3 Moderate: Bending; interfering with standing or walking

4 Extreme: Bending of trunk preventing standing or walking

LEG

0 No dystonia present

1 Slight: Dystonia but not causing impairment; clinically insignificant

2 Mild: Dystonia; walks briskly and unaided

3 Moderate: Dystonia; severely impairs walking or requires assistance

4 Severe: Unable to stand or walk on involved leg

## *Scoring: Movement Scale*

| Region | Provoking Factor (PF) | Severity Factor (SF) | Weight (W) | Weighted Score (PF × SF × W) |
|---|---|---|---|---|
| Eyes | 0–4 | 0–4 | 0.5 | 0–8 |
| Mouth | 0–4 | 0–4 | 0.5 | 0–8 |
| Speech/ swallowing | 0–4 | 0–4 | 1.0 | 0–16 |
| Neck | 0–4 | 0–4 | 0.5 | 0–8 |
| Right arm | 0–4 | 0–4 | 1.0 | 0–16 |
| Left arm | 0–4 | 0–4 | 1.0 | 0–16 |
| Trunk | 0–4 | 0–4 | 1.0 | 0–16 |
| Right leg | 0–4 | 0–4 | 1.0 | 0–16 |
| Left leg | 0–4 | 0–4 | 1.0 | 0–16 |

Total (sum: maximum 120).

*Source:* Ref. 166. Burke RE, Fahn S, Marsden CD, Bressman SB, Moskowitz C, Friedman J. Validity and reliability of a rating scale for the primary torsion dystonias. *Neurology*. 1985;35(1):73–77.

# E

# *Dystonia Discomfort Scale*

The Dystonia Discomfort Scale (DDS) is an assessment tool to measure the severity of symptomatology in patients with cervical dystonia.

Patients are asked to rate their symptomatology in multiples of 5% on a scale ranging from 0% (no complaints) to 100% (maximum subjective severity of the untreated condition). Scores are documented by the patient in a diary on a daily basis.

The DDS has been shown to be a valid and sensitive tool to monitor cervical dystonia symptoms over time. Indeed, in a long-term treatment setting, a positive correlation was shown between DDS scores and scores obtained using the widely accepted Toronto Western Spasmodic Torticollis Rating Scale (TWSTRS). Furthermore, the DDS can be easily performed by patients on a daily basis, and as such may offer advantages over assessments that require attendance at a clinic.

The DDS patient diary, together with further information for clinicians and patients, can be accessed by following the link: www.dds.iabnetz.de/. Please cite this link when referring to this tool.

**Dear Patient,**

Dystonias such as spasmodic torticollis (cervical dystonia, torticollis), blepharospasm, graphospasm and so forth are a group of very different and usually chronic conditions. Until now their treatment has almost always been frustrating.

The situation has changed fundamentally with the introduction of botulinum toxin therapy. This therapy is now by far the most successful method of treating dystonia.

In order to achieve optimal treatment results, the botulinum toxin therapy must be tailored individually to your specific symptoms. It must also take into account changes in your symptoms as your condition progresses. Additional observations can also help to facilitate the management of your condition.

To achieve all of this, your treating physician needs the most accurate overview possible of the course of your treatment. For this, he or she is entirely dependent on your cooperation.

This patient diary should help you record your observations.

The patient diary can of course also be used to record the course of other treatments.

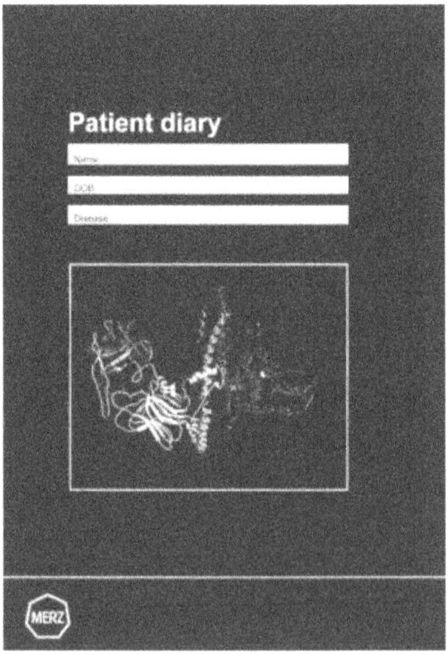


**For further assistance, contact:**

- Deutsche Dystonie Gesellschaft e.V., Rissener Landstr. 85. D-22587 Hamburg, info@dystonie.de
- Bundesverband Torticollis e.V., Eckernkamp 39. D-59077 Hamm, bvtorti@aol.com

Prof. Dr. Dirk Dressier. Professor of Neurology
Head of the Movement Disorders Section
Hannover Medical School
Carl-Neuberg-Str. 1
D-30625 Hannover
Germany
t +49-511-532-3111/3736 f+49-511-532-8110 dressler.dirk@mh-hannover.de



**Instructions for using the patient diary**

1 Please complete the diary every night before going to sleep.

2 Please circle the percentage that best describes your dystonia symptoms today. 0% indicates that you do not feel any dystonia symptoms at all, 100% that your dystonia is at its most extreme and you are not receiving any treatment. For ratings between 0% and 100%, circle the percentage that seems appropriate. Use examples A and B for guidance.

3 You may find it difficult initially to specify your symptoms in intervals of 5%. However, these small increments will help you to record precisely slight changes in your dystonia symptoms occurring from one day to the next.

4 Record everything of note which occurs on that day in the "Comments" column. Use example C for guidance.

5 Please bring your diary to each repeat visit.

6 Your physician can reorder the patient diary.

**Examples:**

A Cervical dystonia has been diagnosed but not yet treated in one female patient. Her dystonia symptoms are at 100%. Following the start of treatment, her dystonia symptoms are usually only 20% on most days. After about three months, the efficacy of the treatment slowly declines and her dystonia symptoms again reach 60%. About one week after repeating the treatment, her dystonia symptoms again decrease to 20% on most days.

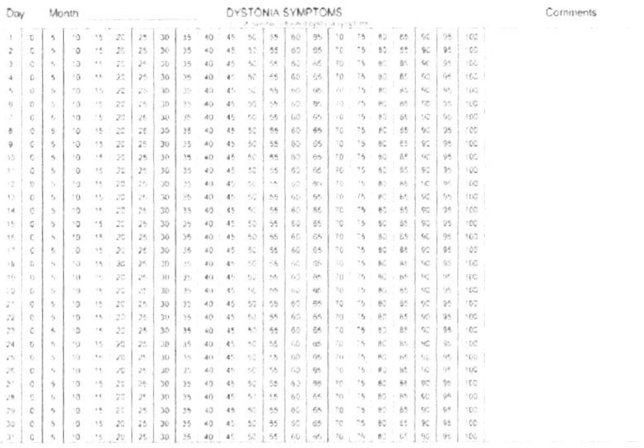


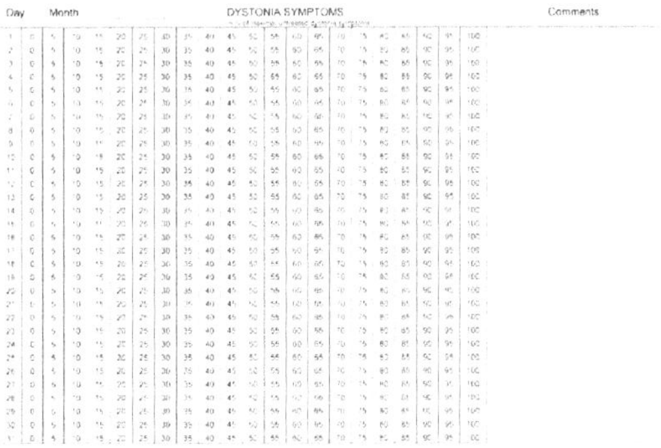


B A male patient has dystonia symptoms of 50% from 7 a.m. to 3 p.m. By the time he goes to bed, symptoms increase to 70%. In terms of the entire day, this corresponds most closely to 60%.

C A female patient plays 2 hours of tennis twice a week. She records this diligently in her patient diary and sees that her dystonia symptoms are twice as severe on these days than on other days. She reduces her tennis sessions to 45 minutes, and her dystonia symptoms no longer indicate any deterioration.

*Source:* Ref. 626. Dressler D, Kupsch A, Paus S, Seitzinger A, Gebhardt B. Sustained efficacy of IncobotulinumtoxinA (Xeomin; botulinum neurotoxin type A, free from complexing proteins) in long-term treatment of cervical dystonia. *Eur J Neurol.* 2011;18(suppl 2):482.

# Reference

Prospective Phase IV study

Principal Investigator: Dirk Dressler, Hannover Medical School, Hannover, Germany

Study funded by Merz Pharmaceuticals GmbH, Frankfurt am Main, Germany

# F

# *Modified Tardieu Scale*

<table>
<tr><th>Purpose</th><th>Modified Tardieu Scale</th></tr>
<tr><td>Assessment of Spasticity<br>The Tardieu scale assesses the response to stretch at slow and fast velocities<br>The scale was first developed by Tardieu and has been revised by several investigators</td><td>Patient is positioned in sitting to test upper and supine to test lower limbs<br>Measurements:<br><br>1. Measurements<br>• Quality of muscle reaction (scored 0–5)<br>• Angle of muscle<br>• Angle of muscle reaction<br><br>2. Speed definitions: Original Tardieu<br>• V1 is slow as possible<br>• V2 speed of limb falling under gravity<br>• V3 moving as fast as possible<br><br>Speed definitions: Modified Tardieu<br>• R1 quick stretch is the catch angle when the muscle reacts at quick speed of stretch, equivalent to V3<br>• R2 slow stretch is equivalent to passive range of motion (PROM) or to V1<br>• R1–R2 = dynamic tone component of the muscle. Measured in degrees (623)<br><br>Quality of Muscle Reaction<br>• 0 = No resistance to PROM<br>• 1 = Slight resistance throughout the course of PROM, no clear catch at a precise angle<br>• 2 = Clear catch at a precise angle, interrupting the passive movement, followed by release<br>• 3 = Fatigable clonus for <10 seconds when maintaining pressure and at a precise angle<br>• 4 = Unfatigable clonus for >10 seconds when maintaining pressure and at a precise angle<br>• 5 = Joint is immobile. (Some versions scored 0–4)</td></tr>
</table>

*Sources:* Refs. 218, 623, 624.

# G

# *Toronto Western Spasmodic Torticollis Severity Scale*

## I. Torticollis Severity Scale

**A. Maximal Excursion**
**1. Rotation** *(turn: right or left)*
0 = None [0°]
1 = Slight [<¼ range, 1°–22°]
2 = Mild [¼–½ range, 23°–45°]
3 = Moderate [½–¾ range, 46°–67°]
4 = Severe [>¾ range, 68°–90°]
**2. Laterocollis** *(tilt: right or left, exclude shoulder elevation)*
0 = None [0°]
1 = Mild [1°–15°]
2 = Moderate [16°–35°]
3 = Severe [>35°]
**3. Anterocollis/Retrocollis** *(a or b)*
**a. Anterocollis**
0 = None
1 = Mild downward deviation of chin
2 = Moderate downward deviation (approximates ½ possible range)
3 = Severe (chin approximates chest)
**b. Retrocollis**
0 = None
1 = Mild backward deviation of vertex with upward deviation of chin
2 = Moderate backward deviation (approximates ½ possible range
3 = Severe (approximates full range)
**4. Lateral shift** *(right or left)*
0 = Absent
1 = Present
**5. Sagittal shift** *(forward or backward)*
0 = Absent
1 = Present

**B. Duration Factor** *(Weighted x 2)*
0 = None
1 = Occasional deviation (<25% of the time, most often submaximal)
2 = Occasional deviation (<25% of the time, often maximal) or Intermittent deviation (25%–50% of the time, most often submaximal)
3 = Intermittent deviation (25% –50% of the time, often maximal) **or** Frequent deviation (50%–75% of the time, most often submaximal)
4 = Frequent deviation (50%–75% of the time, often maximal) **or** Constant deviation (>75% of the time, most often submaximal)
5 = Constant deviation (>75% of the time, often maximal)

**C. Effect of Sensory Tricks**
0 = Complete relief by one or more tricks
1 = Partial or only limited relief by tricks
2 = Little or no benefit from tricks

**D. Shoulder Elevation/Anterior Displacement**
0 = Absent
1 = Mild (<1/3 possible range, intermittent or constant)
2 = Moderate (1/3 – 2/3 possible range and constant, > 75% of the time) or Severe (> 2/3 possible range and intermittent)
3 = Severe and constant

**E. Range of Motion** *(without aid of sensory tricks)*
0 = Able to move to extreme opposite position
1 = Able to move head well past midline but not to extreme opposite position
2 = Able to move head barely past midline
3 = Able to move head toward but not past midline
4 = Barely able to move head beyond abnormal posture

**F. Time** *(up to 60 seconds) for which patient is able to maintain head within 10° of neutral position without using sensory tricks (mean of two attempts)*
0 = > 60 seconds
1 = 46–60 seconds
2 = 31–45 seconds
3 = 16–30 seconds
4 = < 15 seconds

# II. Disability Scale (Maximum = 20)

**A. Work** *(occupation or housework/home management)*
0 = No difficulty
1 = Normal work expectations with satisfactory performance at usual level of occupation but some interference by torticollis
2 = Most activities unlimited, selected activities very difficult and hampered but still possible with satisfactory performance
3 = Working at lower than usual occupation level; most activities hampered, all possible but with less than satisfactory performance in some activities
4 = Unable to engage in voluntary or gainful employment; still able to perform some domestic responsibilities satisfactorily
5 = Marginal or no ability to perform domestic responsibilities

**B. Activities of Daily Living** (e.g., *feeding, dressing, or hygiene, including washing, shaving, makeup*)
0 = No difficulty with any activity
1 = Activities unlimited but some interference by torticollis
2 = Most activities unlimited, selected activities very difficult and hampered but still possible using simple tricks
3 = Most activities hampered or laborious but still possible; may use extreme tricks
4 = All activities impaired; some impossible or require assistance
5 = Dependent on others in most self-care tasks

**C. Driving**
0 = No difficulty (or has never driven a car)
1 = Unlimited ability to drive but bothered by torticollis
2 = Unlimited ability to drive but requires tricks (including touching or holding face, holding head against head rest) to control torticollis
3 = Can drive only short distances
4 = Usually cannot drive because of torticollis
5 = Unable to drive and cannot ride in a car for long stretches as a passenger because of torticollis

**D. Reading**
1 = Unlimited ability to read in normal seated position but bothered by torticollis
2 = Unlimited ability to read in normal seated position but requires use of tricks to control torticollis
3 = Unlimited ability to read but requires extensive measures to control torticollis or is able to read only in nonseated position (e.g., lying down)
4 = Limited ability to read because of torticollis despite tricks
5 = Unable to read more than a few sentences because of torticollis

**E. Television**
0 = No difficulty
1 = Unlimited ability to watch television in normal seated position but bothered by torticollis
2 = Unlimited ability to watch television in normal seated position but requires use of tricks to control torticollis
3 = Unlimited ability to watch television but requires extensive measures to control torticollis or is able to view only in nonseated position (e.g., lying down)
4 = Limited ability to watch television because of torticollis
5 = Unable to watch television more than a few minutes because of torticollis

**F. Activities Outside the Home** *(e.g., shopping, walking about, movies, dining, and other recreational activities)*
0 = No difficulty
1 = Unlimited activities but bothered by torticollis
2 = Unlimited activities but requires simple tricks to accomplish
3 = Accomplishes activities only when accompanied by others because of torticollis
4 = Limited activities outside the home; certain activities impossible or given up because of torticollis
5 = Rarely if ever engages in activities outside the home

*Sources:* Refs. 167, 168.

# III. Pain Scale (Maximum = 20)

**A. Severity of Pain** Rate the severity of neck pain during the last week on a scale of 0–10:
0 = No pain
10 = The most excruciating pain imaginable
**Score calculated as**: (Best + Worst + (2 × Usual))/4
**Best** ____
**Worst** ____
**Usual** ____
**Score**: ____

**B. Duration of Pain**
0 = None
1 = Present <10% of the time
2 = Present 10%–25% of the time
3 = Present 26%–50% of the time
4 = Present 51%–75% of the time
5 = Present >76% of the time

**C. Disability Due to Pain**
0 = No limitation or interference from pain
1 = Pain is quite bothersome but not a source of disability
2 = Pain definitely interferes with some tasks but is not a major contributor to disability
3 = Pain accounts for some (less than half) but not all of disability
4 = Pain is a major source of difficulty with activities; separate from this, head pulling is also a source of some (less than half) disability
5 = Pain is the major source of disability; without it most impaired activities could be performed quite satisfactorily despite the head pulling

*Source:* Ref. 625. Consky ES, Lang AE. Clinical assessments of patients with cervical dystonia. In: Jankovic J, Hallett M, eds. *Therapy with Botulinum Toxin*. New York, NY: Marcel Dekker, Inc; 1994:211–237.

# *References*


1. Rossetto O, Megighian A, Scorzeto M, Montecucco C. Botulinum neurotoxins. *Toxicon*. 2013;67:31–36.
2. Hallett M, Karp B. Pharmacology and physiology. In: Alter KE, Hallett M, Karp B, Lungu C, eds. *Ultrasound-Guided Chemodenervation Procedures: Text and Atlas*. New York, NY: Demos Medical Pub; 2013:2–8.
3. Kaeser PS, Regehr WG. Molecular mechanisms for synchronous, asynchronous, and spontaneous neurotransmitter release. *Annu Rev Physiol*. 2014;76:333–363.
4. Wenzel RG. Pharmacology of botulinum neurotoxin serotype A. *Am J Health Syst Pharm*. 2004;61(22 suppl 6):S5–S10.
5. Tighe AP, Schiavo G. Botulinum neurotoxins: mechanism of action. *Toxicon*. 2013;67:87–93.
6. de Maio M. Therapeutic uses of botulinum toxin: from facial palsy to autonomic disorders. *Expert Opin Biol Ther*. 2008;8(6):791–798.
7. Dressler D. Clinical applications of botulinum toxin. *Curr Opin Microbiol*. 2012a;15(3):325–336.
8. Fischer A, Koriazova L, Oblatt-Montal M, Montal M. Botulinum neurotoxin—a modular nanomachine. In: Jankovic J, Albanese A, Zouhair Atassi M, Dolly JO, Hallett M, Mayer NH. *Botulinum Toxin: Therapeutic Clinical Practice and Science*. Philadelphia, PA: Saunders, Elsevier; 2009:30–40.
9. Hallett M. One man's poison—clinical applications of botulinum toxin. *N Engl J Med*. 1999;341(2):118–120.
10. Abrams SA, Hallett M. Clinical utility of different botulinum neurotoxin preparations. *Toxicon*. 2013;67:81–86.
11. Wheeler A, Smith HS. Botulinum toxins: mechanisms of action, antinociception and clinical applications. *Toxicology*. 2013;306:124–146.
12. Galloux M, Vitrac H, Montagner C, et al. Membrane interaction of botulinum neurotoxin A translocation (T) domain. The belt region is a regulatory loop for membrane interaction. *J Biol Chem*. 2008;283(41):27668–27676.
13. Dolly JO, Meng J, Wang J, et al. Multiple steps in the blockade of exocytosis by botulinum neurotoxins. In: Jankovic J, Albanese A, Zouhair Atassi M, Dolly JO, Hallett M, Mayer NH, eds. *Botulinum Toxin: Therapeutic Clinical Practice and Science*. Philadelphia, PA: Saunders, Elsevier; 2009:1–14.

14. Chen R, Karp BI, Goldstein SR, Bara-Jimenez W, Yaseen Z, Hallett M. Effect of muscle activity immediately after botulinum toxin injection for writer's cramp. *Mov Discord*. 1999;14(2):307–312.
15. Berry MG, Stanek JJ. Botulinum neurotoxin A: a review. *J Plast Reconstr Aesthet Surg*. 2012;65(10):1283–1291.
16. Kennelly J, Jenkins B, Zhou J, Haag-Molkenteller C, Brin M. OnabotulinumtoxinA for the treatment of urinary incontinence due to neurogenic detrusor overactivity. 50th Annual Meeting of the Interagency Botulism Research Coordinating Committee (IBRCC); November 2013; Annapolis, MD:111–112.
17. Elovic EP, Esquenazi A, Alter KE, Lin JL, Alfaro A, Kaelin DL. Chemodenervation and nerve blocks in the diagnosis and management of spasticity and muscle overactivity. *PM R*. 2009;1(9):842–851.
18. Alter KE. High-frequency ultrasound guidance for neurotoxin injections. *Phys Med Rehabil Clin N Am*. 2010;21(3):607–630.
19. Benecke R. Clinical relevance of botulinum toxin immunogenicity. *BioDrugs*. 2012;26(2):e1–e9.
20. Greene P, Fahn S. Development of antibodies to botulinum toxin type A in patients with torticollis treated with injection of botulinum toxin type A. In: DasGupta BR, ed. *Botulinum and Tetanus Neurotoxins: Neurotransmission and Biomedical Aspects*. New York, NY: Plenum Press; 1993:651–654.
21. Naumann M, Carruthers A, Carruthers J, et al. Meta-analysis of neutralizing antibody conversion with onabotulinumtoxinA (Botox) across multiple indications. *Mov Disord*. 2010;25(13):2211–2218.
22. Hong JS, Sathe GG, Niyonkuru C, Munin MC. Elimination of dysphagia using ultrasound guidance for botulinum toxin injections in cervical dystonia. *Muscle Nerve*. 2012;46(4):535–539.
23. Truong DD, Jost WH. Botulinum toxins: clinical use. *Parkinsonism Relat Disord*. 2006;12(6):331–355.
24. Petrou I. Medy-Tox introduces neuronox to the botulinum toxin arena. *Eur Aesth Guide*. 2009 Spring:57.
25. Dressler D, Benecke R. Pharmacology of therapeutic botulinum toxin preparations. *Disabil Rehabil*. 2007;29(23):1761–1768.
26. Neuronox PI [package Insert/prescribing information]. Chungcheongbuk-do, ROK: Medy-tox, Inc. Available at (http://www.mesozon.com/shop/images/Neuronox/Neuronox%20Medical.pdf). Updated August 2005.
27. BTXA PI [package insert/prescribing information]. Lanzhou, Gansu PRC: Lanzhou Institute of Biological Products Co., Ltd (LIBP). Available at http://www.btxa.com/discover/prescribing_information.pdf. 2011.
28. Pickett A, O'Keeffe R, Panjwani N. The protein load of therapeutic botulinum toxins. *Eur J Neurol*. 2007;14(4):e11.
29. Bigalke H. Properties of pharmaceutical products of botulinum neurotoxins. In: Jankovic J, Albanese A, Zouhair Atassi M, Dolly JO, Hallett M, Mayer NH, eds. *Botulinum Toxin: Therapeutic Clinical Practice and Science*. Philadelphia, PA: Saunders, Elsevier; 2009:389–397.

30. Dressler D, Comella C. Comparative clinical trials of botulinum toxins. In: Jankovic J, Albanese A, Zouhair Atassi M, Dolly JO, Hallett M, Mayer NH, eds. *Botulinum Toxin: Therapeutic Clinical Practice and Science*. Philadelphia, PA: Saunders, Elsevier; 2009:398–405.
31. Frevert J. Xeomin is free from complexing proteins. *Toxicon*. 2009;54(5):697–701.
32. Brin MF. Basic and clinical aspects of BOTOX. *Toxicon*. 2009a;54(5):676–682.
33. Brin MF. Development of future indications for BOTOX. *Toxicon*. 2009b;54(5): 668–674.
34. Botox PI [package insert/prescribing information]. Irvine, CA: Allergan. Available at http://www.allergan.com/assets/pdf/botox_cosmetic_pi.pdf. Updated September 2013.
35. Botox MHRA. UK: MHRA Approval Variation Documentation. Revised January 25, 2014. Available at http://www.mhra.gov.uk/home/groups/par/documents/websiteresources/con108643.pdf. Updated July 8, 2010.
36. Dysport PI [package insert/prescribing information]. Basking Ridge, NJ: Ipsen Biopharmaceuticals, Inc. Available at http://pi.medicis.us/printer_friendly/dysport.pdf. Updated March 2012.
37. Pickett A. Dysport: pharmacological properties and factors that influence toxin action. *Toxicon*. 2009;54(5):683–689.
38. Xeomin PI [package insert/prescribing information]. Greensboro, NC: Merz Pharmaceuticals. Available at http://www.xeomin.com/files/Xeomin_PI.pdf. Updated April 2014.
39. Jost WH, Blümel J, Grafe S. Botulinum neurotoxin type A free of complexing proteins (Xeomin) in focal dystonia. *Drugs*. 2007;67(5):669–683.
40. Xeomin 100 units. eMC: MHRA Summary of Product Characteristics Documentation. Revised June 30, 2014. Available at http://www.medicines.org.uk/emc/medicine/20666/SPC. Updated June 30, 2014.
41. Pagan FL, Harrison A. A guide to dosing in the treatment of cervical dystonia and blepharospasm with Xeomin: a new botulinum neurotoxin A. *Parkinsonism Relat Disord*. 2012;18(5):441–445.
42. Grein S, Mander GJ, Taylor HV. Xeomin is stable without refrigeration: complexing proteins are not required for stability of botulinum neurotoxin type A preparations. *Toxicon*. 2008;51(suppl):13.
43. Arezzo JC. NeuroBloc/Myobloc: unique features and findings. *Toxicon*. 2009;54(5):690–696.
44. Myobloc [package insert/prescribing information]. Louisville, KY: Solstice Neurosciences (US WorldMeds). Available at http://www.myobloc.com/hp_about/PI_5-19-10.pdf. Updated May 2010.
45. NeuroBloc SPC. European Medicines Agency (EMA) Summary of Product Characteristics. Available at http://www.ema.europa.eu/docs/en_GB/document_library/EPAR_-_Product_Information/human/000301/WC500026906.pdf. Updated January 22, 2001
46. Atassi MZ. Basic immunological aspects of botulinum toxin therapy. *Mov Disord*. 2004;19(suppl 8):S68–S84.
47. Trindade De Almeida AR, Secco LC, Carruthers A. Handling botulinum toxins: an updated literature review. *Dermatol Surg*. 2011;37(11):1553–1565.

48. Hexsel D, Hexsel C, Siega C, Schilling-Souza J, Rotta FT, Rodrigues TC. Fields of effects of 2 commercial preparations of botulinum toxin type A at equal labeled unit doses: a double-blind randomized trial. *JAMA Dermatol.* 2013;149(12):1386–1391.
49. Ravindra P, Jackson BL, Parkinson RJ. Botulinum toxin type A for the treatment of non-neurogenic overactive bladder: does using onabotulinumtoxinA (Botox) or abobotulinumtoxinA (Dysport) make a difference? *BJU Int.* 2013;112(1):94–99.
50. Pickett A. Evaluating botulinum toxin products for clinical use requires accurate, complete, and unbiased data. *Clin Ophthalmol.* 2011b;5:1287–1290.
51. Wohlfarth K, Sycha T, Ranoux D, Naver H, Caird D. Dose equivalence of two commercial preparations of botulinum neurotoxin type A: time for a reassessment? *Curr Med Res Opin.* 2009;25(7):1573–1584.
52. Wenzel RG, Jones D, Borrego JA. Comparing two botulinum toxin type A formulations using manufacturers' product summaries. *J Clin Pharm Ther.* 2007;32(4):387–402.
53. Bhidayasiri R, Cardoso F, Truong DD. Botulinum toxin in blepharospasm and oromandibular dystonia: comparing different botulinum toxin preparations. *Eur J Neurol.* 2006;13(suppl 1):21–29.
54. Sampaio C, Costa J, Ferreira JJ. Clinical comparability of marketed formulations of botulinum toxin. *Mov Disord.* 2004;19(suppl 8):S129–S136.
55. Ravenni R, De Grandis D, Mazza A. Conversion ratio between Dysport and Botox in clinical practice: an overview of available evidence. *Neurol Sci.* 2013;34(7):1043–1048.
56. Dressler D, Rothwell JC. Electromyographic quantification of the paralysing effect of botulinum toxin in the sternocleidomastoid muscle. *Eur Neurol.* 2000;43(1):13–16.
57. El Kahky HM, Diab HM, Aly DG, Farag NM. Efficacy of onabotulinum toxin A (Botox) versus abobotulinum toxin A (Dysport) using a conversion factor (1 : 2.5) in treatment of primary palmar hyperhidrosis. *Dermatol Res Pract.* 2013;2013(686329):1–6.
58. Kim SB, Ban B, Jung KS, Yang GH. A pharmacodynamic comparison study of different botulinum toxin type A preparations. *Dermatol Surg.* 2013;39(suppl 1 pt 2):150–154.
59. Dressler D, Tacik P, Adib Saberi F. Botulinum toxin therapy of cervical dystonia: comparing onabotulinumtoxinA (Botox) and incobotulinumtoxinA (Xeomin). *J Neural Transm.* 2014b;121(1):29–31.
60. Michaels BM, Csank GA, Ryb GE, Eko FN, Rubin A. Prospective randomized comparison of onabotulinumtoxinA (Botox) and abobotulinumtoxinA (Dysport) in the treatment of forehead, glabellar, and periorbital wrinkles. *Aesthet Surg J.* 2012;32(1):96–102.
61. Bentivoglio AR, Ialongo T, Bove F, De Nigris F, Fasano A. Retrospective evaluation of the dose equivalence of Botox and Dysport in the management of blepharospasm and hemifacial spasm: a novel paradigm for a never ending story. *Neurol Sci.* 2012;33(2):261–267.

62. Rystedt A, Nyholm D, Naver H. Clinical experience of dose conversion ratios between 2 botulinum toxin products in the treatment of cervical dystonia. *Clin Neuropharmacol*. 2012;35(6):278–282.
63. Jandhyala R. Relative potency of incobotulinumtoxinA vs onabotulinumtoxinA a meta-analysis of key evidence. *J Drugs Dermatol*. 2012;11(6):731–736.
64. Prager W, Rappl T. Phase IV study comparing incobotulinumtoxinA and onabotulinumtoxinA using a 1:1.5 dose-conversion ratio for the treatment of glabellar frown lines. *J Cosmet Dermatol*. 2012;11(4):267–271.
65. Park J, Lee MS, Harrison AR. Profile of Xeomin (incobotulinumtoxinA) for the treatment of blepharospasm. *Clin Ophthalmol*. 2011;5:725–732.
66. Guidubaldi A, Fasano A, Ialongo T, et al. Botulinum toxin A versus B in sialorrhea: a prospective, randomized, double-blind, crossover pilot study in patients with amyotrophic lateral sclerosis or Parkinson's disease. *Mov Disord*. 2011;26(2):313–319.
67. Karsai S, Raulin C. Current evidence on the unit equivalence of different botulinum neurotoxin A formulations and recommendations for clinical practice in dermatology. *Dermatol Surg*. 2009;35(1):1–8.
68. Wabbels B, Reichel G, Fulford-Smith A, Wright N, Roggenkämper P. Double-blind, randomised, parallel group pilot study comparing two botulinum toxin type A products for the treatment of blepharospasm. *J Neural Transm*. 2011;118(2):233–239.
69. Odergren T, Hjaltason H, Kaakkola S, et al. A double blind, randomised, parallel group study to investigate the dose equivalence of Dysport and Botox in the treatment of cervical dystonia. *J Neurol Neurosurg Psychiatry*. 1998;64(1):6–12.
70. Schlereth T, Mouka I, Eisenbarth G, Winterholler M, Birklein F. Botulinum toxin A (Botox) and sweating-dose efficacy and comparison to other BoNT preparations. *Auton Neurosci*. 2005;117(2):120–126.
71. Nüssgens Z, Roggenkämper P. Comparison of two botulinum-toxin preparations in the treatment of essential blepharospasm. *Graefes Arch Clin Exp Ophthalmol*. 1997;235(4):197–199.
72. Li M, Goldberger BA, Hopkins C. Fatal case of Botox-related anaphylaxis? *J Forensic Sci*. 2005;50(1):169–172.
73. Ramirez-Castaneda J, Jankovic J, Comella C, Dashtipour K, Fernandez HH, Mari Z. Diffusion, spread, and migration of botulinum toxin. *Mov Disord*. 2013;28(13):1775–1783.
74. Brodsky MA, Swope DM, Grimes D. Diffusion of botulinum toxins. *Tremor Other Hyperkinet Mov (N Y)*. 2012;2. pii:tre-02-85-417-1. Epub 2012 Aug 6.
75. Boyle MH, McGwin G Jr, Flanagan CE, Vicinanzo MG, Long JA. High versus low concentration botulinum toxin A for benign essential blepharospasm: does dilution make a difference? *Ophthal Plast Reconstr Surg*. 2009;25(2):81–84.
76. Kim HS, Hwang JH, Jeong ST, et al. Effect of muscle activity and botulinum toxin dilution volume on muscle paralysis. *Dev Med Child Neurol*. 2003;45(3):200–206.
77. Lee HJ, DeLisa, JA. *Manual of Nerve Conduction Study and Surface Anatomy for Needle Electromyography*. 4th ed. Philadelphia, PA: Lippincott Williams & Wilkins; 2004.

78. Francisco GE, Boake C, Vaughn A. Botulinum toxin in upper limb spasticity after acquired brain injury: a randomized trial comparing dilution techniques. *Am J Phys Med Rehabil.* 2002;81(5):355–363.
79. Prager W, Zschocke I, Reich C, Brocatti L, Henning K, Steinkraus V. Does dilution have an impact on cosmetic results with BoNT/A? Complex-protein-free BoNT/A for treatment of glabella lines. *Hautarzt.* 2009;60(10):815–820.
80. Lungu C, Hallett M. Toxin handling, reconstitution, and dilution. In: Alter KE, Hallett M, Karp B, Lungu C, eds. *Ultrasound-Guided Chemodenervation Procedures: Text and Atlas.* New York, NY: Demos Medical Pub; 2013c: 10–13.
81. Carruthers J, Fagien S, Matarasso SL; Botox Consensus Group. Consensus recommendations on the use of botulinum toxin type A in facial aesthetics. *Plast Reconstr Surg.* 2004;114(suppl 6):1S–22S.
82. Hui JI, Lee WW. Efficacy of fresh versus refrigerated botulinum toxin in the treatment of lateral periorbital rhytids. *Ophthal Plast Reconstr Surg.* 2007;23(6):433–438.
83. Kane M, Donofrio L, Ascher B, et al. Expanding the use of neurotoxins in facial aesthetics: a consensus panel's assessment and recommendations. *J Drugs Dermatol.* 2010;9(suppl 1):s7–s22; quiz s23–s25.
84. Abbasi NR, Durfee MA, Petrell K, Dover JS, Arndt KA. A small study of the relationship between abobotulinum toxin A concentration and forehead wrinkle reduction. *Arch Dermatol.* 2012;148(1):119–121.
85. Hefter H, Kupsch A, Müngersdorf M, Paus S, Stenner A, Jost W; Dysport Cervical Dystonia Study Group. A botulinum toxin A treatment algorithm for de novo management of torticollis and laterocollis. *BMJ Open.* 2011;1(2):e000196.
86. Hu GC, Chuang YC, Liu JP, Chien KL, Chen YM, Chen YF. Botulinum toxin (Dysport) treatment of the spastic gastrocnemius muscle in children with cerebral palsy: a randomized trial comparing two injection volumes. *Clin Rehabil.* 2009;23(1):64–71.
87. Setler P. The biochemistry of botulinum toxin type B. *Neurology.* 2000;55(12 suppl 5):S22–S28.
88. Callaway JE. Botulinum toxin type B (Myobloc): pharmacology and biochemistry. *Clin Dermatol.* 2004;22(1):23–28.
89. Kranz G, Sycha T, Voller B, Gleiss A, Schnider P, Auff E. Pain sensation during intradermal injections of three different botulinum toxin preparations in different doses and dilutions. *Dermatol Surg.* 2006;32(7):886–890.
90. Alter KE, Munin MC. Comparing guidance techniques for chemodenervation procedures. In: Alter KE, Hallett M, Karp B, Lungu C, eds. *Ultrasound-Guided Chemodenervation Procedures: Text and Atlas.* New York, NY: Demos Medical Pub; 2013a:138–153.
91. Fehlings D, Narayanan U, Andersen J, et al. Botulinum toxin-A use in paediatric hypertonia: Canadian practice parameters. *Can J Neurol Sci.* 2012;39(4): 508–515.
92. Lim EC, Quek AM, Seet RC. Accurate targeting of botulinum toxin Injections: how to and why. *Parkinsonism Relat Disord.* 2011;17(suppl 1):S34–S39.

93. Jordan SE, Ahn SS, Gelabert HA. Combining ultrasonography and electromyography for botulinum chemodenervation treatment of thoracic outlet syndrome: comparison with fluoroscopy and electromyography guidance. *Pain Physician*. 2007;10(4):541–546.
94. Perotto AO. *Anatomical Guide for the Electromyographer: The Limbs and Trunk*. 5th ed. Springfield, IL: Charles C. Thomas Publisher LTD; 2011.
95. Chu-Andrews J, Johnson RJ. *Electrodiagnosis: An Anatomical and Clinical Approach*. Philadelphia, PA: J.B. Lippincott Co; 1986.
96. Jost WH, Valerius K-P. *Pictorial Atlas of Botulinum Toxin Injection: Dosage, Localization, Application*. New Malden, Surrey: Quintessence Books; 2008.
97. Alter KE, Bohart Z, Lungu C. Botulinum toxin therapy for the management of sialorrhea. In: Alter KE, Hallett M, Karp B, Lungu C, eds. *Ultrasound-Guided Chemodenervation Procedures: Text and Atlas*. New York, NY: Demos Medical Pub; 2013a:48–53.
98. Boon AJ, Oney-Marlow TM, Murthy NS, Harper CM, McNamara TR, Smith J. Accuracy of electromyography needle placement in cadavers: non-guided vs. ultrasound guided. *Muscle Nerve*. 2011;44(1):45–49.
99. Kwon JY, Hwang JH, Kim JS. Botulinum toxin A injection into calf muscles for treatment of spastic equinus in cerebral palsy: a controlled trial comparing sonography and electric stimulation-guided injection techniques: a preliminary report. *Am J Phys Med Rehabil*. 2010;89(4):279–286.
100. Henzel MK, Munin MC, Niyonkuru C, Skidmore ER, Weber DJ, Zafonte RD. Comparison of surface and ultrasound localization to identify forearm flexor muscles for botulinum toxin injections. *PM R*. 2010;2(7):642–646.
101. Yang EJ, Rha DW, Yoo JK, Park ES. Accuracy of manual needle placement for gastrocnemius muscle in children with cerebral palsy checked against ultrasonography. *Arch Phys Med Rehabil*. 2009;90(5):751–744.
102. Picelli A, Tamburin S, Bonetti P, et al. Botulinum toxin type A injection into the gastrocnemius muscle for spastic equinus in adults with stroke: a randomized controlled trial comparing manual needle placement, electrical stimulation and ultrasonography-guided injection techniques. *Am J Phys Med Rehabil*. 2012;91(11):957–964.
103. Py AG, Zein Addeen G, Perrier Y, Carlier RY, Picard A. Evaluation of the effectiveness of botulinum toxin injections in the lower limb muscles of children with cerebral palsy. Preliminary prospective study of the advantages of ultrasound guidance. *Ann Phys Rehabil Med*. 2009;52(3):215–223.
104. Ploumis A, Varvarousis D, Konitsiotis S, Beris A. Effectiveness of botulinum toxin injection with and without needle electromyographic guidance for the treatment of spasticity in hemiplegic patients: a randomized controlled trial. *Disabil Rehabil*. 2014;36(4):313–318.
105. Molloy FM, Shill HA, Kaelin-Lang A, Karp BI. Accuracy of muscle localization without EMG: implications for treatment of limb dystonia. *Neurology*. 2002;58(5):805–807.
106. Geenen C, Consky E, Ashby P. Localizing muscles for botulinum toxin treatment of focal hand dystonia. *Can J Neurol Sci*. 1996;23(3):194–197.

*107.* Chin TY, Nattrass GR, Selber P, Graham HK. Accuracy of intramuscular injection of botulinum toxin A in juvenile cerebral palsy: a comparison between manual needle placement and placement guided by electrical stimulation. *J Pediatr Orthop*. 2005;25(3):286–291.

*108.* Davisdon J, Jayaraman S. Guided interventions in musculoskeletal ultrasound: what's the evidence? *Clin Radiol*. 2011;66(2):140–152.

*109.* Alter KE. Ultrasound guidance for botulinum neurotoxin therapy: cervical dystonia. In: Truong D, Hallett M, Zachary CB, Dressler D, eds. *Manual of Botulinum Toxin Therapy*. 2nd ed. Cambridge, UK: Cambridge University Press; 2013a:46–59.

*110.* Marina MB, Sani A, Hamzaini AH, Hamidon BB. Ultrasound-guided botulinum toxin A injection: an alternative treatment for dribbling. *J Laryngol Otol*. 2008;122(6):609–614.

*111.* Alter KE, Skurow SM. Instrumentation and knobology. In: Alter KE, Hallett M, Karp B, Lungu C, eds. *Ultrasound-Guided Chemodenervation Procedures: Text and Atlas*. New York, NY: Demos Medical Pub; 2013:84–107.

*112.* Chen SL, Bih LI, Chen GD, Huang YH, You YH. Comparing a transrectal ultrasound-guided with a cystoscopy-guided botulinum toxin A injection in treating detrusor external sphincter dyssynergia in spinal cord injury. *Am J Phys Med Rehabil*. 2011;90(9):723–730.

*113.* Nowakowski P, Bieryło A, Duniec L, Kosson D, Łazowski T. The substantial impact of ultrasound-guided regional anaesthesia on the clinical practice of peripheral nerve blocks. *Anaesthesiol Intensive Ther*. 2013;45(4):223–229.

*114.* Schnabel A, Meyer-Frießem CH, Zahn PK, Pogatzki-Zahn EM. Ultrasound compared with nerve stimulation guidance for peripheral nerve catheter placement: a meta-analysis of randomized controlled trials. *Br J Anaesth*. 2013;111(4):564–572.

*115.* Alter KE, Lin JL. Ultrasound guidance for nerve and motor point blocks. In: Alter KE, Hallett M, Karp B, Lungu C, eds. *Ultrasound-Guided Chemodenervation Procedures: Text and Atlas*. New York, NY: Demos Medical Pub; 2013:170–183.

*116.* Lee IH, Yoon YC, Sung DH, Kwon JW, Jung JY. Initial experience with imaging-guided intramuscular botulinum toxin injection in patients with idiopathic cervical dystonia. *AJR Am J Roentgenol*. 2009;192(4):996–1001.

*117.* Gormley ME Jr. Management of spasticity in children: part 1: chemical denervation. *J Head Trauma Rehabil*. 1999;14(1):97–99.

*118.* Wood KM. The use of phenol as a neurolytic agent: a review. *Pain*. 1978;5(3):205–229.

*119.* Alter KE, Childers MK, Ivanhoe CP. Localized pharmacologic therapeutic options: current and novel treatments to optimize upper- and lower-limb spasticity outcomes. *Medscape CME/CE Course*. 2011.

*120.* Awad EA, Awad OE. *Injection techniques for spasticity: A practical guide to treatment of cerebral palsy, hemiplegia, multiple sclerosis, and spinal cord injury*. Minneapolis, MN: EA Awad Publisher; 1993.

*121.* Koyyalagunta D, Burton AW. The role of chemical neurolysis in cancer pain. *Curr Pain Headache Rep*. 2010;14(4):261–267.

122. On AY, Kirazli Y, Kismali B, Akset R. Mechanisms of action of phenol block and botulinus toxin type A in relieving spasticity: electrophysiologic investigation and follow-up. *Am J Phys Med Rehabil.* 1999;78(4):344–349.
123. Ghai A, Garg N, Hooda S, Gupta T. Spasticity—pathogenesis, prevention, and treatment strategies. *Saudi J Anaesth.* 2013;7(4):453–460.
124. Lennard TA. *Physiatric Procedures in Clinical Practice.* Philadelphia, PA: Hanley & Belfus; 1995.
125. Mayer NH, Esquenazi A, Childers MK. Common patterns of clinical motor dysfunction. *Muscle Nerve Suppl.* 1997;6:S21–S35.
126. Mayer NH. Clinicophysiologic concepts of spasticity and motor dysfunction in adults with an upper motor neuron lesion. *Muscle Nerve Suppl.* 1997;6:S1–S13.
127. Lee J, Lee YS. Percutaneous chemical nerve block with ultrasound-guided intraneural injection. *Eur Radiol.* 2008;18(7):1506–1512.
128. Mahakkanukrauh P, Somsarp V. Dual innervation of the brachialis muscle. *Clin Anat.* 2002;15(3):206–209.
129. Keenan MA, Tomas ES, Stone L, Gerstén LM. Percutaneous phenol block of the musculocutaneous nerve to control elbow flexor spasticity. *J Hand Surg Am.* 1990;15(2):340–346.
130. Meierhofer JT, Anetseder M, Roewer N, Wunder C, Schwemmer U. Guidance of axillary multiple injection technique for plexus anesthesia: ultrasound versus nerve stimulation. *Anaesthesist.* 2014;63:568–573.
131. Flack S, Anderson C. Ultrasound guided lower extremity blocks. *Paediatr Anaesth.* 2012;22(1):72–80.
132. Kocabas H, Salli A, Demir AH, Ozerbil OM. Comparison of phenol and alcohol neurolysis of tibial nerve motor branches to the gastrocnemius muscle for treatment of spastic foot after stroke: a randomized controlled pilot study. *Eur J Phys Rehabil Med.* 2010;46(1):5–10.
133. Kenney C, Jankovic J. Botulinum neurotoxin treatment of cranial-cervical dystonia. In: Jankovic J, Albanese A, Zouhair Atassi M, Dolly JO, Hallett M, Mayer NH, eds. *Botulinum Toxin: Therapeutic Clinical Practice and Science.* Philadelphia, PA: Saunders, Elsevier; 2009:92–101.
134. Defazio G, Livrea P. Epidemiology of primary blepharospasm. *Mov Disord.* 2002;17(1):7–12.
135. Blackburn MK, Lamb RD, Digre KB, et al. FL-41 tint improves blink frequency, light sensitivity, and functional limitations in patients with benign essential blepharospasm. *Ophthalmology.* 2009;116(5):997–1001.
136. Jankovic J, Schwartz K, Clemence W, Aswad A, Mordaunt J. A randomized, double-blind, placebo-controlled study to evaluate botulinum toxin type A in essential hand tremor. *Mov Disord.* 1996;11(3):250–256.
137. Jankovic J, Kenney C, Grafe S, Goertelmeyer R, Comes G. Relationship between various clinical outcome assessments in patients with blepharospasm. *Mov Disord.* 2009;24(3):407–413.
138. Gronseth GS, Woodroffe LM, Getchius TSD. Appendix 4: Narrative classification of evidence schemes and appendix 6: Tools for building conclusions and recommendations. In: Gronseth GS, Woodroffe LM, Getchius TSD, eds. *Clinical Practice Guideline Process Manual,* 2011 Edition. St. Paul, MN: American

Academy of Neurology; 2011:38–40, 42–44. Available at http://tools.aan.com/globals/axon/assets/9023.pdf

139. Price J, Farish S, Taylor H, O'Day J. Blepharospasm and hemifacial spasm. Randomized trial to determine the most appropriate location for botulinum toxin injections. *Ophthalmology*. 1997;104(5):865–868.

140. Wang A, Jankovic J. Hemifacial spasm: clinical findings and treatment. *Muscle Nerve*. 1998;21(12):1740–1747.

141. Digre K, Corbett JJ. Hemifacial spasm: differential diagnosis, mechanism, and treatment. *Adv Neurol*. 1988;49:151–176.

142. Tan EK, Chan LL. Clinico-radiologic correlation in unilateral and bilateral hemifacial spasm. *J Neurol Sci*. 2004;222(1–2):59–64.

143. Costa J, Espírito-Santo C, Borges A, et al. Botulinum toxin type A therapy for hemifacial spasm. *Cochrane Database Syst Rev*. 2005b;(1):CD004899.

144. Cillino S, Raimondi G, Guépratte N, et al. Long-term efficacy of botulinum toxin A for treatment of blepharospasm, hemifacial spasm, and spastic entropion: a multicentre study using two drug-dose escalation indexes. *Eye (Lond)*. 2010;24(4):600–607.

145. Lungu C, Hallett M. Hemifacial spasm. In: Alter KE, Hallett M, Karp B, Lungu C. *Ultrasound-Guided Chemodenervation Procedures: Text and Atlas*. New York, NY: Demos Medical Pub; 2013b:28–29.

146. Choi SI, Kim MW, Park DY, Huh R, Jang DH. Electrophysiologic investigation during facial motor neuron suppression in patients with hemifacial spasm: possible pathophysiology of hemifacial spasm: a pilot study. *Ann Rehabil Med*. 2013;37(6):839–847.

147. Yaltho TC, Jankovic J. The many faces of hemifacial spasm: differential diagnosis of unilateral facial spasm. *Mov Disord*. 2011;26(9):1582–1592.

148. Kenney C, Jankovic J. Botulinum toxin in the treatment of blepharospasm and hemifacial spasm. *J Neural Transm*. 2008;115(4):585–591.

149. Ababneh OH, Cetinkaya A, Kulwin DR. Long-term efficacy and safety of botulinum toxin A injections to treat blepharospasm and hemifacial spasm. *Clin Experiment Ophthalmol*. 2014;42(3):254–261.

150. Trosch RM, Adler CH, Pappert EJ. Botulinum toxin type B (Myobloc) in subjects with hemifacial spasm: results from an open label, dose-escalation safety study. *Mov Disord*. 2007;22(9):1258–1264.

151. Persaud R, Garas G, Silva S, Stamatoglou C, Chatrath P, Patel K. An evidence-based review of botulinum toxin (Botox) applications in non-cosmetic head and neck conditions. *JRSM Short Rep*. 2013;4(2):10.

152. Bentivoglio AR, Fasano A, Albanese A. Botulinum neurotoxin in tremors, tics, hemifacial spasm, spasmodic dysphonia, and stuttering. In: Jankovic J, Albanese A, Zouhair Atassi M, Dolly JO, Hallett M, Mayer NH, eds. *Botulinum Toxin: Therapeutic Clinical Practice and Science*. Philadelphia, PA: Saunders, Elsevier; 2009:112–130.

153. Sinclari CF, Gurey LE, Blitzer A. Oromandibular dystonia: long-term management with botulinum toxin. *Laryngoscope*. 2013;123(12):3078–3083.

154. Young N, Blitzer. Treatment of oromandibular dystonia, bruxism, and temporomandibular disorders with botulinum neurotoxin. In: Jankovic J, Albanese A, Zouhair Atassi M, Dolly JO, Hallett M, Mayer NH, eds. *Botulinum*

*Toxin: Therapeutic Clinical Practice and Science*. Philadelphia, PA: Saunders, Elsevier; 2009:204–213.

155. Lee DH, Jin SP, Cho S, et al. RimabotulinumtoxinB versus OnabotulinumtoxinA in the treatment of masseter hypertrophy: a 24-week double-blind randomized split-face study. *Dermatology*. 2013;226(3):227–232.
156. Alter KE, Munin MC. US-guided neurotoxin (BoNT) injections: clinical applications. In: Alter KE, Hallett M, Karp B, Lungu C, eds. *Ultrasound-Guided Chemodenervation Procedures: Text and Atlas*. New York, NY: Demos Medical Pub; 2013b:154–169.
157. Karp BI. Botulinum toxin physiology in focal hand and cranial dystonia. *Toxins (Basel)*. 2012;4(11):1404–1414.
158. Reichel G, Stenner A, Jahn A. The phenomenology of cervical dystonia. *Fortschr Neurol Psychiatr*. 2009;77(5):272–277.
159. LeDoux MS. Dystonia: phenomenology. *Parkinsonism Relat Disord*. 2012;18(suppl 1):S162–S164.
160. Costa J, Espírito-Santo C, Borges A, et al. Botulinum toxin type A for cervical dystonia. *Cochrane Database Syst Rev*. 2005a;(1):CD003633.
161. Chan J, Brin MF, Fahn S. Idiopathic cervical dystonia: clinical characteristics. *Mov Disord*. 1991;6(2):119–126.
162. Fletcher NA, Harding AE, Marsden CD. The relationship between trauma and idiopathic torsion dystonia. *J Neurol Neurosurg Psychiatry*. 1991;54(8):713-717.
163. Sheehy MP, Marsden CD. Trauma and pain in spasmodic torticollis. *Lancet*. 1980;1(8171):777-778.
164. Lungu C, Hallett M. Cervical dystonia. In: Alter KE, Hallett M, Karp B, Lungu C, eds. *Ultrasound-Guided Chemodenervation Procedures: Text and Atlas*. New York, NY: Demos Medical Pub; 2013a:24-27.
165. Jankovic J, Tsui J, Bergeron C. Prevalence of cervical dystonia and spasmodic torticollis in the United States general population. *Parkinsonism Relat Disord*. 2007;13(7):411–416.
166. Burke RE, Fahn S, Marsden CD, Bressman SB, Moskowitz C, Friedman J. Validity and reliability of a rating scale for the primary torsion dystonias. *Neurology*. 1985;35(1):73–77.
167. Comella CL, Stebbins GT, Goetz CG, Chmura TA, Bressman SB, Lang AE. Teaching tape for the motor section of the Toronto Western Spasmodic Torticollis Scale. *Mov Disord*. 1997;12(4):570–575.
168. Consky ES, Basinski A, Belle L, Ranawaya R, Lang AE. The Toronto Western Spasmodic Torticollis Rating Scale (TWSTRS): assessment of validity and inter-rater reliability [abstract]. *Neurology*. 1990;40(suppl 1):445.
169. Tsui JK, Eisen A, Stoessl AJ, Calne S, Calne DB. Double-blind study of botulinum toxin in spasmodic torticollis. *Lancet*. 1986;2(8501):245–247.
170. Tsui JK, Fross RD, Calne S, Calne DB. Local treatment of spasmodic torticollis with botulinum toxin. *Can J Neurol Sci*. 1987;14(3 suppl):533–535.
171. Dressler D, Kupsch A, Seitzinger A, Paus S. The dystonia discomfort scale (DDS): a novel instrument to monitor the temporal profile of botulinum toxin therapy in cervical dystonia. *Eur J Neurol*. 2014a;21(3):459–462.

172. Quagliato EM, Carelli EF, Viana MA. A prospective, randomized, double-blind study comparing the efficacy and safety of type A botulinum toxins botox and prosigne in the treatment of cervical dystonia. *Clin Neuropharmacol.* 2010;33(1):22–26.
173. Chapman MA, Barron R, Tanis DC, Gill CE, Charles PD. Comparison of botulinum neurotoxin preparations for the treatment of cervical dystonia. *Clin Ther.* 2007;29(7):1325–1337.
174. Frevert J. Content of botulinum neurotoxin in Botox/Vistabel, Dysport/Azzalure, and Xeomin/Bocouture. *Drugs R D.* 2010;10(2):67–73.
175. Pickett A. Consistent biochemical data are essential for comparability of botulinum toxin type A products. *Drugs R D.* 2011a;11(1):97–98.
176. Albanese A, Lalli S. Update on dystonia. *Curr Opin Neurol.* 2012;25(4):483–490.
177. Karp BI. Botulinum neurotoxin treatment of limb and occupational dystonias. In: Jankovic J, Albanese A, Zouhair Atassi M, Dolly JO, Hallett M, Mayer NH, eds. *Botulinum Toxin: Therapeutic Clinical Practice and Science.* Philadelphia, PA: Saunders, Elsevier; 2009:102–111.
178. Katz M, Byl NN, San Luciano M, Ostrem JL. Focal task-specific lower extremity dystonia associated with intense repetitive exercise: a case series. *Parkinsonism Relat Disord.* 2013;19(11):1033–1038.
179. Alter KE, Nahab FB. Lower limb dystonia. In: Alter KE, Hallett M, Karp B, Lungu C, eds. *Ultrasound-Guided Chemodenervation Procedures: Text and Atlas.* New York, NY: Demos Medical Pub; 2013a:30–35.
180. McKeon A, Matsumoto JY, Bower JH, Ahlskog JE. The spectrum of disorders presenting as adult-onset focal lower extremity dystonia. *Parkinsonism Relat Disord.* 2008;14(8):613–619.
181. Steeves TD, Day L, Dykeman J, Jette N, Pringsheim T. The prevalence of primary dystonia: a systematic review and meta-analysis. *Mov Disord.* 2012;27(14):1789–1796.
182. Butler AG, Duffey PO, Hawthorne MR, Barnes MP. The socioeconomic implications of dystonia. *Adv Neurol.* 1998;78:349–358.
183. McClinton S, Heiderscheit BC. Diagnosis of primary task-specific lower extremity dystonia in a runner. *J Orthop Sports Phys Ther.* 2012;42(8):688–697.
184. García-Ruiz PJ, del Val J, Losada M, Campos JM. Task-specific dystonia of the lower limb in a flamenco dancer. *Parkinsonism Relat Disord.* 2011;17(3):221–222.
185. Karp BI, Cole RA, Cohen LG, Grill S, Lou JS, Hallett M. Long-term botulinum toxin treatment of focal hand dystonia. *Neurology.* 1994;44(1):70–76.
186. Kruisdijk JJM, Koelman JHTM, Ongerboer de Visser BW, de Haan RJ, Speelman JD. Botulinum toxin for writer's cramp: a randomised, placebo-controlled trial and 1-year follow-up. *J Neurol Neurosurg Psychiatry.* 2007;78(3):264–270.
187. Charles D, Gill CE. Neurotoxin injection for movement disorders. *Continuum (Minneap Minn).* 2010;16(1 Movement Disorders):131–157.
188. Karp B, Hallett M. Focal dystonia of the upper extremity. In: Alter KE, Hallett M, Karp B, Lungu C, eds. *Ultrasound-Guided Chemodenervation Procedures: Text and Atlas.* New York, NY: Demos Medical Pub; 2013:16–19.

189. Lungu C, Karp BI, Alter KE, Zolbrod R, Hallett M. Long-term follow-up of botulinum toxin therapy for focal hand dystonia: outcome at 10 years or more. *Mov Disord*. 2011;26(4):750–753.
190. Hanson M. Use of chemodenervation in dystonic conditions. *Cleve Clin J Med*. 2012;79(suppl 2):S25–S29.
191. Thenganatt MA, Jankovic J. Treatment of dystonia. *Neurotherapeutics*. 2014;11(1):139–152.
192. Quartarone A. Transcranial magnetic stimulation in dystonia. *Handb Clin Neurol*. 2013;116:543–553.
193. Dykstra DD, Mendez A, Chappuis D, Baxter R, DesLauriers L, Stuckey M. Treatment of cervical dystonia and focal hand dystonia by high cervical continuously infused intrathecal baclofen: a report of 2 cases. *Arch Phys Med Rehabil*. 2005;86(4):830–833.
194. Truong DD. Botulinum toxins in the treatment of primary focal dystonias. *J Neurol Sci*. 2012;316(1-2):9–14.
195. Dressler D. Botulinum toxin for treatment of dystonia. *Eur J Neurol*. 2010a;17(suppl 1):88–96.
196. Schuele S, Jabusch HC, Lederman RJ, Altenmüller E. Botulinum toxin injections in the treatment of musician's dystonia. *Neurology*. 2005;64(2):341–343.
197. Hallett M, Albanese A, Dressler D, et al. Evidence-based review and assessment of botulinum neurotoxin for the treatment of movement disorders. *Toxicon*. 2013;67:94–114.
198. Simpson DM, Blitzer A, Brashear A, et al, and Therapeutics and Technology Assessment Subcommittee of the American Academy of Neurology. Assessment: Botulinum neurotoxin for the treatment of movement disorders (an evidence-based review): report of the Therapeutics and Technology Assessment Subcommittee of the American Academy of Neurology. *Neurology*. 2008;70(19):1699–1706.
199. Pullman SL, Greene P, Fahn S, Pedersen SF. Approach to the treatment of limb disorders with botulinum toxin A. Experience with 187 patients. *Arch Neurol*. 1996;53(7):617–624.
200. Cole R, Hallett M, Cohen LG. Double-blind trial of botulinum toxin for treatment of focal hand dystonia. *Mov Disord*. 1995;10(4):466–471.
201. Tsui JK, Bhatt M, Calne S, Calne DB. Botulinum toxin in the treatment of writer's cramp: a double-blind study. *Neurology*. 1993;43(1):183–185.
202. Yoshimura DM, Aminoff MJ, Olney RK. Botulinum toxin therapy for limb dystonias. *Neurology*. 1992;42(3 pt 1):627–630.
203. Contarino MF, Kruisdijk JJM, Koster L, Ongerboer de Visser BW, Speelman JD, Koelman JHTM. Sensory integration in writer's cramp: comparison with controls and evaluation of botulinum toxin effect. *Clin Neurophysiol*. 2007a;118(10):2195–2206.
204. Lance JW. The control of muscle tone, reflexes, and movement: Robert Wartenberg Lecture. *Neurology*. 1980a;30(12):1303–1313.
205. Lance JW. Symposium synopsis. In: Feldman RG, Young RR, Koella WP, eds. *Spasticity: Disordered Motor Control*. Ann Arbor, MI: Symposia Specialists, University of Michigan; 1980b:17–24.

206. Lance JW. Pyramidal and extrapyramidal disorders. In: Shahani BT, ed. *Electromyography in CNS Disorders: Central EMG*. Stoneham, MA: Butterworth Publishers; 1984:1–18.
207. Alter KE, Nahab FB. Upper motor neuron syndromes. In: Alter KE, Hallett M, Karp B, Lungu C, eds. *Ultrasound-Guided Chemodenervation Procedures: Text and Atlas*. New York, NY: Demos Medical Pub; 2013b:36–45.
208. Sheean G, McGuire JR. Spastic hypertonia and movement disorders: pathophysiology, clinical presentation, and quantification. *PM R*. 2009;(9):827–833.
209. Messina C. Pathophysiology of muscle tone. *Funct Neurol*. 1990;5(3): 217–223.
210. Burke D. Spasticity as an adaptation to pyramidal tract injury. *Adv Neurol*. 1988;47:401–423.
211. Mayer NH. Clinicophysiologic concepts of spasticity and motor dysfunction in adults with an upper motorneuron lesion. In: Mayer NH, Simpson DM, eds. *Spasticity: Etiology, Evaluation, Management and the Role of Botulinum Toxin*. Bronx, NY: We Move [Worldwide Education and Awareness for Movement Disorders]; 2002:1–11.
212. Gracies JM, Lugassy M, Weisz DJ, Vecchio M, Flanagan S, Simpson DM. Botulinum toxin dilution and endplate targeting in spasticity: a double-blind controlled study. *Arch Phys Med Rehabil*. 2009;90(1):9–16.e2.
213. Sanger TD, Delgado MR, Gaebler-Spira D, Hallett M, Mink JW; Task Force on Childhood Motor Disorders. Classification and definition of disorders causing hypertonia in childhood. *Pediatrics*. 2003;111(1):e89–e97.
214. Esquenazi A, Albanese A, Chancellor MB, et al. Evidenced-based review and assessment of bolulinum neurotoxin for the treatment of adult spasticity in the upper motor neuron syndrome. *Toxicon*. 2013;67:115–128.
215. Mayer NH, Esquenazi A. Muscle overactivity and movement dysfunction in the upper motoneuron syndrome. *Phys Med Rehabil Clin N Am*. 2003;14(4):855–883,vii–viii.
216. Mayer NH. Choosing upper limb muscles for focal intervention after traumatic brain injury. *J Head Trauma Rehabil*. 2004;19(2):119–142.
217. Ansari NN, Naghdi S, Arab TK, Jalaie S. The interrater and intrarater reliability of the Modified Ashworth Scale in the assessment of muscle spasticity: limb and muscle group effect. *NeuroRehabilitation*. 2008a;23(3):231–237.
218. Ansari NN, Naghdi S, Hasson S, Azarsa MH, Azarnia S. The Modified Tardieu Scale for the measurement of elbow flexor spasticity in adult patients with hemiplegia. *Brain Inj*. 2008b;22(13–14):1007–1012.
219. Morris S. Ashworth and Tardieu Scales: their clinical relevance for measuring spasticity in adult and paediatric neurological populations. *Phys Ther Rev*. 2002;7(1):53–62.
220. Collin C, Wade DT, Davies S, Home V. The Barthel ADL Index: a reliability study. *Int Disabil Stud*. 1988;10(2):61–63.
221. Dodds TA, Martin DP, Stolov WC, Deyo RA. A validation of the functional independence measurement and its performance among rehabilitation inpatients. *Arch Phys Med Rehabil*. 1993;74(5):531–536.

222. Jethwa A, Mink J, Macarthur C, Knights S, Fehlings T, Fehlings D. Development of the Hypertonia Assessment Tool (HAT): a discriminative tool for hypertonia in children. *Dev Med Child Neurol*. 2010;52(5):e83–e87.
223. Gilmore R, Sakzewski L, Boyd R. Upper limb activity measures for 5- to 16-year-old children with congenital hemiplegia: a systematic review. *Dev Med Child Neurol*. 2010;52(1):14–21.
224. Fowler EG, Staudt LA, Greenberg MB, Oppenheim WL. Selective Control Assessment of the Lower Extremity (SCALE): development, validation, and interrater reliability of a clinical tool for patients with cerebral palsy. *Dev Med Child Neurol*. 2009;51(8):607614.
225. Ashford S, Turner-Stokes L. Goal attainment for spasticity management using botulinum toxin. *Physiother Res Int*. 2006;11(1):24–34.
226. Esquenazi A, Mayer N. Botulinum toxin for the management of muscle overactivity and spasticity after stroke. *Curr Atheroscler Rep*. 2001;3(4):295–298.
227. Chung CY, Chen CL, Wong AM. Pharmacotherapy of spasticity in children with cerebral palsy. *J Formos Med Assoc*. 2011;110(4):215–222.
228. Graham HK. Botulinum toxin type A management of spasticity in the context of orthopaedic surgery for children with spastic cerebral palsy. *Eur J Neurol*. 2001;8(suppl 5):S30–S39.
229. Gormley ME Jr, O'Brien CF, Yablon SA. A clinical overview of treatment decisions in the management of spasticity. *Muscle Nerve Suppl*. 1997;6:S14–S20.
230. Chancellor MB, Elovic E, Esquenazi A, et al. Evidence-based review and assessment of botulinum neurotoxin for the treatment of urologic conditions. *Toxicon*. 2013;67:129–140.
231. Jost WH, Hefter H, Reissig A, Kollewe K, Wissel J. Efficacy and safety of botulinum toxin type A (Dysport) for the treatment of post-stroke arm spasticity: results of the German-Austrian open-label post-marketing surveillance prospective study. *J Neurol Sci*. 2014;337(1–2):86–90.
232. Quality Standards Subcommittee of the American Academy of Neurology and the Practice Committee of the Child Neurology Society, Delgado MR, Hirtz D, Aisen M, et al. Practice parameter: pharmacologic treatment of spasticity in children and adolescents with cerebral palsy (an evidence-based review): report of the Quality Standards Subcommittee of the American Academy of Neurology and the Practice Committee of the Child Neurology Society. *Neurology*. 2010;74(4):336–343.
233. van Campenhout A, Molenaers G. Localization of the motor endplate zone in human skeletal muscles of the lower limb: anatomical guidelines for injection with botulinum toxin. *Dev Med Child Neurol*. 2011;53(2):108–119.
234. Phadke CP, Davidson C, Ismail F, Boulias C. The effect of neural lesion type on botulinum toxin dosage: a retrospective chart review. *PM R*. 2014;6(5):406–411.
235. Wissel J, Ward AB, Erztgaard P, et al. European consensus table on the use of botulinum toxin A in adult spasticity. *J Rehabil Med*. 2009;41(1):13–25.

236. Damiano DL, Alter KE, Chambers H. New clinical and research trends in lower extremity management for ambulatory children with cerebral palsy. *Phys Med Rehabil Clin N Am*. 2009;20(3):469–491.
237. Dressler D. Clinical applications of botulinum toxin. *Curr Opin Microbiol*. 2012c;15(3):325–336.
238. Barnes MP, Best D, Kidd L, et al. The use of botulinum toxin type-B in the treatment of patients who have become unresponsive to botulinum toxin type-A—initial experiences. *Eur J Neurol*. 2005;12(12):947–955.
239. Francisco GE. Botulinum toxin: dosing and dilution. *Am J Phys Med Rehabil*. 2004;83(suppl 10):S30–S37.
240. Botox NZ Data Sheet Version 11. Medsafe: New Zealand Medicines and Medical Devices Safety Authority. Available at http://www.medsafe.govt.nz/profs/datasheet/b/Botoxinj.pdf. Updated December 2013.
241. Botox HC (DIN 01981501) DPD Product Monograph from Health Canada. Available at (www.hc-sc.gc.ca) http://webprod5.hc-sc.gc.ca/dpd-bdpp/item-iteme.do?pm-mp=00025717. Updated July 7, 2014.
242. Botox SPC (European Medicines Agency (EMA) Article 29 Referral Appendices Including Summary of Product Characteristics). Available at http://www.ema. europa.eu/docs/en_GB/document_library/Referrals_document/Botox_29/WC500010942.pdf. Updated Febraury 2003.
243. Dysport MHRA. UK: MHRA Approval Extension Documentation. Revised May 1, 2011. Available at http://www.mhra.gov.uk/home/groups/par/documents/websiteresources/con108612.pdf. Updated January 5, 2011.
244. Dysport NZ Data Sheet Version 11. Medsafe: New Zealand Medicines and Medical Devices Safety Authority. Available at http://www.medsafe.govt.nz/profs/datasheet/d/Dysportinj.pdf. Updated December 17, 2013.
245. Dysport 300 Units, Dysport 500 Units. eMC: MHRA Summary of Product Characteristics Documentation. Revised December 23, 2013. Available at https://www.medicines.org.uk/emc/medicine/870/SPC/Dysport+300+units+Dysport+500+units/. Updated December 23, 2013.
246. Xeomin HC (DIN 02324032) DPD Product Monograph from Health Canada. Available at (www.hc-sc.gc.ca) http://webprod5.hc-sc.gc.ca/dpd-bdpp/item-iteme.do?pm-mp=00021812. Updated June 28, 2013.
247. Xeomin SPC (European Medicines Agency (EMA) Article 29 Referral Appendicies Including Summary of Product Characteristics). Available at http://www.ema.europa.eu/docs/en_GB/document_library/Referrals_document/Xeomin_29/WC500008796.pdf. Updated July 21, 2013.
248. Xeomin is not currently registered/approved for use in New Zealand.
249. Guettard E, Roze E, Abada G, et al. Management of spasticity and dystonia in children with acquired brain injury with rehabilitation and botulinum toxin A. *Dev Neurorehabil*. 2009;12(3):128–138.
250. Heinen F, Desloovere K, Schroeder AS, et al. The updated European Consensus 2009 on the use of botulinum toxin for children with cerebral palsy. *Eur J Paediatr Neurol*. 2010;14(1):45–66.

251. Barwood S, Baillieu C, Boyd R, et al. Analgesic effects of botulinum toxin A: a randomized, placebo-controlled clinical trial. *Dev Med Child Neurol.* 2000;42(2):116–121.
252. Copeland L, Edwards P, Thorley M, et al. Botulinum toxin A for nonambulatory children with cerebral palsy: a double blind randomized controlled trial. *J Pediatr.* 2014;165:140–146.e4.
253. Heinen F, Molenaers G, Fairhurst C, et al. European Consensus Table 2006 on botulinum toxin for children with cerebral palsy. *Eur J Paediatr Neurol.* 2006a;10(5-6):215–225.
254. Papavasiliou AS, Nikaina I, Foska K, Bouros P, Mitsou G, Filiopoulos C. Safety of botulinum toxin A in children and adolescents with cerebral palsy in a pragmatic setting. *Toxins (Basel).* 2013;5(3):524–536.
255. Rousseaux M, Daveluy W. The risk-benefit of high doses of botulinum toxin injections for muscle spasticity. *Ann Readapt Med Phys.* 2007;50(suppl 1):S1–S3.
256. Pascual-Pascual SI, Pascual-Castroviejo I. Safety of botulinum toxin type A in children younger than 2 years. *Eur J Paediatr Neurol.* 2009;13(6):511–515.
257. Novak I, McIntyre S, Morgan C, et al. A systemic review of interventions for children with cerebral palsy: state of the evidence. *Dev Med Child Neurol.* 2013;55(10):885–910.
258. Fitz-Henry J. The ASA classification and peri-operative risk. *Ann R Coll Surg Engl.* 2011;93(3):185–187.
259. Brucki S, Nitrini R. Camptocormia in Alzheimer's disease: an association? *Mov Disord.* 2008;23(1):156–157.
260. Finsterer J, Strobl W. Causes of camptocormia. *Disabil Rehabil.* 2011;33(17-18):1702–1703.
261. Ashour R, Jankovic J. Joint and skeletal deformities in Parkinson's disease, multiple system atrophy, and progressive supranuclear palsy. *Mov Disord.* 2006;21(11):1856–1863.
262. Jankovic J, Leder S, Warner D, Schwartz K. Cervical dystonia: clinical findings and associated movement disorders. *Neurology.* 1991;41(7):1088–1091.
263. Doménech J, Tormos JM, Barrios C, Pascual-Leone A. Motor cortical hyperexcitability in idiopathic scoliosis: could focal dystonia be a subclinical etiological factor? *Eur Spine J.* 2010;19(2):223–230.
264. Finsterer J, Strobl W. Presentation, etiology, diagnosis, and management of camptocormia. *Eur Neurol.* 2010;64(1):1–8.
265. Gómez-Puerta JA, Peris P, Grau JM, Martinez MA, Guañabens N. Camptocormia as a clinical manifestation of mitochondrial myopathy. *Clin Rheumatol.* 2007;26(6):1017–1019.
266. Delcey V, Hachulla E, Michon-Pasturel U, et al. Camptocormia: a sign of axial myopathy. Report of 7 cases. *Rev Med Interne.* 2002;23(2):144–154.
267. Serratrice J, Weiller PJ, Pouget J, Serratrice G. An unrecognized cause of camptocormia: proximal myotonic myopathy. *Presse Med.* 2000;29(20):1121–1123.
268. Jankovic J. Disease-oriented approach to botulinum toxin use. *Toxicon.* 2009b;54(5):614–623.
269. Margraf NG, Wrede A, Rohr A, et al. Camptocormia in idiopathic Parkinson's disease: a focal myopathy of the paravertebral muscles. *Mov Disord.* 2010;25(5):542–551.

270. Schäbitz WR, Glatz K, Schuhan C, et al. Severe forward flexion of the trunk in Parkinson's disease: focal myopathy of the paraspinal muscles mimicking camptocormia. *Mov Disord.* 2003;18(4):408–414.
271. von Coelln R, Raible A, Gasser T, Asmus F. Ultrasound-guided injection of the iliopsoas muscle with botulinum toxin in camptocormia. *Mov Disord.* 2008;23(6):889–892.
272. Azher SN, Jankovic J. Camptocormia: pathogenesis, classification and response to therapy. *Neurology.* 2005;65(3):355–359.
273. Fietzek UM, Schroeteler FE, Ceballos-Baumann AO. Goal attainment after treatment of parkinsonian camptocormia with botulinum toxin. *Mov Disord.* 2009b;24(13):2027–2028.
274. Colosimo C, Salvatori FM. Injection of the iliopsoas muscle with botulinum toxin in camptocormia. *Mov Disord.* 2009;24(2):316–317.
275. Benecke R, Dressler D. Botulinum toxin treatment of axial and cervical dystonia. *Disabil Rehabil.* 2007;29(23):1769–1777.
276. Comella CL, Shannon KM, Jaglin J. Extensor truncal dystonia: successful treatment with botulinum toxin injections. *Mov Disord.* 1998;13(3):552–555.
277. Ghika J, Nater B, Henderson J, Bogousslavsky J, Regli F. Delayed segmental axial dystonia of the trunk on standing after lumbar disc operation. *J Neurol Sci.* 1997;152(2):193–197.
278. Rosales RL, Ng AR, Santos MM, Fernandez HH. The broadening application of chemodenervation in X-linked dystonia-parkinsonism (Part II): an open-label experience with botulinum toxin-A (Dysport) injections for oromandibular, lingual, and truncal-axial dystonias. *Int J Neurosci.* 2011;121(suppl 1):44–56.
279. Bonanni L, Thomas A, Varanese S, Scorrano V, Onofrj M. Botulinum toxin treatment of lateral axial dystonia in Parkinsonism. *Mov Disord.* 2007;22(14):2097–2103.
280. Quirk JA, Sheean GL, Marsden CD, Lees AJ. Treatment of nonoccupational limb and trunk dystonia with botulinum toxin. *Mov Disord.* 1996;11(4):377–383.
281. Alter KE, Hallett M, Karp BI, Lungu C. Advances in toxin therapy: Utilizing ultrasound guidance for botulinum toxin injections *Toxicon.* 2013b;68:68–69.
282. Gironell A, Kulisevsky J. Diagnosis and management of essential tremor and dystonic tremor. *Ther Adv Neurol Disord.* 2009;2(4):215–222.
283. Deuschl G, Krack P, Lauk M, Timmer J. Clinical neurophysiology of tremor. *J Clin Neurophysiol.* 1996;13(2):110–121.
284. Gironell A, Kulisevsky J, Pascual-Sedano B, Barbanoj M. Routine neurophysiological tremor analysis as a diagnostic tool for essential tremor: a prospective study. *J Clin Neurophysiol.* 2004;21(6):446–450.
285. Schneider SA, Deuschl G. The treatment of tremor. *Neurotherapeutics.* 2014;11(1):128–138.
286. Zappia M, Albanese A, Bruno E, et al. Treatment of essential tremor: a systematic review of evidence and recommendations from the Italian Movement Disorders Association. *J Neurol.* 2013;260(3):714–740.
287. Pal PK, Samii A, Schulzer M, Mak E, Tsui JK. Head tremor in cervical dystonia. *Can J Neurol Sci.* 2000;27(2):137–142.

288. Jankovic J, Fahn S. Physiologic and pathologic tremor. Diagnosis, mechanisms, and managagement. *Ann Intern Med.* 1980;93(3):460–465.
289. Deuschl G, Bain P, Brin MF. Consensus statement of the Movement Disorder Society on Tremor. *Ad Hoc Scientific Committee. Mov Disord.* 1998;13(suppl3):2–23.
290. Zesiewicz TA, Shaw JD, Allison KG, Staffetti JS, Okun MS, Sullivan KL. Update on treatment of essential tremor. *Curr Treat Options Neurol.* 2013;15(4):410–423.
291. Lyons M, Shneyder N, Evidente V. Primary writing tremor responds to unilateral thalamic deep brain stimulation. *Turk Neurosurg.* 2013;23(1):122–124.
292. Fasano A, Bove F, Lang AE. The treatment of dystonic tremor: a systematic review. *J Neurol Neurosurg Psychiatry.* 2014;85:759–769.
293. Boghen D, Flanders M. Effectiveness of botulinum toxin in the treatment of spasmodic torticollis. *Eur Neurol.* 1993;33(3):199–203.
294. Borodic GE, Mills L, Joseph M. Botulinum A toxin for the treatment of adult-onset spasmodic torticollis. *Plast Reconstr Surg.* 1991;87(2):285–289.
295. Rahimi F, Bee C, Debicki D, Roberts AC, Bapat P, Jog M. Effectiveness of BoNT A in Parkinson's disease upper limb tremor management. *Can J Neurol Sci.* 2013;40(5):663–669.
296. Henderson JM, Ghika JA, Van Melle G, Haller E, Einstein R. Botulinum toxin A in non-dystonic tremors. *Eur Neurol.* 1996;36(1):29-35.
297. Trosch RM, Pullman SL. Botulinum toxin A injections for the treatment of hand tremors. *Mov Disord.* 1994;9(6):601–609.
298. Jankovic J, Schwartz K. Botulinum toxin treatment of tremors. *Neurology.* 1991;41(8):1185–1188.
299. Brin MF, Lyons KE, Doucette J, et al. A randomized, double masked, controlled trial of botulinum toxin type A in essential hand tremor. *Neurology.* 2001;56(11):1523–1528.
300. Jankovic J. Pretarsal injection of botulinum toxin for blepharospasm and apraxia of eyelid opening. *J Neurol Neurosurg Psychiatry.* 1996;60(6):704.
301. Tan EK. Botulinum toxin treatment of sialorrhea: comparing different therapeutic preparations. *Eur J Neurol.* 2006;13(suppl 1):60–64.
302. Ellies M, Laskawi R, Rohrbach-Volland S, Arglebe C. Up-to-date report of botulinum toxin therapy in patients with drooling caused by different etiologies. *J Oral Maxillofac Surg.* 2003;61(4):454–457.
303. Naumann M, Dressler D, Hallett M, et al. Evidence-based review and assessment of botulinum neurotoxin for the treatment of secretory disorders. *Toxicon.* 2013;67:141–152.
304. Blackhall LJ. Amyotrophic lateral sclerosis and palliative care: where we are, and the road ahead. *Muscle Nerve.* 2012;45(3):311-318.
305. Seppi K, Weintraub D, Coelho M, et al. The Movement Disorder Society Evidence-Based Medicine Review Update: Treatments for the non-motor symptoms of Parkinson's disease. *Mov Disord.* 2011;26(suppl 3):S42–S80.
306. Benson J, Daugherty KK. Botulinum toxin A in the treatment of sialorrhea. *Ann Pharmacother.* 2007;41(1):79–85.

*307.* Tahmassebi JF, Curzon MEJ. The cause of drooling in children with cerebral palsy—hypersalivation or swallowing defect? *Int J Paediatr Dent.* 2003;13(2):106–111.

*308.* Harris SR, Purdy AH. Drooling and its management in cerebral palsy. *Dev Med Child Neurol.* 1987;29(6):807–811.

*309.* Jongerius PH, van den Hoogen FJA, van Limbeek J, Gabreëls FJ, van Hulst K, Rotteveel JJ. Effect of botulinum toxin in the treatment of drooling: a controlled clinical trial. *Pediatrics.* 2004;114(3):620–627.

*310.* Dogu O, Apaydin D, Sevim S, Talas DU, Aral M. Ultrasound-guided versus 'blind' intraparotid injections of botulinum toxin-A for the treatment of sialorrhoea in patients with Parkinson's disease. *Clin Neurol Neurosurg.* 2004;106(2): 93–96.

*311.* Silvestre-Rangil J, Silvestre FJ, Puente-Sandoval A, Requeni–Bernal J, Simó-Ruiz JM. Clinical-therapeutic management of drooling: review and update. *Med Oral Patol Oral Cir Bucal.* 2011;16(6):e763–e766.

*312.* Eiland LS. Glycopyrrolate for chronic drooling in children. *Clin Ther.* 2012;34(4):735–742.

*313.* Usta MG, Tufan AE, CüceloĐlu EA. Diphenhydramine use in the treatment of risperidone-induced sialorrhea. *J Child Adolesc Psychopharmacol.* 2012;22(3):254–255.

*314.* Levy NS, Lowenthal DT. Application of botulinum toxin to clinical therapy: advances and cautions. *Am J Ther.* 2012;19(4):281–286.

*315.* Hornibrook J, Cochrane N. Contemporary surgical management of severe sialorrhea in children. *ISRN Pediatr.* 2012;2012:364875.

*316.* Truong DD, Bhidayasiri R. Evidence for the effectiveness of botulinum toxin for sialorrhoea. *J Neural Transm.* 2008;115(4):631–635.

*317.* Chinnapongse R, Gullo K, Nemeth P, Zhang Y, Griggs L. Safety and efficacy of botulinum toxin type B for treatment of sialorrhea in Parkinson's disease: a prospective double-blind trial. *Mov Disord.* 2012;27(2):219–226.

*318.* Intiso D. Therapeutic use of botulinum toxin in neurorehabilitation. *J Toxicol.* 2012;2012:802893.

*319.* Reddihough D, Erasmus CE, Johnson H, McKellar GM, Jongerius PH, and Cerebral Palsy Institute. Botulinum toxin assessment, intervention and after-care for paediatric and adult drooling: international consensus statement. *Eur J Neurol.* 2010;17(suppl 2):109–121.

*320.* Ondo WG, Hunter C, Moore W. A double-blind placebo-controlled trial of botulinum toxin B for sialorrhea in Parkinson's disease. *Neurology.* 2004;62(1):37–40.

*321.* Young CA, Ellis C, Johnson J, Sathasivam S, Pih N. Treatment for sialorrhea (excessive saliva) in people with motor neuron disease/amyotrophic lateral sclerosis. *Cochrane Database Syst Rev.* 2011;(5):CD006981.

*322.* Gilio F, Iacovelli E, Frasca V, et al. Botulinum toxin type A for the treatment of sialorrhoea in amyotrophic lateral sclerosis: a clinical and neurophysiological study. *Amyotroph Lateral Scler.* 2010;11(4):359–363.

*323.* Jackson CE, Gronseth G, Rosenfeld J, et al; Muscle Study Group. Randomized double-blind study of botulinum toxin type B for sialorrhea in ALS patients. *Muscle Nerve.* 2009;39(2):137–143.

324. Basciani M, Di Rienzo F, Fontana A, Copetti M, Pellegrini F, Intiso D. Botulinum toxin type B for sialorrhoea in children with cerebral palsy: a randomized trial comparing three doses. *Dev Med Child Neurol.* 2011;53(6):559-564.
325. Wu KP, Ke JY, Chen CY, Chen CL, Chou MY, Pei YC. Botulinum toxin type A on oral health in treating sialorrhea in children with cerebral palsy: a randomized, double-blind, placebo-controlled study. *J Child Neurol.* 2011; 26(7):838-843.
326. Rodriguez-Murphy E, Marti-Bonmati E, Camps-Seguí E, Bagán JV. Manually guided botulinum toxin type A submandibular injections for the treatment of sialorrhea in tube-fed patients with advanced amyotrophic lateral sclerosis. *Am J Health Syst Pharm.* 2011;68(18):1680–1681.
327. Lee JH, Lee BN, Kwon SO, Chung RH, Han SH. Anatomical localization of submandibular gland for botulinum toxin injection. *Surg Radiol Anat.* 2010a;32(10):945–949.
328. Contarino MF, Pompili M, Tittoto P, et al. Botulinum toxin B ultrasound-guided injections for sialorrhea in amyotrophic lateral sclerosis and Parkinson's disease. *Parkinsonism Relat Disord.* 2007b;13(5):299–303.
329. Ellies M, Laskawi R, Rohrbach-Volland S, Arglebe C, Beuche W. Botulinum toxin to reduce saliva flow: selected indications for ultrasound-guided toxin application into salivary glands. *Laryngoscope.* 2002;112(1):82–86.
330. Strutton DR, Kowalski JW, Glaser DA, Stang PE. US prevalence of hyperhidrosis and impact on individuals with axillary hyperhidrosis: results from a national survey. *J Am Acad Dermatol.* 2004;51(2):241–248.
331. Lakraj AA, Moghimi N, Jabbari B. Hyperhidrosis: anatomy, pathophysiology and treatment with emphasis on the role of botulinum toxins. *Toxins (Basel).* 2013;5(4):820–840.
332. Del Sorbo F, Brancati F, De Joanna G, Valente EM, Lauria G, Albanese A. Primary focal hyperhidrosis in a new family not linked to known loci. *Dermatology.* 2011;223(4):335–342.
333. Hornberger J, Grimes K, Naumann M, et al, and Multi-Specialty Working Group on the Recognition, Diagnosis, and Treatment of Primary Focal Hyperhidrosis. Recognition, diagnosis, and treatment of primary focal hyperhidrosis. *J Am Acad Dermatol.* 2004;51(2):274–286.
334. Eckardt A, Kuettner C. Treatment of gustatory sweating (Frey's syndrome) with botulinum toxin A. *Head Neck.* 2003;25(8):624–628.
335. Glaser DA, Naumann M. Botulinum neurotoxin in the management of hyperhidrosis and other hypersecretory disorders. In: Jankovic J, Albanese A, Zouhair Atassi M, Dolly JO, Hallett M, Mayer NH, eds. *Botulinum Toxin: Therapeutic Clinical Practice and Science.* Philadelphia, PA: Saunders, Elsevier; 2009.
336. Cohen JL, Cohen G, Solish N, Murray CA. Diagnosis, impact, and management of focal hyperhidrosis: treatment review including botulinum toxin therapy. *Facial Plast Surg Clin North Am.* 2007;15(1):17-30,v–vi.
337. Vadoud-Seyedi J, Heenen M, Simonart T. Treatment of idiopathic palmar hyperhidrosis with botulinum toxin. Report of 23 cases and review of the literature. *Dermatology.* 2001;203(4):318–321.

338. Pena MA, Alam M, Yoo SS. Complications with the use of botulinum toxin type A for cosmetic applications and hyperhidrosis. *Semin Cutan Med Surg*. 2007;26(1):29–33.
339. Baumann LS, Halem ML. Systemic adverse effects after botulinum toxin type B (myobloc) injections for the treatment of palmar hyperhidrosis. *Arch Dermatol*. 2003;139(2):226–227.
340. Cardarelli WJ. Managed care aspects of managing neurogenic bladder/neurogenic detrusor overactivity. *Am J Manag Care*. 2013;19(suppl 10):S205–S208.
341. Ginsberg D. Optimizing therapy and management of neurogenic bladder. *Am J Manag Care*. 2013a;19(suppl 10):S197-S204.
342. Milsom I, Abrams P, Cardozo L, Roberts RG, Thüroff, Wein AJ. How widespread are the symptoms of an overactive bladder and how are they managed? A population-based prevalence study. *BJU Int*. 2001;87(9):760–766.
343. Haylen BT, de Ridder D, Freeman RM, et al, and International Urogynecological Association; International Continence Society. An International Urogynecological Association (IUGA)/International Continence Society (ICS) joint report on the terminology for female pelvic floor dysfunction. *Neurourol Urodyn*. 2010;29(1):4–20.
344. Maman K, Aballea S, Nazir J, et al. Comparative efficacy and safety of medical treatments for the management of overactive bladder: a systematic literature review and mixed treatment comparison. *Eur Urol*. 2014;65(4):755–765.
345. Roehrborn CG. Male lower urinary tract symptoms (LUTS) and benign prostatic hyperplasia (BPH). *Med Clin North Am*. 2011;95(1):87–100.
346. Ginsberg D. The epidemiology and pathophysiology of neurogenic bladder. *Am J Manag Care*. 2013b;19(suppl 10):S191–S196.
347. Mangera A, Chapple C. Modern evaluation of lower urinary tract symptoms in 2014. *Curr Opin Urol*. 2014;24(1):15–20.
348. Oelke M, Bachmann A, Descazeaud A, et al, and European Association of Urology. EAU guidelines on the treatment and follow-up of non-neurogenic male lower urinary tract symptoms including benign prostatic obstruction. *Eur Urol*. 2013;64(1):118–140.
349. Marberger M. Medical management of lower urinary tract symptoms in men with benign prostatic enlargement. *Adv Ther*. 2013;30(4):309-319.
350. Andersson KE. Pharmacotherapy of the overactive bladder. *Discov Med*. 2009;8(42):118–124.
351. Mangera A, Andersson KE, Apostolidis A, et al. Contemporary management of lower urinary tract disease with botulinum toxin A: a systematic review of botox (onabotulinumtoxinA) and dysport (abobotulinumtoxinA). *Eur Urol*. 2011;60(4):784–795.
352. Cantoro U, Minardi D, Lacetera V, Conti A, Catanzariti F, Muzzonigro G. Repeated injection of botulinum toxin A in patients with neurogenic bladder: our experience. *Urologia*. 2012;79(suppl 19):9–14.
353. Maneckshа RP, Cullen IM, Ahmad S, et al. Prospective randomised controlled trial comparing trigone-sparing versus trigone-including intradetrusor injection of abobotulinumtoxina for refractory idiopathic detrusor overactivity. *Eur Urol*. 2012;61(5):928–935.

354. Grise P, Ruffion A, Denys P, Egon G, Chartier Kastler E. Efficacy and tolerability of botulinum toxin type A in patients with neurogenic detrusor overactivity and without concomitant anticholinergic therapy: comparison of two doses. *Eur Urol*. 2010;58(5):759–766.
355. Ehren I, Volz D, Farrelly E, et al. Efficacy and impact of botulinum toxin A on quality of life in patients with neurogenic detrusor overactivity: a randomised, placebo-controlled, double-blind study. *Scand J Urol Nephrol*. 2007;41(4):335–340.
356. Ghei M, Maraj BH, Miller R, et al. Effects of botulinum toxin B on refractory detrusor overactivity: a randomized, double-blind, placebo controlled, crossover trial. *J Urol*. 2005;174(5):1873–1877; discussion 1877.
357. Habchi H, Galaup JP, Morel-Journel N, Ruffion A. Botulinum A toxin and detrusor sphincter dyssynergia: retrospective study of 47 patients. *Prog Urol*. 2014;24(4):234–239.
358. Safari S, Jamali S, Habibollahi P, Arshadi H, Nejat F, Kajbafzadeh AM. Intravesical injections of botulinum toxin type A for management of neuropathic bladder: a comparison of two methods. *Urology*. 2010;76(1):225–230.
359. Nikoobakht M, Daneshpajooh A, Ahmadi H, et al. Intraprostatic botulinum toxin type A injection for the treatment of benign prostatic hyperplasia: Initial experience with Dysport. *Scand J Urol Nephrol*. 2010;44(3):151–157.
360. Crawford ED, Hirst K, Kusek JW, et al. Effects of 100 and 300 units of onabotulinumtoxinA on lower urinary tract symptoms of benign prostatic hyperplasia: a phase II randomized clinical trial. *J Urol*. 2011;186(3): 965–970.
361. Smitherman TA, Burch R, Sheikh H, Loder E. The prevalence, impact, and treatment of migraine and severe headaches in the United States: a review of statistics from national surveillance studies. *Headache*. 2013;53(3):427–436.
362. Jackson JL, Kuriyama A, Hayashino Y. Botulinum toxin A for prophylactic treatment of migraine and tension headaches in adults: a meta-analysis. *JAMA*. 2012;307(16):1736–1745.
363. Headache Classification Committee of the International Headache Society. Classification and diagnostic criteria for the headache disorders, cranial neuralgias and facial pain. *Cephalalgia*. 1988;8(suppl 7):1–96.
364. Headache Classification Subcommittee of the International Headache Society. The International Classification of Headache Disorders: 2nd edition. *Cephalalgia*. 2004;24(suppl 1):9–160.
365. Silberstein SD. Botulinum toxin in headache management. In: Jankovic J, Albanese A, Zouhair Atassi M, Dolly JO, Hallett M, Mayer NH, eds. *Botulinum Toxin: Therapeutic Clinical Practice and Science*. Philadelphia, PA: Saunders, Elsevier; 2009.
366. Proietti Cecchini A, Grazzi L. Emerging therapies for chronic migraine. *Curr Pain Headache Rep*. 2014;18(4):408.
367. Silberstein SD. Migraine. *Lancet*. 2004;363(9406):381–391.
368. Schwartz BS, Stewart WF, Simon D, Lipton RB. Epidemiology of tension-type headache. *JAMA*. 1998;279(5):381–383.

*369.* Blumenfeld AM, Binder W, Silberstein SD, Blitzer A. Procedures for administering botulinum toxin type A for migraine and tension-type headache. *Headache.* 2003;43(8):884–891.
*370.* Schulte-Mattler WJ, Krack P, and BoNTTH Study Group. Treatment of chronic tension-type headache with botulinum toxin A: a randomized, double-blind, placebo-controlled multicenter study. *Pain.* 2004;109(1–2):110–114.
*371.* Jabbari B, Machado D. Treatment of refractory pain with botulinum toxins—an evidence-based review. *Pain Med.* 2011;12(11):1595–1606.
*372.* Blumenfeld AM, Dodick DW, Silberstein SD. Botulinum neurotoxin for the treatment of migrain and other primary headache disorders. *Dermatol Clin.* 2004;22(2):167–175.
*373.* Naumann M, So Y, Argoff CE, et al, and Therapeutics and Technology Assessment Subcomittee of the American Academy of Neurology. Assessment: botulinum neurotoxin in the treatment of autonomic disorders and pain (an evidence-based review): report of the Therapeutics and Technology Assessment Subcommittee of the American Academy of Neurology. *Neurology.* 2008;70(19):1707–1714.
*374.* Chankrachang S, Arayawichanont A, Poungvarin N, et al. Prophylactic botulinum type A toxin complex (Dysport) for migraine without aura. *Headache.* 2011;51(1):52–63.
*375.* Petri S, Tölle T, Straube A, Pfaffenrath V, Stefenelli U, Ceballos-Baumann A, and Dysport Migraine Study Group. Botulinum toxin as preventive treatment for migraine: a randomized double-blind study. *Eur Neurol.* 2009;62(4):204–211.
*376.* Menezes C, Rodrigues B, Magalhães E, Melo A. Botulinum toxin type A in refractory chronic migraine: an open-label trial. *Arq Neuropsiquiatr.* 2007;65(3A):596–598.
*377.* Straube A, Empl M, Ceballos-Baumann, Tölle T, Stefenelli U, Pfaffenrath V, and Dysport Tension-Type Headache Study Group. Pericranial injection of botulinum toxin type A (Dysport) for tension-type headache—a multicentre, double-blind, randomized, placebo-controlled study. *Eur J Neurol.* 2008;15(3):205–213.
*378.* Rollnik JD, Tanneberger O, Schubert M, Schneider U, Dengler R. Treatment of tension-type headache with botulinum toxin type A: a double-blind, placebo-controlled study. *Headache.* 2000b;40(4):300–305.
*379.* Grogan PM, Alvarez MV, Jones L. Headache direction and aura predict migraine responsiveness to rimabotulinumtoxinB. *Headache.* 2013;53(1):126–136.
*380.* Royal MA. Botulinum toxins in pain management. *Phys Med Rehabil Clin N Am.* 2003;14(4):805–820.
*381.* Soares A, Andriolo RB, Atallah AN, da Silva EM. Botulinum toxin for myofascial pain syndromes in adults. *Cochrane Database Syst Rev.* 2012;4:CD007533.
*382.* Simons DG, Travell JG, Simons LS. *Travell and Simons' Myofascial Pain and Dysfunction: The Trigger Point Manual.* 2nd ed. Vol 1: *Upper Half of Body.* Baltimore, MD: Lippincott, Williams & Wilkins; 1999.
*383.* Porta M. A comparative trial of botulinum toxin type A and methylprednisolone for the treatment of myofascial pain syndrome and pain from chronic muscle spasm. *Pain.* 2000;85(1–2):101–105.

*384.* Zhou JY, Wang D. An update on botulinum toxin A injections of trigger points for myofascial pain. *Curr Pain Headache Rep.* 2014;18(1):386.

*385.* Chou LW, Hong CZ, Wu ES, Hsueh WH, Kao MJ. Serial ultrasonographic findings of plantar fasciitis after treatment with botulinum toxin A: a case study. *Arch Phys Med Rehabil.* 2011;92(2):316–319.

*386.* Miller D, Richardson, Eisa M, Bajwa RJ, Jabbari B. Botulinum neurotoxin-A for treatment of refractory neck pain: a randomized, double-blind study. *Pain Med.* 2009;10(6):1012–1017.

*387.* Lew HL, Lee EH, Castaneda A, Klima R, Date E. Therapeutic doses of botulinum toxin A in treating neck and upper back pain of myofascial origin: a pilot study. *Arch Phys Med Rehabil.* 2008;89(1):75–80.

*388.* Ojala T, Arokoski JP, Partanen J. The effect of small doses of botulinum toxin A on neck-shoulder myofascial pain syndrome: a double-blind, randomized, and controlled crossover trial. *Clin J Pain.* 2006;22(1):90–96.

*389.* Qerama E, Fuglsang-Frederiksen A, Kasch H, Bach FW, Jensen TS. A double-blind, controlled study of botulinum toxin A in chronic myofascial pain. *Neurology.* 2006;67(2):241–245.

*390.* Ferrante FM, Bearn L, Rothrock R, King L. Evidence against trigger point injection technique for the treatment of cervicothoracic myofascial pain with botulinum toxin type A. *Anesthesiology.* 2005;103(2):377–383.

*391.* Wheeler AH, Goolkasian P, Gretz SS. Botulinum toxin A for the treatment of chronic neck pain. *Pain.* 2001;94(3):255–260.

*392.* Freund BJ, Schwartz M. Treatment of whiplash associated neck pain [corrected] with botulinum toxin-A: a pilot study. *J Rheumatol.* 2000;27(2):481–484.

*393.* Lang AM. A preliminary comparison of the efficacy and tolerability of botulinum toxin serotypes A and B in the treatment of myofascial pain syndrome: a retrospective, open-label chart review. *Clin Ther.* 2003;25(8):2268–2278.

*394.* Müller-Schwefe GHH, Überall MA. Dysport® for the treatment of myofascial back pain: Results from an open-label, Phase II, randomized, multicenter, dose-ranging study. *Scand J Pain.* 2011;2(1):25–33.

*395.* Carroll A, Barnes M, Comiskey C. A prospective randomized controlled study of the role of botulinum toxin in whiplash-associated disorder. *Clin Rehabil.* 2008;22(6):513–519.

*396.* Göbel H, Heinze A, Reichel G, Hefter H, Benecke R; Dysport myofascial pain study group. Efficacy and safety of a single botulinum type A toxin complex treatment (Dysport) for the relief of upper back myofascial pain syndrome: results from a randomized double-blind placebo-controlled multicentre study. *Pain.* 2006;125(1–2):82–88.

*397.* Jabbari B. Botulinum neurotoxins in the treatment of refractory pain. *Nat Clin Pract Neurol.* 2008;4(12):676–685.

*398.* Childers MK, Wilson DJ, Gnatz SM, Conway RR, Sherman AK. Botulinum toxin type A use in piriformis muscle syndrome: a pilot study. *Am J Phys Med Rehabil.* 2002;81(10):751–759.

*399.* Fishman LM, Anderson C, Rosner B. BOTOX and physical therapy in the treatment of piriformis syndrome. *Am J Phys Med Rehabil.* 2002;81(12):936–942.

400. Lang AM. Botulinum toxin type B in piriformis syndrome. *Am J Phys Med Rehabil*. 2004;83(3):198–202.
401. Fowler IM, Tucker AA, Weimerskirch BP, Moran TJ, Mendez RJ. A randomized comparison of the efficacy of 2 techniques for piriformis muscle injection: ultrasound-guided versus nerve stimulator with fluoroscopic guidance. *Reg Anesth Pain Med*. 2014;39(2):126–132.
402. Michel F, Decavel P, Toussirot E, et al. Piriformis muscle syndrome: diagnostic criteria and treatment of a monocentric series of 250 patients. *Ann Phys Rehabil Med*. 2013;56(5):371–383.
403. Yoon SJ, Ho J, Kang HY, et al. Low-dose botulinum toxin type A for the treatment of refractory piriformis syndrome. *Pharmacotherapy*. 2007;27(5):657–665.
404. Fishman LM, Konnoth C, Rozner B. Botulinum neurotoxin type B and physical therapy in the treatment of piriformis syndrome: a dose-finding study. *Am J Phys Med Rehabil*. 2004;83(1):42–50; quiz 51–53.
405. Behnam A, Mahyar S, Ezzati K, Rad SM. The use of dry needling and myofascial meridians in a case of plantar fasciitis. *J Chiropr Med*. 2014;13(1):43–18.
406. Neufeld SK, Cerrato R. Plantar fasciitis: evaluation and treatment. *J Am Acad Orthop Surg*. 2008;16(6):338–346.
407. Huang YC, Wei SH, Wang HK, Lieu FK. Ultrasonographic guided botulinum toxin type A treatment for plantar fasciitis: an outcome-based investigation for treating pain and gait changes. *J Rehabil Med*. 2010;42(2):136–140.
408. Babcock MS, Foster L, Pasquina P, Jabbari B. Treatment of pain attributed to plantar fasciitis with botulinum toxin A: a short-term, randomized, placebo-controlled, double-blind study. *Am J Phys Med Rehabil*. 2005;84(9):649–654.
409. Peterlein CD, Funk JF, Hölscher A, Schuh A, Placzek R. Is botulinum toxin A effective for the treatment of plantar fasciitis? *Clin J Pain*. 2012;28(6): 527–533.
410. Placzek R, Hölscher A, Deuretzbacher G, Meiss L, Perka C. Treatment of chronic plantar fasciitis with botulinum toxin A—an open pilot study on 25 patients with a 14-week-follow-up. *Z Orthop Ihre Grenzgeb*. 2006;144(4):405–409.
411. Singh JA. Botulinum toxin therapy for osteoarticular pain: an evidence-based review. *Ther Adv Musculoskel Dis*. 2010;2(2):105–118.
412. Centers for Disease Control and Prevention (CDC). Prevalence and most common causes of disability among adults—United States, 2005. *MMWR* 2009;58(16):421–426.
413. Brander VA, Stulberg SD, Adams AD, et al. Predicting total knee replacement pain: a prospective, observational study. *Clin Orthop Relat Res*. 2003;(416):416–427.
414. Bellamy N, Campbell J, Robinson V, Gee T, Bourne R, Wells G. Intraarticular corticosteroid for treatment of osteoarthritis of the knee. *Cochrane Database Syst Rev*. 2006a;(2):CD005328.
415. Bellamy N, Campbell J, Robinson V, Gee T, Bourne R, Wells G. Viscosupplementation for the treatment of osteoarthritis of the knee. *Cochrane Database Syst Rev*. 2006b;(2):CD005321.
416. Singh JA. Use of botulinum toxin in musculoskeletal pain. *Version 2 F1000Res*. 2013;2:52.

417. Singh JA, Mahowald ML, Noorbaloochi S. Intraarticular botulinum toxin a for refractory painful total knee arthroplasty: a randomized controlled trial. *J Rheumatol*. 2010;37(11):2377–2386.
418. Singh JA, Mahowald ML, Noorbaloochi S. Intra-articular botulinum toxin type A for refractory shoulder pain: a randomized, double-blinded, placebo-controlled trial. *Transl Res*. 2009;153(5):205–216.
419. Mahowald ML, Singh JA, Dykstra D. Long term effects of intra-articular botulinum toxin A for refractory joint pain. *Neurotox Res*. 2006;9(2–3):179–188.
420. Singer BJ, Silbert PL, Dunne JW, Song S, Singer KP. An open label pilot investigation of the efficacy of botulinum toxin type A [Dysport] injection in the rehabilitation of chronic anterior knee pain. *Disabil Rehabil*. 2006;28(11):707–113.
421. Marchini C, Acler M, Bolognari MA, et al. Efficacy of botulinum toxin type A treatment of functional impairment of degenerative hip joint: Preliminary results. *J Rehabil Med*. 2010;42(7):691–693.
422. Singh JA, Mahowald ML. Intra-articular botulinum toxin A as an adjunctive therapy for refractory joint pain in patients with rheumatoid arthritis receiving biologics: a report of two cases. *Joint Bone Spine*. 2009;76(2):190–194.
423. Dykstra DD, Stuckey MW, Schimpff SN, Singh JA, Mahowald ML. The effects of intra-articular botulinum toxin on sacroiliac, cervical/lumbar facet and sternoclavicular joint pain and C-2 root and lumbar disc pain: a case series of 11 patients. *Pain Clinic*. 2007;19(1):27–32.
424. Singh JA, Fitzgerald PM. Botulinum toxin for shoulder pain: a cochrane systematic review. *J Rheumatol*. 2011;38(3):409–318.
425. Joo YJ, Yoon SJ, Kim CW, et al. A comparison of the short-term effects of a botulinum toxin type A and triamcinolone acetate injection on adhesive capsulitis of the shoulder. *Ann Rehabil Med*. 2013;37(2):208–214.
426. Wilson NA, Press JM, Zhang LQ. In vivo strain of the medial vs. lateral quadriceps tendon in patellofemoral pain. *J Appl Physiol*. 2009;107(2):422–428.
427. Sheehan FT, Babushkina A, Alter KE. Kinematic determinants of anterior knee pain in cerebral palsy: a case-control study. *Arch Phys Med Rehabil*. 2012a;93(8):1431–1440.
428. Sheehan FT, Borotikar BS, Behnam AJ, Alter KE. Alterations in in vivo knee joint kinematics following a femoral nerve branch block of the vastus medialis: implications for patellofemoral pain syndrome. *Clin Biomech (Bristol, Avon)*. 2012b;27(6):525–631.
429. Silbert BI, Singer BJ, Silbert PL, Gibbons JT, Singer KP. Enduring efficacy of botulinum toxin type A injection for refractory anterior knee pain. *Disabil Rehabil*. 2012;34(1):62–68.
430. Ahmad Z, Siddiqui N, Malik SS, et al. Lateral epicondylitis: a review of pathology and management. *Bone Joint J*. 2013b;95-B(9):1158–1164.
431. Ahmad Z, Brooks R, Kang SN, et al. The effect of platelet-rich plasma on clinical outcomes in lateral epicondylitis. *Arthroscopy*. 2013a;29(11):1851–1862.

432. Hayton MJ, Santini AJ, Hughes PJ, Frostick SP, Trail IA, Stanley JK. Botulinum toxin injection in the treatment of tennis elbow. A double-blind, randomized, controlled, pilot study. *J Bone Joint Surg Am.* 2005;87(3):503–507.
433. Lin YC, Tu YK, Chen SS, Lin IL, Chen SC, Guo HR. Comparison between botulinum toxin and corticosteroid injection in the treatment of acute and subacute tennis elbow: a prospective, randomized, double-blind, active drug-controlled pilot study. *Am J Phys Med Rehabil.* 2010;89(8):653–659.
434. Lim EC, Seet RC, Cheah AE, Lim AY. Injection of botulinum toxin to the extensor carpi radialis brevis for tennis elbow. *J Hand Surg Eur Vol.* 2010;35(5):425–426.
435. Placzek R, Drescher W, Deuretzbacher G, Hempfing A, Meiss AL. Treatment of chronic radial epicondylitis with botulinum toxin A. A double-blind, placebo-controlled, randomized multicenter study. *J Bone Joint Surg Am.* 2007;89(2):255–260.
436. Wong SM, Hui AC, Tong PY, Poon DW, Yu E, Wong LK. Treatment of lateral epicondylitis with botulinum toxin: a randomized, double-blind, placebo-controlled trial. *Ann Intern Med.* 2005;143(11):793–797.
437. Waseem Z, Boulias C, Gordon A, Ismail F, Sheean G, Furlan AD. Botulinum toxin injections for low-back pain and sciatica. *Cochrane Database Syst Rev.* 2011;(1):CD008257.
438. Jabbari B, Ney J, Sichani A, Monacci W, Foster L, Difazio M. Treatment of refractory, chronic low back pain with botulinum neurotoxin A: an open-label, pilot study. *Pain Med.* 2006;7(3):260–264.
439. Ney JP, Difazio M, Sichani A, Monacci W, Foster L, Jabbari B. Treatment of chronic low back pain with successive injections of botulinum toxin A over 6 months: a prospective trial of 60 patients. *Clin J Pain.* 2006;22(4):363–369.
440. Foster L, Clapp L, Erickson M, Jabbari B. Botulinum toxin A and chronic low back pain: a randomized, double-blind study. *Neurology.* 2001;56(10):1290–1293.
441. Lee JH, Lee SH, Song SH. Clinical effectiveness of botulinum toxin A compared to a mixture of steroid and local anesthetics as a treatment for sacroiliac joint pain. *Pain Med.* 2010b;11(5):692–700.
442. Sanders RJ, Hammond SL, Rao NM. Thoracic outlet syndrome: a review. *Neurologist.* 2008;14(6):365–373.
443. Foley JM, Finlayson H, Travlos A. A review of thoracic outlet syndrome and the possible role of botulinum toxin in the treatment of thoracic outlet syndrome. *Toxins (Basel).* 2012;4(11):1223–2235.
444. Alter KE. Ultrasound-guided botulinum neurotoxin injections for thoracic outlet syndrome. In: Truong D, Hallett M, Zachary CB, Dressler D, eds. *Manual of Botulinum Toxin Therapy.* 2nd ed. Cambridge, UK: Cambridge University Press; 2013b: 269–277.
445. Watson LA, Pizzari T, Balster S. Thoracic outlet syndrome part 2: conservative management of thoracic outlet. *Man Ther.* 2010;15(4):305–314.
446. Jordan SE, Ahn SS, Freischlag JA, Gelabert HA, Machleder HI. Selective botulinum toxin chemodenervation of the scalene muscles for treatment of neurogenic thoracic outlet syndrome. *Ann Vasc Surg.* 2000;14(4):365–369.

447. Finlayson HC, O'Connor RJ, Brasher PM, Travlos A. Botulinum toxin injection for management of thoracic outlet syndrome: a double-blind, randomized, controlled trial. *Pain*. 2011;152(9):2023–2028.

448. Christo PJ, Christo DK, Carinci AJ, Freischlag JA. Single CT-guided chemodenervation of the anterior scalene muscle with botulinum toxin for neurogenic thoracic outlet syndrome. *Pain Med*. 2010;11(4):504–511.

449. Torriani M, Gupta R, Donahue DM. Botulinum toxin injection in neurogenic thoracic outlet syndrome: results and experience using a ultrasound-guided approach. *Skeletal Radiol*. 2010;39(10):973–980.

450. Brown EA, Schütz SG, Simpson DM. Botulinum toxin for neuropathic pain and spasticity: an overview. *Pain Manag*. 2014;4(2):129–151.

451. Viana R, Pereira S, Mehta S, Miller T, Teasell R. Evidence for therapeutic interventions for hemiplegic shoulder pain during the chronic stage of stroke: a review. *Top Stroke Rehabil*. 2012;19(6):514–622.

452. Rawicki B, Sheean G, Fung VS, Goldsmith S, Morgan C, Novak I, and Cerebral Palsy Institute. Botulinum toxin assessment, intervention and aftercare for paediatric and adult niche indications including pain: international consensus statement. *Eur J Neurol*. 2010;17(suppl 2):122–134.

453. Castiglione A, Bagnato S, Boccagni C, Romano MC, Galardi G. Efficacy of intra-articular injection of botulinum toxin type A in refractory hemiplegic shoulder pain. *Arch Phys Med Rehabil*. 2011;92(7):1034–1037.

454. Kong KH, Neo JJ, Chua KS. A randomized controlled study of botulinum toxin A in the treatment of hemiplegic shoulder pain associated with spasticity. *Clin Rehabil*. 2007;21(1):28–35.

455. de Boer KS, Arwert HJ, de Groot JH, Meskers CG, Mishre AD, Arendzen JH. Shoulder pain and external rotation in spastic hemiplegia do not improve by injection of botulinum toxin A into the subscapular muscle. *J Neurol Neurosurg Psychiatry*. 2008;79(5):581–583.

456. Yelnik AP, Colle FM, Bonan IV, Vicaut E. Treatment of shoulder pain in spastic hemiplegia by reducing spasticity of the subscapular muscle: a randomised, double blind, placebo controlled study of botulinum toxin A. *J Neurol Neurosurg Psychiatry*. 2007;78(8):845–848.

457. Marciniak CM, Harvey RL, Gagnon CM, et al. Does botulinum toxin type A decrease pain and lessen disability in hemiplegic survivors of stroke with shoulder pain and spasticity?: a randomized, double-blind, placebo-controlled trial. *Am J Phys Med Rehabil*. 2012;91(12):1007–1019.

458. Marco E, Duarte E, Vila J, et al. Is botulinum toxin type A effective in the treatment of spastic shoulder pain in patients after stroke? A double-blind randomized clinical trial. *J Rehabil Med*. 2007;39(6):440–447.

459. Singh JA, Fitzgerald PM. Botulinum toxin for shoulder pain. *Cochrane Database Syst Rev*. 2010;(9):CD008271.

460. Koog YH, Jin SS, Yoon K, Min BI. Interventions for hemiplegic shoulder pain: systematic review of randomised controlled trials. *Disabil Rehabil*. 2010;32(4):282–291.

461. Dutton JJ, White JJ, Richard MJ. Myobloc for the treatment of benign essential blepharospasm in patients refractory to botox. *Ophthal Plast Reconstr Surg*. 2006;22(3):173–177.

462. Girlanda P, Quartarone A, Sinicropi S, Nicolosi C, Messina C. Unilateral injection of botulinum toxin in blepharospasm: single fiber electromyography and blink reflex study. *Mov Disord*. 1996;11(1):27–31.
463. Jankovic J. Clinical efficacy and tolerability of Xeomin in the treatment of blepharospasm. *Eur J Neurol*. 2009a;16(suppl 2):14–18.
464. Jankovic J, Orman J. Botulinum A toxin for cranial-cervical dystonia: a double-blind, placebo-controlled study. *Neurology*. 1987;37(4):616–623.
465. Dressler D. Routine use of Xeomin in patients previously treated with Botox: long term results. *Eur J Neurol*. 2009;16(suppl 2):2–5.
466. Gil Polo C, Rodríguez Sanz MF, Berrocal Izquierdo N, et al. Blepharospasm and hemifacial spasm: long-term treatment with botulinum toxin. *Neurologia*. 2013;28(3):131–136.
467. Jitpimolmard S, Tiamkao S, Laopaiboon M. Long term results of botulinum toxin type A (Dysport) in the treatment of hemifacial spasm: a report of 175 cases. *J Neurol Neurosurg Psychiatry*. 1998;64(6):751–757.
468. Pang AL, O'Day J. Use of high-dose botulinum A toxin in benign essential blepharospasm: is too high too much? *Clin Experimental Ophthalmol*. 2006;34(5):441–444.
469. Rollnik JD, Matzke M, Wohlfarth K, Dengler R, Bigalke H. Low-dose treatment of cervical dystonia, blepharospasm and facial hemispasm with albumin-diluted botulinum toxin type A under EMG guidance. An open label study. *Eur Neurol*. 2000a;43(1):9–12.
470. Sampaio C, Ferreira JJ, Simões F, et al. DYSBOT: a single-blind, randomized parallel study to determine whether any differences can be detected in the efficacy and tolerability of two formulations of botulinum toxin type A—Dysport and Botox—assuming a ratio of 4:1. *Mov Disord*. 1997;12(6):1013–1018.
471. Tsai CP, Chiu MC, Yen DJ, Guo YC, Yuan CL, Lee TC. Quantitative assessment of efficacy of Dysport (botulinum toxin type A) in the treatment of idiopathic blepharospasm and hemifacial spasm. *Acta Neurol Taiwan*. 2005;14(2):61–68.
472. Van den Bergh P, Francart J, Mourin S, Kollmann P, Laterre EC. Five-year experience in the treatment of focal movement disorders with low-dose Dysport botulinum toxin. *Muscle Nerve*. 1995;18(7):720–729.
473. Tan EK, Jankovic J. Botulinum toxin A in patients with oromandibular dystonia: long-term follow-up. *Neurology*. 1999;53(9):2102–2107.
474. Brin MF, Comella CL, Jankovic J, Lai F, Naumann M, and CD-017 BoNTA Study Group. Long-term treatment with botulinum toxin type A in cervical dystonia has low immunogenicity by mouse protection assay. *Mov Disord*. 2008;23(10):1353–1360.
475. Chinnapongse R, Pappert EJ, Evatt M, Freeman A, Birmingham W. An open-label, sequential dose-escalation, safety, and tolerability study of rimabotulinumtoxinb in subjects with cervical dystonia. *Int J Neurosci*. 2010;120(11):703–710.
476. Dressler D, Paus S, Seitzinger A, Gebhardt B, Kupsch A. Long-term efficacy and safety of incobotulinumtoxinA injections in patients with cervical dystonia. *J Neurol Neurosurg Psychiatry*. 2013;84(9):1014–1019.

477. Evidente VG, Fernandez HH, LeDoux MS, et al. A randomized, double-blind study of repeated incobotulinumtoxinA (Xeomin) in cervical dystonia. *J Neural Transm*. 2013;120(12):1699–1707.
478. Fernandez HH, Pagan F, Danisi F, et al, and XCiDaBLE Study Group. Prospective study evaluating incobotulinumtoxinA for cervical dystonia or blepharospasm: interim results from the first 145 subjects with cervical dystonia. *Tremor Other Hyperkinet Mov (N Y)*. 2013;3. pii: tre-03-139-2924-1.
479. Flowers JM, Hicklin LA, Marion MH. Anterior and posterior sagittal shift in cervical dystonia: a clinical and electromyographic study, including a new EMG approach of the longus colli muscle. *Mov Disord*. 2011;26(13):2409–2414.
480. Gill CE, Manus ND, Pelster MW, et al. Continuation of long-term care for cervical dystonia at an academic movement disorders clinic. *Toxins (Basel)*. 2013;5(4):776–783.
481. Hauser RA, Truong D, Hubble J, et al. AbobotulinumtoxinA (Dysport) dosing in cervical dystonia: an exploratory analysis of two large open-label extension studies. *J Neural Transm*. 2013;120(2):299–307.
482. Herting B, Wunderlich S, Glöckler T, et al. Computed tomographically controlled injection of botulinum toxin into the longus colli muscle in severe anterocollis. *Mov Disord*. 2004;19(5):588–590.
483. Kaji R, Shimizu H, Takase T, Osawa M, Yanagisawa N. A double-blind comparative study to evaluate the efficacy and safety of NerBloc (rimabotulinumtoxinB) administered in a single dose to patients with cervical dystonia. *Brain Nerve*. 2013;65(2):203–211.
484. Pappert EJ, Germanson T, and Myobloc/Neurobloc European Cervical Dystonia Study Group. Botulinum toxin type B vs. type A in toxin-naïve patients with cervical dystonia: randomized, double-blind, noninferiority trial. *Mov Disord*. 2008;23(4):510–517.
485. Poewe W, Deuschl G, Nebe A, et al, and for the German Dystonia Study Group. What is the optimal dose of botulinum toxin A in the treatment of cervical dystonia? Results of a double blind, placebo controlled, dose ranging study using Dysport. *J Neurol Neurosurg Psychiatry*. 1998;64(1):13–17.
486. Ruiz PJ, Castrillo JC, Burguera JA, et al. Evolution of dose and response to botulinum toxin A in cervical dystonia: a multicenter study. *J Neurol*. 2011;258(6):1055–1057.
487. Kim SD, Yiannikas C, Mahant N, Vucic S, Fung VS. Treatment of proximal upper limb tremor with botulinum toxin therapy. *Mov Disord*. 2014;29(6):835–838.
488. Wu LJ, Jankovic J. Runner's dystonia. *J Neurol Sci*. 2006;251(1-2):73–76.
489. Rosenberg NS, Odderson IR. Diagnosis and treatment of abductor hallucis focal dystonia with botulinum toxin injection: a case presentation. *PM R*. 2013;5(8):726–728.
490. Singer C, Papapetropoulos S. Adult-onset primary focal foot dystonia. *Parkinsonism Relat Disord*. 2006;12(1):57–60.
491. Dysport HC (DIN 02387735) DPD Product Monograph from Health Canada. Available at (www.hc-sc.gc.ca) http://webprod5.hc-sc.gc.ca/dpd-bdpp/item-iteme.do?pm-mp=00024641. Updated November 11, 2013.

492. Intiso D, Simone V, Di Rienzo F, et al. High doses of a new botulinum toxin type A (NT-201) in adult patients with severe spasticity following brain injury and cerebral palsy. *NeuroRehabilitation*. 2014;34(3):515–522. doi:10.3233/NRE-141052.
493. Santamato A, Panza F, Ranieri M, et al. Efficacy and safety of higher doses of botulinum toxin type A NT 201 free from complexing proteins in the upper and lower limb spasticity after stroke. *J Neural Transm*. 2013b;120(3):469–476.
494. Dressler S, Adib Saberi F. First high dose use of complex free botulinum toxin type A. *Mov Disord*. 2006;21(suppl 15):S640.
495. Pathak MS, Nguyen HT, Graham HK, Moore AP. Management of spasticity in adults: practical application of botulinum toxin. *Eur J Neurol*. 2006;13 (suppl 1):42–50.
496. Hubble J, Schwab J, Hubert C, Abbott CC. Dysport (botulinum toxin type A) in routine therapeutic usage: a telephone needs assessment survey of European physicians to evaluate current awareness and adherence to product labeling changes. *Clin Neuropharmacol*. 2013;36(4):122–127.
497. Smith SJ, Ellis E, White S, Moore AP. A double-blind placebo controlled study of botulinum toxin in upper limb spasticity after stroke or head injury. *Clin Rehabil*. 2000;14(1):5–13.
498. Ashford S, Turner-Stokes L. Management of shoulder and proximal upper limb spasticity using botulinum toxin and concurrent therapy interventions: a preliminary analysis of goals and outcomes. *Disabil Rehabil*. 2009;31(3):220–226.
499. Baker R, Jasinski M, Maciag-Tymecka I, et al. Botulinum toxin treatment of spasticity in diplegic cerebral palsy: a randomized, double-blind, placebo-controlled, dose-ranging study. *Dev Med Child Neurol*. 2002;44(10):666–675.
500. Bakheit AM, Fedorova NV, Skoromets AA, Timerbaeva SL, Bhakta BB, Coxon L. The beneficial antispasticity effect of botulinum toxin type A is maintained after repeated treatment cycles. *J Neurol Neurosurg Psychiatry*. 2004;75(11):1558–1561.
501. Bakheit AM, Pittock S, Moore AP, et al. A randomized, double-blind, placebo-controlled study of the efficacy and safety of botulinum toxin type A in upper limb spasticity in patients with stroke. *Eur J Neurol*. 2001;8(6): 559–565.
502. Bakheit AM, Thilmann AF, Ward AB, et al. A randomized, double-blind, placebo-controlled, dose-ranging study to compare the efficacy and safety of three doses of botulinum toxin type A (Dysport) with placebo in upper limb spasticity after stroke. *Stroke*. 2000;31(10):2402–2406.
503. Barnes MP, Schnitzler A, Medeiros L, Aguilar M, Lehnert-Batar A, Minnasch P. Efficacy and safety of NT 201 for upper limb spasticity of various etiologies—a randomized parallel-group study. *Acta Neurol Scand*. 2010;122(4):295–302.
504. Berweck S, Heinen F. Use of botulinum toxin in pediatric spasticity (cerebral palsy). *Mov Disord*. 2004;19(suppl 8):S162–S167.
505. Bhakta BB, Cozens JA, Chamberlain MA, Bamford JM. Impact of botulinum toxin type A on disability and carer burden due to arm spasticity after stroke: a randomised double blind placebo controlled trial. *J Neurol Neurosurg Psychiatry*. 2000;69(2):217–221.

*506.* Brashear A, Gordon MF, Elovic E, et al, and Botox Post-Stroke Spasticity Study Group. Intramuscular injection of botulinum toxin for the treatment of wrist and finger spasticity after a stroke. *N Engl J Med.* 2002;347(6):395–400.

*507.* Brashear A, McAfee AL, Kuhn ER, Fyffe J. Botulinum toxin type B in upper-limb poststroke spasticity: a double-blind, placebo-controlled trial. *Arch Phys Med Rehabil.* 2004;85(5):705–709.

*508.* Childers MK, Brashear A, Jozefczyk P, et al. Dose-dependent response to intramuscular botulinum toxin type A for upper-limb spasticity in patients after a stroke. *Arch Phys Med Rehabil.* 2004;85(7):1063–1069.

*509.* Corry IS, Cosgrove AP, Walsh EG, McClean D, Graham HK. Botulinum toxin A in the hemiplegic upper limb: a double-blind trial. *Dev Med Child Neurol.* 1997;39(3):185–193.

*510.* Esquenazi A, Novak I, Sheean G, Singer BJ, Ward AB. International consensus statement for the use of botulinum toxin treatment in adults and children with neurological impairments—introduction. *Eur J Neurol.* 2010;17(suppl 2):1–8.

*511.* Falso M, Galluso R, Malvicini A. Functional influence of botulinum neurotoxin type A treatment (Xeomin) of multifocal upper and lower limb spasticity on chronic hemiparetic gait. *Neurol Int.* 2012;4(2):e8.

*512.* Fietzek UM, Kossmehl P, Barthels A, Ebersbach G, Zynda B, Wissel J. Botulinum toxin B increases mouth opening in patients with spastic trismus. *Eur J Neurol.* 2009a;16(12):1299–1304.

*513.* Gracies JM, Bayle N, Goldberg S, Simpson DM. Botulinum toxin type B in the spastic arm: a randomized, double-blind, placebo-controlled, preliminary study. *Arch Phys Med Rehabil.* 2014;95:1303–1311.

*514.* Hesse S, Reiter F, Konrad M, Jahnke MT. Botulinum toxin type A and short-term electrical stimulation in the treatment of upper limb flexor spasticity after stroke: a randomized, double-blind, placebo-controlled trial. *Clin Rehabil.* 1998;12(5):381–388.

*515.* Kaňovský P, Slawek J, Denes Z, et al. Efficacy and safety of botulinum neurotoxin NT 201 in poststroke upper limb spasticity. *Clin Neuropharmacol.* 2009b;32(5):259–265.

*516.* Mayer NH, Simpson DM. Dosing, administration, and a treatment algorithm for use of botulinum toxin a for adult-onset muscle overactivity in patients with an upper motoneuron lesion. In: Mayer NH, Simpson DM, eds. *Spasticity: Etiology, Evaluation, Management and the Role of Botulinum Toxin.* Bronx, NY: We Move [Worldwide Education and Awareness for Movement Disorders]; 2002:154–165.

*517.* Muller F, Cugy E, Ducerf C, et al. Safety and self-reported efficacy of botulinum toxin for adult spasticity in current clinical practice: a prospective observational study. *Clin Rehabil.* 2012;26(2):174–179.

*518.* Nalysnyk L, Papapetropoulos S, Rotella P, Simeone JC, Alter KE, Esquenazi A. OnabotulinumtoxinA muscle injection patterns in adult spasticity: a systematic literature review. *BMC Neurol.* 2013;13:118.

*519.* Richardson D, Sheean G, Werring D, et al. Evaluating the role of botulinum toxin in the management of focal hypertonia in adults. *J Neurol Neurosurg Psychiatry.* 2000;69(4):499–506.

520. Royal College of Physicians, British Society of Rehabilitation Medicine, Chartered Society of Physiotherapy, Association of Chartered Physiotherapists Interested in Neurology. *Spasticity in Adults: Management Using Botulinum Toxin. National Guidelines*. London, UK: RCP; 2009.
521. Santamato A, Ranieri M, Panza F, et al. Effectiveness of switching therapy from complexing protein-containing botulinum toxin type A to a formulation with low immunogenicity in spasticity after stroke: a case report. *J Rehabil Med*. 2012;44(9):795–797.
522. Sheean G, Lannin NA, Turner-Stokes L, Rawicki B, Snow BJ, and Cerebral Palsy Institute. Botulinum toxin assessment, intervention and after-care for upper limb hypertonicity in adults: international consensus statement. *Eur J Neurol*. 2010;17(suppl 2):74–93.
523. Simpson DM, Alexander DN, O'Brien CF, et al. Botulinum toxin type A in the treatment of upper extremity spasticity: a randomized, double-blind, placebo controlled trial. *Neurology*. 1996;46(5):1306–1310.
524. Simpson DM, Gracies JM, Yablon SA, Barbano R, Brashear A, and BoNT/TZD Study Team. Botulinum neurotoxin versus tizanidine in upper limb spasticity: a placebo-controlled study. *J Neurol Neurosurg Psychiatry*. 2009;80(4):380–385.
525. Snow BJ, Tsui JK, Bhatt MH, Varelas M, Hashimoto SA, Calne DB. Treatment of spasticity with botulinum toxin: a double-blind study. *Ann Neurol*. 1990;28(4):512–515.
526. Suputtitada A, Suwanwela NC. The lowest effective dose of botulinum A toxin in adult patients with upper limb spasticity. *Disabil Rehabil*. 2005;27(4):176–184.
527. Teasell R, Foley N, Salter K, Bhogal S. *Botulinum Toxin in the Treatment of Upper and Lower Limb Spasticity Post Stroke*. London, Ontario: The Evidence-Based Review of Stroke Rehabilitation. Available at (www.ebrsr.com) http://www.ebrsr.com/sites/default/files/Appendix-spasticity.pdf. Updated 2012.
528. Burbaud P, Wiart L, Dubos JL, et al. A randomised, double blind, placebo controlled trial of botulinum toxin in the treatment of spastic foot in hemiparetic patients. *J Neurol Neurosurg Psychiatry*. 1996;61(3):265–269.
529. Caty GD, Detrembleur C, Bleyenheuft C, Deltombe T, Lejeune TM. Effect of simultaneous botulinum toxin injections into several muscles on impairment, activity, participation, and quality of life among stroke patients presenting with a stiff knee gait. *Stroke*. 2008;39(10):2803–2808.
530. Gaber TA, Basu B, Shakespeare D, Singh R, Salam S, McFarlane J. Botulinum toxin in the management of hitchhiker's toe. *NeuroRehabilitation*. 2011;28(4):395–399.
531. Gusev YI, Banach M, Simonow A, et al. Efficacy and safety of botulinum type A toxin in adductor spasticity due to multiple sclerosis. *J Musculoskelet Pain*. 2008;16(3):175–188.
532. Hyman N, Barnes M, Bhakta B, et al. Botulinum toxin (Dysport) treatment of hip adductor spasticity in multiple sclerosis: a prospective, randomised, double blind, placebo controlled, dose ranging study. *J Neurol Neurosurg Psychiatry*. 2000;68(6):707–712.
533. Intiso D, Basciani M. Botulinum toxin type A in the healing of a chronic buttock ulcer in a patient with spastic paraplegia after spinal cord injury. *J Rehabil Med*. 2009;41(13):1100–1102.

534. Kaji R, Osako Y, Suyama K, Maeda T, Uechi Y, Iwasaki M, and GSK1358820 Spasticity Study Group. Botulinum toxin type A in post-stroke lower limb spasticity: a multicenter, double-blind, placebo-controlled trial. *J Neurol.* 257(8):1330–1337.
535. Kurtis MM, Floyd AG, Yu QP, Pullman SL. High doses of botulinum toxin effectively treat disabling up-going toe. *J Neurol Sci.* 2008;264(1-2):118-120.
536. Lippert-Grüner M, Svestkova O. Early use of Xeomin neurotoxin for local antispasticity therapy for pes equines after acquired brain injury (ABI). *Brain Inj.* 2011;25(12):1266–1269.
537. Oechsner M. Treatment of hip adductor spasticity with botulinum toxin type B. *Nervenarzt.* 2002;73(12):1179–1182.
538. Pittock SJ, Moore AP, Hardiman O, et al. A double-blind randomised placebo-controlled evaluation of three doses of botulinum toxin type A (Dysport) in the treatment of spastic equinovarus deformity after stroke. *Cerebrovasc Dis.* 2003;15(4):289–300.
539. Santamato A, Micello MF, Panza F, et al. Safety and efficacy of incobotulinum toxin type A (NT 201-Xeomin) for the treatment of post-stroke lower limb spasticity: a prospective open-label study. *Eur J Phys Rehabil Med.* 2013a;49(4):483–489.
540. Papavasiliou AS, Nikaina I, Bouros P, Rizou I, Filiopoulos C. Botulinum toxin treatment in upper limb spasticity: treatment consistency. *Eur J Paediatr Neurol.* 2012;16(3):237–242.
541. Molenaers G, Fagard K, Van Campenhout A, Desloovere K. Botulinum toxin A treatment of the lower extremities in children with cerebral palsy. *J Child Orthop.* 2013;7(5):383–387.
542. Brandenburg JE, Krach LE, Gormley ME Jr. Use of rimabotulinum toxin for focal hypertonicity management in children with cerebral palsy with nonresponse to onabotulinum toxin. *Am J Phys Med Rehabil.* 2013;92(10):898–904.
543. Sanger TD, Kukke SN, Sherman-Levine S. Botulinum toxin type B improves the speed of reaching in children with cerebral palsy and arm dystonia: an open-label, dose-escalation pilot study. *J Child Neurol.* 2007;22(1):116–122.
544. Heinen F, Schroeder AS, Fietzek U, Berweck S. When it comes to botulinum toxin, children and adults are not the same: multi-muscle option for children with cerebral palsy. *Mov Disord.* 2006b;21(11):2029–2030.
545. Wallen MA, O'Flaherty SJ, Waugh MCA. Functional outcomes of intramuscular botulinum toxin type A in the upper limbs of children with cerebral palsy: a phase II trial. *Arch Phys Med Rehabil.* 2004;85(2):192–200.
546. Schwerin A, Berweck S, Fietzek UM, Heinen F. Botulinum toxin B treatment in children with spastic movement disorders: a pilot study. *Pediatr Neurol.* 2004;31(2):109–113.
547. Kaňovský P, Bares M, Severa S, Richardson A, and Dysport Paediatric Limb Spasticity Study Group. Long-term efficacy and tolerability of 4-monthly versus yearly botulinum toxin type A treatment for lower-limb spasticity in children with cerebral palsy. *Dev Med Child Neurol.* 2009a;51(6):436–445.

548. Zonta MB, Bruck I, Puppi M, Muzzolon S, de Carvalho Neto A, Coutinho dos Santos LH. Effects of early spasticity treatment on children with hemiplegic cerebral palsy: a preliminary study. *Arq Neuropsiquiatr*. 2013;71(7):453–461.
549. Goldstein EM. Safety of high-dose botulinum toxin type A therapy for the treatment of pediatric spasticity. *J Child Neurol*. 2006;21(3):189–192.
550. Graham HK, Aoki KR, Autti-Rämö I, et al. Recommendations for the use of botulinum toxin type A in the management of cerebral palsy. *Gait Posture*. 2000;11(1):67–79.
551. Heinen F, Wissel J, Philipsen A, et al. Interventional neuropediatrics: treatment of dystonic and spastic muscular hyperactivity with botulinum toxin A. *Neuropediatrics*. 1997;28(6):307–313.
552. Koman LA, Smith BP, Williams R, et al. Upper extremity spasticity in children with cerebral palsy: a randomized, double-blind, placebo-controlled study of the short-term outcomes of treatment with botulinum A toxin. *J Hand Surg Am*. 2013;38(3):435–446.e1.
553. Scholtes VA, Dallmeijer AJ, Knol DL, et al. The combined effect of lower-limb multilevel botulinum toxin type A and comprehensive rehabilitation on mobility in children with cerebral palsy: a randomized clinical trial. *Arch Phys Med Rehabil*. 2006;87(12):1551–1558.
554. Jung NH, Heinen F, Westhoff B, et al; German Abo Study Group. Hip lateralisation in children with bilateral spastic cerebral palsy treated with botulinum toxin type A: a 2-year follow-up. *Neuropediatrics*. 2011;42(1):18–23.
555. Polak F, Morton R, Ward C, Wallace WA, Doderlein L, Siebel A. Double-blind comparison study of two doses of botulinum toxin A injected into calf muscles in children with hemiplegic cerebral palsy. *Dev Med Child Neurol*. 2002;44(8):551–555.
556. Mall V, Heinen F, Siebel A, et al. Treatment of adductor spasticity with BTX-A in children with CP: a randomized, double-blind, placebo-controlled study. *Dev Med Child Neurol*. 2006;48(1):10–13.
557. Engström P, Bartonek Å, Tedroff K, Orefelt C, Haglund-Åkerlind Y, Gutierrez-Farewik EM. Botulinum toxin A does not improve the results of cast treatment for idiopathic toe-walking: a randomized controlled trial. *J Bone Joint Surg Am*. 2013;95(5):400–407.
558. Tedroff K, Löwing K, Haglund-Åkerlind Y, Gutierrez-Farewik E, Forssberg H. Botulinum toxin A treatment in toddlers with cerebral palsy. *Acta Paediatr*. 2010;99(8):1156–1162.
559. Deleplanque B, Lagueny A, Flurin V, et al. Botulinum toxin in the management of spastic hip adductors in non-ambulatory cerebral palsy children. *Rev Chir Orthop Reparatrice Appar Mot*. 2002;88(3):279–285.
560. Moore AP, Ade-Hall RA, Smith CT, et al. Two-year placebo-controlled trial of botulinum toxin A for leg spasticity in cerebral palsy. *Neurology*. 2008;71(2):122–128.
561. Pascual-Pascual SI, Pascual-Castroviejo I, Ruiz PJ. Treating spastic equinus foot from cerebral palsy with botulinum toxin type A: what factors influence

the results?: an analysis of 189 consecutive cases. *Am J Phys Med Rehabil.* 2011;90(7):554–563.

562. Sławek J, Klimont L. Functional improvement in cerebral palsy patients treated with botulinum toxin A injections—preliminary results. *Eur J Neurol.* 2003;10(3):313–317.
563. Steenbeek D, Meester-Delver A, Becher JG, Lankhorst GJ. The effect of botulinum toxin type A treatment of the lower extremity on the level of functional abilities in children with cerebral palsy: evaluation with goal attainment scaling. *Clin Rehabil.* 2005;19(3):274–282.
564. van Campenhout A, Verhaegen A, Pans S, Molenaers G. Botulinum toxin type A injections in the psoas muscle of children with cerebral palsy: muscle atrophy after motor end plate-targeted injections. *Res Dev Disabil.* 2013;34(3)1052–1058.
565. Pahwa R, Busenbark K, Swanson-Hyland EF, et al. Botulinum toxin treatment of essential head tremor. *Neurology.* 1995;45(4):822–824.
566. Levin OS, Vasechkin SV. Dysport in the treatment of essential tremor. *Zh Nevrol Psikhiatr Im S S Korsakova.* 2011;111(12):21–24.
567. Wissel J, Masuhr F, Schelosky L, Ebersbach G, Poewe W. Quantitative assessment of botulinum toxin treatment in 43 patients with head tremor. *Mov Disord.* 1997;12(5):722–726.
568. Papapetropoulos S, Singer C. Treatment of primary writing tremor with botulinum toxin type A injections: report of a case series. *Clin Neuropharmacol.* 2006;29(6):364–367.
569. Bain PG, Findley LJ, Britton TC, et al. Primary writing tremor. *Brain.* 1995;118 (pt 6):1461–1472.
570. Atkins JL, Butler PE. Hyperhidrosis: a review of current management. *Plast Reconstr Surg.* 2002;110(1):222–228.
571. Baumann LS, Slezinger A, Halem M, et al. Double-blind, randomized, placebo-controlled pilot study of the safety and efficacy of Myobloc (botulinum toxin type B) for the treatment of palmar hyperhidrosis. *Dermatol Surg.* 2005a;31(3):263–270.
572. Baumann LS, Slezinger A, Halem M, et al. Pilot Study of the safety and efficacy of Myobloc (botulinum toxin type B) for treatment of axillary hyperhidrosis. *Int J Dermatol.* 2005b;44(5):418–424.
573. Bhidayasiri R, Truong DD. Evidence for effectiveness of botulinum toxin for hyperhidrosis. *J Neural Transm.* 2008;115(4):641–645.
574. Campanati A, Giuliodori K, Martina E, Giuliano A, Ganzetti G, Offidani A. Onabotulinumtoxin type A (Botox) versus incobotulinumtoxin type A (Xeomin) in the treatment of focal idiopathic palmar hyperhidrosis: results of a comparative double-blind clinical trial. *J Neural Transm.* 2014;121(1):21–26.
575. Dressler D. Comparing Botox and Xeomin for axillar hyperhidrosis. *J Neural Transm.* 2010b;117(3):317–319.
576. Heckmann M, Ceballos-Baumann AO, Plewig G, and Hyperhidrosis Study Group. Botulinum toxin A for axillary hyperhidrosis (excessive sweating). *N Engl J Med.* 2001;344(7):488–493.

577. Lowe NJ, Yamauchi PS, Lask GP, Patnaik R, Iyer S. Efficacy and safety of botulinum toxin type A in the treatment of palmar hyperhidrosis: a double-blind, randomized, placebo-controlled study. *Dermatol Surg*. 2002;28(9):822–827.
578. Lowe NJ, Glaser DA, Eadie N, Daggett S, Kowalski JW, Lai PY, and North American Botox in Primary Axillary Hyperhidrosis Clinical Study Group. Botulinum toxin type A in the treatment of primary axillary hyperhidrosis: a 52-week multicenter double-blind, randomized, placebo-controlled study of efficacy and safety. *J Am Acad Dermatol*. 2007;56(4):604–611.
579. Naumann M, Lowe NJ. Botulinum toxin type A in treatment of bilateral primary axillary hyperhidrosis: randomised, parallel group, double blind, placebo controlled trial. *BMJ*. 2001;323(7313):596–599.
580. Naumann M, Zellner M, Toyka KV, Reiners K. Treatment of gustatory sweating with botulinum toxin. *Ann Neurol*. 1997;42(6):973–975.
581. Odderson IR. Long-term quantitative benefits of botulinum toxin type A in the treatment of axillary hyperhidrosis. *Dermatol Surg*. 2002;28(6):480–483.
582. Rosell K, Hymnelius K, Swartling C. Botulinum toxin type A and B improve quality of life in patients with axillary and palmar hyperhidrosis. *Acta Derm Venereol*. 2013;93(3):335–339.
583. Saadia D, Voustianiouk A, Wang AK, Kaufmann H. Botulinum toxin type A in primary palmar hyperhidrosis: randomized, single-blind, two-dose study. *Neurology*. 2001;57(11):2095–2099.
584. Schnider P, Binder M, Auff E, Kittler H, Berger T, Wolff K. Double-blind trial of botulinum A toxin for the treatment of focal hyperhidrosis of the palms. *Br J Dermatol*. 1997;136(4):548–552.
585. Simonetta Moreau M, Cauhepe C, Magues JP, Senard JM. A double-blind, randomized, comparative study of Dysport vs. Botox in primary palmar hyperhidrosis. *Br J Dermatol*. 2003;149(5):1041–1045.
586. Talarico-Filho S, Mendonça do Nascimento M, Sperandeo de Macedo F, De Sanctis Pecora C. A double-blind, randomized, comparative study of two type A botulinum toxins in the treatment of primary axillary hyperhidrosis. *Dermatol Surg*. 2007;33(suppl 1):S44–S50.
587. Vadoud-Seyedi J, Simonart T. Treatment of axillary hyperhidrosis with botulinum toxin type A reconstituted in lidocaine or in normal saline: a randomized, side-by-side, double-blind study. *Br J Dermatol*. 2007;156(5):986–989.
588. Abdel-Meguid TA. Botulinum toxin-A injections into neurogenic overactive bladder–to include or exclude the trigone? A prospective, randomized, controlled trial. *J Urol*. 2010;184(6):2423–2428.
589. Apostolidis A, Dasgupta P, Fowler CJ. Proposed mechanism for the efficacy of injected botulinum toxin in the treatment of human detrusor overactivity. *Eur Urol*. 2006;49(4):644-650.
590. Brubaker L, Richter HE, Visco A, et al, and Pelvic Floor Disorders Network. Refractory idiopathic urge urinary incontinence and botulinum A injection. *J Urol*. 2008;180(1):217–222.
591. Cohen BL, Barboglio P, Rodriguez D, Gousse AE. Preliminary results of a dose-finding study for botulinum toxin-A in patients with idiopathic overactive bladder: 100 versus 150 units. *Neurourol Urodyn*. 2009;28(3):205–208.

592. Cruz F, Herschorn S, Aliotta P, et al. Efficacy and safety of onabotulinumtoxinA in patients with urinary incontinence due to neurogenic detrusor overactivity: a randomised, double-blind, placebo-controlled trial. *Eur Urol.* 2011;60(4):742–750
593. de Sèze M, Petit H, Gallien P, et al. Botulinum A toxin and detrusor sphincter dyssynergia: a double-blind lidocaine-controlled study in 13 patients with spinal cord disease. *Eur Urol.* 2002;42(1):56–62.
594. Dmochowski R, Chapple C, Nitti VW, et al. Efficacy and safety of onabotulinumtoxinA for idiopathic overactive bladder: a double-blind, placebo controlled, randomized, dose ranging trial. *J Urol.* 2010;184(6):2416–2422.
595. Dykstra DD, Sidi AA. Treatment of detrusor–sphincter dyssynergia with botulinum A toxin: a double-blind study. *Arch Phys Med Rehabil.* 1990;71(1):24–26.
596. Gallien P, Reymann JM, Amarenco G, Nicolas B, de Sèze M, Bellissant E. Placebo controlled, randomized, double blind study of the effects of botulinum A toxin on detrusor sphincter dyssynergia in multiple sclerosis patients. *J Neurol Neurosurg Psychiatry.* 2005;76(12):1670–1676.
597. Giannantoni A, Di Stasi SM, Stephen RL, Bini V, Costantini E, Porena M. Intravesical resiniferatoxin versus botulinum-A toxin injections for neurogenic detrusor overactivity: a prospective randomized study. *J Urol.* 2004;172(1):240–243.
598. Herschorn S, Gajewski J, Ethans K, et al. Efficacy of botulinum toxin A injection for neurogenic detrusor overactivity and urinary incontinence: a randomized, double-blind trial. *J Urol.* 2011;185(6):2229–2235.
599. Hirst GR, Watkins AJ, Guerrero K, et al. Botulinum toxin B is not an effective treatment of refractory overactive bladder. *Urology.* 2007;69(1):69-73.
600. Kuo HC, Liu HT. Therapeutic effects of add-on botulinum toxin A on patients with large benign prostatic hyperplasia and unsatisfactory response to combined medical therapy. *Scand J Urol Nephrol.* 2009;43(3):206–211.
601. Maria G, Brisinda G, Civello IM, Bentivoglio AR, Sganga G, Albanese A. Relief by botulinum toxin of voiding dysfunction due to benign prostatic hyperplasia: results of a randomized, placebo-controlled study. *Urology.* 2003;62(2):259–264; discussion 264–265.
602. Sahai A, Khan MS, Dasgupta P. Efficacy of botulinum toxin-A for treating idiopathic detrusor overactivity: results from a single center, randomized, double-blind, placebo controlled trial. *J Urol.* 2007;177(6):2231–2236.
603. Schurch B, de Sèze M, Denys P, et al, and Botox Detrusor Hyperreflexia Study Team. Botulinum toxin type A is a safe and effective treatment for neurogenic urinary incontinence: results of a single treatment, randomized, placebo controlled 6-month study. *J Urol.* 2005;174(1):196–200.
604. Fadeyi MO, Adams QM. Use of botulinum toxin type B for migraine and tension headaches. *Am J Health Syst Pharm.* 2002;59(19):1860–1862.
605. Goadsby PJ, Lipton RB, Ferrari MD. Migraine–current understanding and treatment. *N Engl J Med.* 2002;346(4):257–270.
606. Gwynn MW, English JB, Baker TS. Double-blind, placebo-controlled study of Myobloc (botulinum toxin type B) for the treatment of chronic headache. *Headache.* 2003;43(5):577–578.

*607.* Padberg M, de Bruijn SF, de Haan RJ, Tavy DL. Treatment of chronic tension-type headache with botulinum toxin: a double-blind, placebo-controlled clinical trial. *Cephalalgia.* 2004;24(8):675–680.

*608.* Schulte-Mattler WJ, Martinez-Castrillo JC. Botulinum toxin therapy of migraine and tension-type headache: comparing different botulinum toxin preparations. *Eur J Neurol.* 2006;13(suppl 1):51–54.

*609.* Winner P. Open-label study of Myobloc (botulinum toxin B) for chronic daily headache. *Headache.* 2003;43:576–577.

*610.* Lim JY, Koh JH, Paik NJ. Intramuscular botulinum toxin-A reduces hemiplegic shoulder pain: a randomized, double-blind, comparative study versus intraarticular triamcinolone acetonide. *Stroke.* 2008;39(1):126–131.

*611.* Al-Al-Shaikh M, Michel F, Parratte B, Kastler B, Vidal C, Aubry S. An MRI evaluation of changes in piriformis muscle morphology induced by botulinum toxin injections in the treatment of piriformis syndrome. *Diagn Interv Imaging.* 2014. Apr 3. pii: S2211-5684(14)00046–1. doi: 10.1016/j.diii.2014.02.015. [Epub ahead of print]

*612.* Baker JA, Pereira G. The efficacy of botulinum toxin A for spasticity and pain in adults: a systematic review and meta-analysis using the Grades of Recommendation, Assessment, Development and Evaluation approach. *Clin Rehabil.* 2013;27(12):1084–1096.

*613.* Benecke R, Heinze A, Reichel G, Hefter H, Göbel H, and Dysport Myofascial Pain Study Group. Botulinum type A toxin complex for the relief of upper back myofascial pain syndrome: how do fixed-location injections compare with trigger point-focused injections? *Pain Med.* 2011;12(11):1607–1614.

*614.* Boon AJ, Smith J, Dahm DL, et al. Efficacy of intra-articular botulinum toxin type A in painful knee osteoarthritis: a pilot study. *PM R.* 2010;2(4):269–276.

*615.* Le EN, Freischlag JA, Christo PJ, Chhabra A, Wigley FM. Thoracic outlet syndrome secondary to localized scleroderma treated with botulinum toxin injection. *Arthritis Care Res (Hoboken).* 2010;62(3):430–433.

*616.* Fahn S, Jankovic J, Hallett M. *Principles and Practice of Movement Disorders.* Philadelphia, PA: Saunders, Elsevier; 2007.

*617.* Morgante F, Klein C. Dystonia. *Continuum (Minneap Minn).* 2013;19(5 movement disorders):1225–1241.

*618.* Strader S, Rodnitzky RL, Gonzalez-Alegre P. Secondary dystonia in a botulinum toxin clinic: clinical characteristics, neuroanatomical substrate and comparison with idiopathic dystonia. *Parkinsonism Relat Disord.* 2011;17(10):749–752.

*619.* van Doornik J, Kukke S, Sanger TD. Hypertonia in childhood secondary dystonia due to cerebral palsy is associated with reflex muscle activation. *Mov Disord.* 2009;24(7):965–971.

*620.* Göertelmeyer R, Brinkmann S, Comes G, Delcker A. The Blepharospasm Disability Index (BSDI) for the assessment of functional health in focal dystonia. *Clin Neurophysiol.* 2002;113(suppl 1):S77–S78.

*621.* Roggenkämper P, Jost WH, Bihari K, Comes G, Grafe S, and NT 201 Blepharospasm Study Team. Efficacy and safety of a new botulinum toxin type A free of complexing proteins in the treatment of blepharospasm. *J Neural Transm.* 2006;113(3):303– 312.

622. Fahn S, List T, Moslowitz C, et al. Double-blind controlled study of botulinum toxin for blepharospasm. *Neurology*. 1985;35(suppl 1):271–272.
623. Boyd RN, Graham HK. Objective measurement of clinical findings in the use of botulinum toxin type A for the management of children with cerebral palsy. *Eur J Neurol*. 1999;6(suppl 1):S23–S35.
624. Haugh AB, Pandyan AD, Johnson GR. A systematic review of the Tardieu Scale for the measurement of spasticity. *Disabil Rehabil*. 2006;28(15):899–907.
625. Consky ES, Lang AE. Clinical assessments of patients with cervical dystonia. In: Jankovic J, Hallett M, eds. *Therapy with Botulinum Toxin*. New York, NY: Marcel Dekker, Inc; 1994:211–237.
626. Dressler D, Kupsch A, Paus S, Seitzinger A, Gebhardt B. Sustained efficacy of IncobotulinumtoxinA (Xeomin; botulinum neurotoxin type A, free from complexing proteins) in long-term treatment of cervical dystonia. *Eur J Neurol*. 2011;18(suppl 2):482.
627. Speelman JD, Brans JW. Cervical dystonia and botulinum treatment: is electromyographic guidance necessary? *Mov Disord*. 1995;10(6):802.

## Suggested Readings

Aoki KR. Review of a proposed mechanism for the antinociceptive action of botulism toxin type A. *Neurotoxicology*. 2005;25(5):785–793.

Benner JS, Nichol MB, Rovner ES, et al. Patient-reported reasons for discontinuing overactive bladder medication. *BJU Int*. 2010;105(9):1276–1282.

Comella CL, Leurgans S, Wuu J, Stebbins GT, Chmura T, and Dystonia Study Group. Rating scales for dystonia: a multicenter assessment. *Mov Disord*. 2003;18(3):303-312.

Costa J, Espírito-Santo C, Borges A, et al. Botulinum toxin type B for cervical dystonia. *Cochrane Database Syst Rev*. 2005c;(1):CD004315.

Dressler D. Five-year experience with incobotulinumtoxinA (Xeomin): the first botulinum toxin drug free of complexing proteins. *Eur J Neurol*. 2012b;19(3): 385–389.

Dressler D, Dirnberger G. Botulinum toxin therapy: risk factors for therapy failure. *Mov Disord*. 2000;15(suppl 2):51.

Dysport SRI *(Simple Reconstitution Information)*. Basking Ridge, NJ: Ipsen Biopharmaceuticals, Inc. Available at http://www.dysport.com/hcp/Reconstitution-Storage-Handling.php. Updated March 2012.

Epidemiological Study of Dystonia in Europe (ESDE) Collaborative Group. A prevalence study of primary dystonia in eight European countries. *J Neurol*. 2000;247(10):787–792.

Karp B, Hallett M. Truncal dystonia and other truncal dyskinesias. In: Alter KE, Hallett M, Karp B, Lungu C, eds. *Ultrasound-Guided Chemodenervation Procedures: Text and Atlas*. New York, NY: Demos Medical Pub; 2013:20–23.

Koman LA, Smith BP, Balkrishnan R. Spasticity associated with cerebral palsy in children: guidelines for the use of botulinum A toxin. *Paediatr Drugs*. 2003;5(1): 11–23.

Lee LR, Chuang YC, Yang BJ, Hsu MJ, Liu YH. Botulinum toxin for lower limb spasticity in children with cerebral palsy: a single-blinded trial comparing dilution techniques. *Am J Phys Med Rehabil.* 2004;83(10):766–773.

Mense S. Neurobiological basis for the use of botulinum toxin in pain therapy. *J Neurol.* 2004;251(suppl 1):i1–i7.

Olvey EL, Armstrong EP, Grizzle AJ. Contemporary pharmacologic treatments for spasticity of the upper limb after stroke: a systematic review. *Clin Ther.* 2010;32(14):2282–2303.

Shin HJ, Shin JC, Kim WS, Chang WH, Lee SC. Application of ultrasound-guided trigger point injection for myofascial trigger points in the subscapularis and pectoralis muscles to post-mastectomy patients: a pilot study. *Yonsei Med J.* 2014;55(3):792–799.

Stacy M. Epidemiology, clinical presentation, and diagnosis of cervical dystonia. *Neurol Clin.* 2008;26(suppl 1):23–42.

Truong DD, Comella C, Fernandez HH, Ondo WG, and Dysport Benign Essential Blepharospasm Study Group. Efficacy and safety of purified botulinum toxin type A (Dysport) for the treatment of benign essential blepharospasm: a randomized, placebo-controlled, phase II trial. *Parkinsonism Relat Disord.* 2008;14(5):407–414.

Tsui JK, Eisen A, Mak E, Carruthers J, Scott A, Calne DB. A pilot study on the use of botulinum toxin in spasmodic torticollis. *Can J Neurol Sci.* 1985;12(4): 314–316.

Wheeler AH, Goolkasian P, Gretz SS. A randomized, double-blind, prospective pilot study of botulinum toxin injection for refractory, unilateral, cervicothoracic, paraspinal, myofascial pain syndrome. *Spine (Phila Pa 1976).* 1998;23(15): 1662–1666.

# Index

CPSIA information can be obtained
at www.ICGtesting.com
Printed in the USA
BVHW041942181121
621973BV00002B/3

9 781620 700426